S0-CEE-577

ANTITUMOR NATURAL PRODUCTS

Gann Monograph on Cancer Research

The "Gann Monograph on Cancer Research" series is promoted by the Japanese Cancer Association. This semiannual series of monographs was initiated in 1966 by the late Dr. Tomizo Yoshida (1903–1973) and is now published jointly by Japan Scientific Societies Press, Tokyo and Taylor & Francis Ltd., London and Philadelphia. Each volume consists of collected contributions on current topics in cancer problems and allied research fields. The planning for each volume is done by the Monograph Committee of the Japanese Cancer Association, with the final approval of the Board of Directors. It is hoped that the series will serve as an important source of information in the field of cancer research.

The publication of these monographs owes much to the financial support given by the late Professor Kazushige Higuchi, the Jikei University School of Medicine.

Japanese Cancer Association

Monograph Committee of the Japanese Cancer Association

Goro Kosaki	Susumu Nishimura	Tetsuo Ono
Haruo Sugano	Shozo Takayama	Kumao Toyoshima
Shigeru Tsukagoshi	Tadashi Utakoji	

Tomoyuki Kitagawa (Executive Secretary)

JAPANESE CANCER ASSOCIATION

Gann Monograph on Cancer Research No. 36

ANTITUMOR NATURAL PRODUCTS

BASIC AND CLINICAL RESEARCH

IN MEMORY OF PROFESSOR HAMAO UMEZAWA

TOMIO TAKEUCHI
Edited by   KAZUO NITTA
NOBUO TANAKA

RC261
A2
G198
no.36
1989

JAPAN SCIENTIFIC SOCIETIES PRESS, Tokyo
TAYLOR & FRANCIS LTD., London and Bristol

© Japan Scientific Societies Press, 1989
All rights reserved. No part of this publication may be reproduced or transmitted in any form or by any means, electronic or mechanical, including photocopy, recording, or any information storage and retrieval system, without permission in writing from the publisher.

December 1989

Published jointly by
Japan Scientific Societies Press
2-10 Hongo, 6-chome, Bunkyo-ku, Tokyo 113, Japan
ISBN 4-7622-3604-7
          and
Taylor & Francis Ltd.
4 John Street, London WC1N 2ET, UK
1900 Frost Road, Suite 101, Bristol, Pennsylvania 19007, U.S.A.
ISBN 0-85066-854-9

Distributed in all areas outside Japan and Asia between Pakistan and Korea by Taylor & Francis Ltd., London and Bristol.

Printed in Japan

PREFACE

Cancer is one of the greatest enemies of human beings and its extermination is a long-cherished hope of mankind. Many eradication strategies have been developed: surgical operation, radiotherapy, chemotherapy, immunotherapy, hyperthermia and others. During the last two decades, cancer chemotherapy has greatly progressed with occasional healings of neoplastic diseases.

Modern cancer chemotherapy began with the discovery of the antileukemic effect of mechlorethamine (nitrogen mustard) during World War II, followed by similar findings on nitrogen mustard-N-oxide, methotrexate, and 6-mercaptopurine. Although earlier researchers utilized bacterial or fungal culture filtrates on cancer patients or tumor-bearing animals, the late Professor Hamao Umezawa was the pioneer in the field of antitumor antibiotics.

Professor Umezawa started his antibiotic research in 1944 and found many useful substances including kanamycin, an anti-tuberculosis antibiotic effective against both streptomycin-resistant and streptomycin-sensitive bacteria. In 1951, with certainty that antitumor activities must exist in microbial products which had shown a variety of chemical structures and peculiar modes of action, he initiated a systematic search for these antitumor substances. He demonstrated in 1952 that such antibiotics did exist in microorganisms by testing culture filtrates against experimental animal tumors. He found substance No. 289, caryomycin and sarkomycin in 1952 and reported them the following year. The same year (1952), Hackmann reported the antitumor activity of actinomycin C which had been identified as an antibacterial antibiotic by Brockmann in 1951. Thereafter, Professor Umezawa and his coworkers found numerous antitumor antibiotics, such as pluramycins, bleomycins, macromomycin, aclacinomycins, neothramycins, peplomycin, pirarubicin (THP-adriamycin), bactobolin, spergualin, oxanosine, ditrisarubicins, liblomycin and many others.

In 1965, in the hope of exploiting a new area, Professor Umezawa and his colleagues initiated the screening of enzyme inhibitors found in culture filtrates of microorganisms. Among the more than sixty kinds of enzyme inhibitors he found, bestatin (1976), an inhibitor of aminopeptidase B, and forphenicin (1978), an inhibitor of alkaline phosphatase of chicken small intestine, exhibited marked immunomodulating activity, and the former is now clinically used as an adjuvant drug in combination with chemotherapy for cancer patients.

In response to the recent advances in oncogene study, Professor Umezawa and his collaborators started the screening of microbial products which inhibited oncogene expression. By this means he determined that herbimycin inhibited *src* gene expression. He also found a new antibiotic, erbstatin, which inhibited the expression of *erb* B gene.

The field of antibiotic research thus sustained a tremendous loss when this distinguished scientist passed from its midst on the 25th of December, 1986. The Japanese Cancer Association, having issued a series of Gann Monographs on Cancer Research, decided to prepare a volume on recent advances in antitumor natural products dedicated to the memory of Professor Hamao Umezawa.

The title is "Antitumor Natural Products—Basic and Clinical Research—in Memory of Professor Hamao Umezawa". The monograph consists of three parts: survey of development of antitumor natural products, advances in antitumor antibiotics, and new approaches. Although most of the reports are closely related to Dr. Umezawa's research, the contents also deal with broader surveys, particularly in the first part.

In Part I a brief history and characteristics of the antitumor antibiotics discovered in Japan and currently either in clinical use or under development are described. A few useful immunomodulators of microbial origin are included. Similarly, the present status and development of antitumor natural products at the National Cancer Institute in the United States are reported, and other developing antitumor natural products are described.

Basic research and the clinical application of some useful antitumor antibiotics in common use are covered in Part II, together with the involvement of the relationship of structure to anticancer activity and toxicity in anthracyclines. This field is very important and a huge and assiduous effort has been made to reduce the cardiotoxicity and skin toxicity of adriamycin without lessening its antitumor activity; this has not yet, however, been successful.

Part III outlines new antitumor antibiotics found by recent screening methods based on novel concepts. Cadeguomycin, 2-crotonyloxymethyl-4, 5, 6-trihydroxycyclohex-5-enon, lactoquinomycins, spergualins, oxanosine, herbimycin A and erbstatin are described.

This monograph, then, reviews some of the research of the late Professor Umezawa in recognition of his notable contributions to this field, and also presents some of the recent progress made in cancer chemotherapy in the continuing effort to overcome this malignant disease.

We express our sincere gratitude to all contributors to this volume whose reports represent work being done in various parts of the world. We are honored to be able to include remembrances of Professor Umezawa from five distinguished scientists involved in basic and clinical research on cancer chemotherapy: Dr. George Mathé of France, Dr. Irwin H. Krakoff and Dr. Matthew Suffness of the United States of America, and Dr. Tokuji Ichikawa and Dr. Toju Hata of Japan. We also express our appreciation to the Japanese Cancer Association, to Dr. Haruo Sugano of the Cancer Research Institute and to Dr. Takashi Sugimura of the National Cancer Center for suggesting this monograph and for their encouragement during the pre-publication stage. Additionally, we are indebted to Dr. Tomoyuki Kitagawa of the Cancer Research Institute and to Dr. Morimasa Yagisawa of the Japan Antibiotics Research Association for their kind advice and help.

January 1989

T. TAKEUCHI
K. NITTA
N. TANAKA

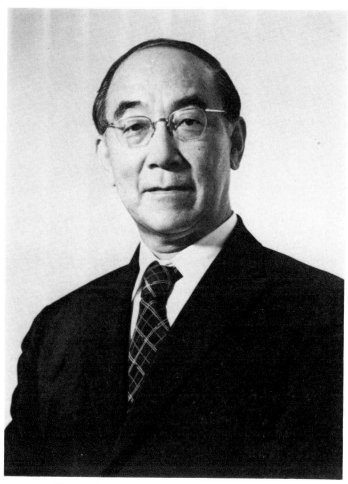

Hamao Umezawa, M. D., Ph. D. (1914–1986)

1914	Born in Fukui, Japan on the 1st of October.
1937	Graduated from University of Tokyo (M.D.).
1944–1947	Associate Professor of University of Tokyo.
1945	Ph. D. in Medicine, University of Tokyo.
1947–1978	Director of the Department of Antibiotics of the National Institute of Health of Japan.
1954–1975	Professor of University of Tokyo.
1959	Asahi Prize.
1959	Prize from the Minister of Science and Technology of Japan.
1960	Commandeur de l'Ordre de la Sante Publique.
1962–1986	Director of the Institute of Microbial Chemistry.
1962	Japan Academy Award.
1962	Order of Culture (Bunka-Kunsho) conferred by the Emperor of Japan.
1971	Ordre Nationale de la Legion d'Honneur (Chevaller).
1971	Fujiwara Prize.
1977	Princess Takamatsu Cancer Research Prize.
1977	Windsor C. Cutting Lectureship Award, University of Hawaii.
1977	Karle-August Forster Prize, Mainz Academy.
1977	Honorary Doctorship from University of Santiago de Compostella.
1978	Honorary Doctorship from Royal Karolinska Institute.
1980	Paul-Ehrlich und Ludwig-Darmstaedter-Preis (Haupt Prize).
1981	Griffuel Prize, L'Associacion pour le Development de la Recherche sur le Cancer.
1981	Honorary Doctorship from University of Oxford.
1983	Smissman Award (American Chemical Society).
1984	Honorary Doctorship from South-Paris University.
1986	First Order of the Sacred Treasure (Kun Itto, Zuihosho) conferred by the Emperor of Japan.
1986	Died in Tokyo on the 25th of December.

Dedication to Professor Hamao Umezawa

HAMAO UMEZAWA

A Polydisciplinary Scientist and a Giant in Human Discovery.

The late Professor Hamao Umezawa was a medical doctor who became a microbiologist and organic chemist through his research carrier. Throughout his scientific life, he has never limited his role to one discipline of medical sciences. He just worked at the rightest place, with the rightest method, to attain the target designed by the medical need.

He thus worked on *antibiotics* and discovered *kanamycin* in 1952.

He was not satisfied by this victory, the first world-wide antibiotic discovered and registered in Japan. Prof. Hamao Umezawa was preoccupied by possible secondary failure, and foresaw the stumbling block which secondary resistance of germs to antibiotics would represent, for the cure of infected patients.

He discovered *dibekacin* which works on aminoglycoside resistant germs, because he had first studied and understood the enzymatic mechanisms of the resistance to kanamycin in 1965. Those mechanisms suggested him the chemical structure of the derivatives he had to produce.

It was as soon as 1953, that he adventured himself in his following main foresight: molecules which would be toxic for cancer cells could be found in microbes. And he discovered the first *antitumor antibiotic*, *sarkomycin*. The cancer pharmacologists and organic chemists followed him all over the world, especially in the United States.

After 1953, he discovered no less than 50 anticancer antibiotics, almost two per year.

None of them was discovered by chance; all were accomplished according to biochemical basis.

In 1956, he produced *phleomycin*, which was active against both tuberculosis bacteria and cancer. Because of its renal toxicity, he screened numerous analogs and convinced that some loose the side effect.

This work led him to discover *bleomycin*, of which effectiveness was shown in Japan by great experts in clinical trials to work in Hodgkin's disease, non Hodgkin's lymphomas, head and neck tumors, and shown by the EORTC Clinical Screening Group in which I was the chairman, to work in testis cancer: this tumor became curable by a bleomycin combination with other therapies soon after its availability.

Bleomycin also opened the door to chemotherapy efficacy against lymphomas and epidermoid tumors. With this antibiotic, he had discovered and introduced a new cytostatic mechanism, less naively conceived than "alkylation" and "intercalation". This antibiotic is working *via* DNA breaks made by bleomycin-iron-oxygen complexes. He discovered that human non-malignant cells produce bleomycin hydrolase which destroys it to be less toxic. The terminal amines of bleomycin having appeared to Hamao Umezawa to play a significant role in its effect, promoted him to produce 500 derivatives, and he offered us *peplomycin* which interested many clinicians for its less riskfull sclerosis effect, but also interested us because of its activity in breast cancer.

Discovery of *baumycin* which appeared to be more active than adriamycin brought him to produce a new anthracycline, aclacinomycin. We were happy to study simultaneously with Japanese friends, its oncostatic effects in rapidly dividing cell tumors, and we observed its highly frequent efficiency in acute myeloid leukemia, even in adriamycin-resistant patients. We consider it as the best drug for reinforcement therapy, especially because the lack of cardiotoxicity. Moreover, aclacinomycin, contrary to the pre-existing anthracyclines, is not mutagenic. But the most interesting effect of aclacinomycin is its *immunopharmacologic* action which we have demonstrated: a) it activates the monocytic-macrophagic series of cells; b) it decreases the increased suppressor cells; c) it can break immunologic tolerance.

The *bestatin* discovery was not only remarkable because it gave to immunopharmacologists a potent $CD4^+$ $CD8^-$ specific activating agent, but it was interesting because, based on Hamao Umezawa's genius recognition that *coriolin*, discovered from a mushroom in 1972, was working by inhibiting Na-K-ATPase at the cell surface, he searched enzyme inhibitors, especially of aminopeptidases which bestatin inhibits.

The most remarkable of his discovered oncostatics in the series of anthracyclines, is *THP-adriamycin*, which may be more active than adriamycin and is much less toxic on hair and on myocardium, as we saw with our hamster test and in our clinical trials. THP-adriamycin also exerts some immunologic actions.

Scientists as artists are learning and practicing more and more often only a restricted part of a speciality, as a music performer plays only one instrument. However, conductors play often with several instruments and have to know all of them.

Prof. Hamao Umezawa was able to work: a) in chemistry, and to discuss about the structure of a substance as well as about the most sophisticated apparatus; b) in biology, and to discuss about the role of an enzyme as well as about the value of a screening test, and c) in medicine, and to discuss about a disease pathophysiology as well as about the bias of a therapeutic trial.

He was indeed more than an orchestra conductor. He was a composer. Though he belonged to the hierarchic level of a Leonardo da Vinci and a Picasso, he did not seem to be satisfied by the latter sentence: "I do not search; I do discover". He was enjoying by searching.

He has been one of the most brilliant citizens who, when Japan was at its nadir, offered an indefectible patriotic faith, an incredible courage, an unsurmountable effort to help his country avoiding to reclose, but to fully open to the World. He has been one of those giant pacific samourais who have conducted his country to today's Zenith.

I regret him passed away, and regret too that we have no Umezawa in our country, France.

Georges MATHÉ
Villejuif, France

DEDICATION TO PROFESSOR HAMAO UMEZAWA

It is a pleasure and an honor to participate in this memorial volume to the late Professor Hamao Umezawa. He had many friends at the National Cancer Institute and they all miss his advice and guidance very much. His expertise in discovery of new antibiotic substances was well known in the U.S. for many years, but the close relationship with the NCI came from his discovery of bleomycin which has become widely used in treatment of various kinds of squamous cell carcinoma. His innovative approaches to screening for enzyme inhibitors of microbial origin and low molecular weight immunomodifiers led to a contract with the NCI in 1975 to support his work on development of new assays and discovery of new antitumor drugs. For the following ten years there was a very close relationship between Professor Umezawa and the Institute of Microbial Chemistry and the Developmental Therapeutics Program of the National Cancer Institute, particularly with Dr. John Douros; later I had the privilege of being the NCI representative to work with the IMC and Professor Umezawa. A very important link between the two Institutes was the friendship between Professor Umezawa and Dr. Vincent DeVita, a pioneer in combination chemotherapy for cancer, who was then the Director of the Division of Cancer Treatment at the NCI and later became Director of the full Institute. Professor Umezawa was extraordinary in his breadth and depth of knowledge. It was most amazing to listen to him discuss in detail such diverse fields as clinical treatment of cancer, organic and medicinal chemistry, biology of actinomycetes, immunology, and molecular biology. Furthermore, he was very kind and thoughtful in his personal relationships and always strove to make the visit of every guest to his Institute memorable. All of his many friends at the National Cancer Institute miss him deeply.

Matthew SUFFNESS
Bethesda, Maryland, U.S.A.

DEDICATION TO PROFESSOR HAMAO UMEZAWA

It is a great privilege to be permitted to participate in the dedication of this mono-graph to Professor Umezawa. Others will address his contributions to laboratory science —indeed, many of the essayists in this monograph are doing just that. I should like to consider his influence on clinical medicine and to express some personal reminiscences.

Foremost among his contributions to clinical oncology is bleomycin. Umezawa's painstaking scientific pursuit of a group of substances with demonstrable antitumor activity led to the identification and characterization of that mixture of peptides. His leadership qualities enabled him to assemble a team that was uniquely qualified to ex-plore its properties. The mass of data developed in his laboratories led to clinical trials in Japan; the unusual properties of bleomycin led to further studies throughout the world and its enthusiastic recognition as an active drug for clinical use. Countless pa-tients are alive because of the inclusion of bleomycin in *curative* combination regimens.

Recognizing the limiting toxicities of bleomycin, Umezawa devoted much of the latter portion of his life to the attempt to develop newer bleomycins with different pro-perties—an effort in which there appears at this time to have been considerable prog-ress. In the same vein, he devoted major effort to the synthesis of new anthracyclines, an effort that has brought new agents to the clinic and that may modify the limiting toxicities of established members of that group of drugs.

I cannot resist the opportunity to record a personal appreciation of Professor Ume-zawa. I first met him at a Japan-US interchange in Hawaii. His warmth and informality in that setting contrasted markedly with my preconceived notion of stiffness and aus-terity. It became clear that his eminence was based on his giant intellect and scientific accomplishments but he was able to meet with those of us who were much his junior in the relaxed give and take that facilitates true progress. I last saw him during the last year of his life when he paid us a two-day visit to the M. D. Anderson Cancer Center in order to talk about our mutual interests in antitumor antibiotic development. He approached our discussions with a genuine sense of inquiry. In those discussions and in a formal lecture, he showed freshness and enthusiasm that might have been expected of a post-doctoral fellow, along with the wisdom and knowledge of the seasoned scientist that he was. That visit was an inspiration to me and my colleagues. We will remember it for many years to come just as we and our patients will benefit from his contributions for many years to come.

Irwin H. Krakoff
Houston, Texas, U.S.A.

PROFESSOR HAMAO UMEZAWA

Although many often become mediocre later in life even if they were a genius in their youth, the late Professor Hamao Umezawa was famed as a boy genius and remained a rare genius throughout his life. He contributed greatly to the welfare of humanity through his talent. It is said that a man of genius is a man of endeavour, and Prof. Umezawa was truly typical of such a one. This can be easily realized by his bibliographic trail of education and occupation, and more distinctly by his awards and decorations such as the Cultural Medal (Bunka Kunsho) and the First Order of the Rising Sun (Kun Itto) as well as by the many honorary titles given by governments, universities, and academic societies both in Japan and in many foreign countries.

He was inducted into the Army once during the World War II but released after a short term to direct his effort toward the task of penicillin production. This was really the start of his research on antibiotics, which continued on until the end of his life. When the Committee for Penicillin Production during the War was succeeded by the Japan Penicillin Research Association after the conflict, he was nominated to and did become its active manager and was a leader of the Association even after the name of the Association was changed to the Japan Antibiotics Research Association. His leadership led Japan to become one of the world's biggest producers of antibiotics, and he himself became acknowledged as the foremost researcher in the world in the field of antibiotics research. He was not only a great discoverer of many useful antibiotics but also a great fosterer of many excellent antibiotics researchers by his heading the Antibiotics Research Division at the National Institute of Health and through his positions as Professor of the Institute of Applied Microbiology and of the Institute of Medical Sciences at the University of Tokyo.

As the Chairman of the Board of Directors of the Japan Antibiotics Research Association, whose members include academic persons and also antibiotic manufacturers, he displayed strong leadership, promoting not only both basic and applied research on antibiotics but also the manufacturing activity of antibiotic drugs. His detailed consultation with government administrators and his valuable advice regarding the minimum governmental requirements for antibiotic drugs were absolutely indispensable.

Prof. Umezawa's name first became famous throughout the world by his discovery of kanamycin; and, of course, this event had a big impact on his later life. Based on royalties incoming from the production of kanamycin, he decided to establish the Microbial Chemistry Research Foundation (the President: T. Ichikawa) by which he was able to operate the Institute of Microbial Chemistry (Director: H. Umezawa). In this Institute, he pursued his own research with full freedom without any obligations to others. After the start of the Institute, he worked diligently day by day without taking rest 365 days a year, and his continuous endeavor was extraordinarily remarkable. Under this brave general, no weak soldiers were gathered, and many excellent scientific achievements were reported continuously. The number of his scientific papers which have been referred in scientific articles became the top in the world-rank and he was famed as the number one person in antibiotics research in the world.

His last research activity was concentrated on the discovery of anticancer drugs, and its motivation was derived from his strong confidence that inhibitory substances against cancer cells can be found among antibiotics of microbial origin. Based on his perspective and persistence, he discovered the potent anticancer antibiotic agent, bleomycin, and this discovery has had a great impact on the world-wide effort to search for anticancer agents among antibiotics.

As Prof. Umezawa was extremely healthy and had never been ill, many of his friends were astonished by the sudden incidence of brain stroke which he suffered 4 years ago. Fortunately, only a little physical disturbance remained and he was released from the hospital. After this, many people wished and hoped that he would assume a less strenuous life style, but again they were astonished by his every endeavour as before to continue his research activity. With his strong desire and will, he travelled and lectured at academic meeting both domestically and abroad.

Unfortunately, in the summer of 1986 he was hospitalized again, this time due to chronic bronchitis, a disease from which he never recovered. Sadly, he passed away on December 25th, 1986, after his last outgoing from the hospital to the Imperial Palace where the First Order Award was conferred upon him by the Emperor on November 5th, 1986.

Tokuji ICHIKAWA
Tokyo, Japan

DEDICATION TO PROFESSOR HAMAO UMEZAWA

Professor Hamao Umezawa passed away on the 25th December, 1986 at the Kita-sato Institute Hospital. It is a great loss to the research in science, and medicine, especially in antibiotic field.

He was born on October 1st, 1914, graduated from the Medical School of Tokyo University in 1937. After the military service, he entered to the Institute for Infectious Diseases in 1944 and engaged in the research of penicillin as the associate professor. Three years later he became the director of the Department of Antibiotics of the National Institute of Health, and presided over the national certification of antibiotic substances. In 1956 he discovered kanamycin. This aminoglycosidic antibiotic showed a high activity against many kinds of pathogenic bacteria and has been widely used in practice specially in tuberculosis. As a result, the Minister of Health and Welfare decided to establish a non-profit organization "Microbial Chemistry Research Foundation" using the profit from the patent, and to construct the Institute of Microbial Chemistry. When the institute was completed in 1962, he was appointed to the director of the Institute and remained throughout his life. Under his direction, researches of the Institute led to a continual stream of publications on secondary metabolites of microorganisms.

The number of new antibiotics, antitumor substances and enzyme inhibitors discovered by him and his associates were counted as many as 57, 35 and 50 respectively. These were reported mainly in the Journal of Antibiotics. He had started much earlier the systematic search of antitumor substances and a number of antitumor substances were found in the culture filtrate of Streptomycetes. Firstly sarkomycin was found in 1953 and glycopeptid antibiotic, bleomycin was found in 1962, and the latter proved to be effective for the treatment of squamous cell carcinomas of the skin. According to Dr. T. Ichikawa, one of the coworkers of Dr. Umezawa, a case of the squamous cell carcinoma of the penis was cured by the treatment with bleomycin. This fact might encourage the researchers engaged in this field. In 1972 the structure of bleomycin was determined, and more than 200 bleomycin analogues differing from one another in the N terminal amine group were obtained by the addition of various amines to the fermentation medium. Concerning the side-effect of bleomycin, though myelo-toxicity was not observed pulmonary fibrosis was reported. Clinically, peplomycin was applied as one of the derivatives having less side-effect than bleomycin.

In 1975, aclarubicin which is effective for blood cancer, was discovered. This substance belongs to anthracycline group and is closely related to doxorubicin (ADM). However, cardiotoxicity of aclarubicin was proved to be less than that of ADM.

In the 1960's he also initiated the screening of culture filtrates for enzyme inhibitors of low molecular weight. This led to the discovery of a variety of compounds. Among them bestatin which binds to cells, stimulates the cell mediated immune system, and is active against certain tumors in experiments. Clinical studies suggested that the use of this substance together with antitumor agents is able to prolong the life of patients of non-lymphatic leukemia, melanoma and of tumor of the head and neck.

He was appointed to the president of the International Society of Chemotherapy from 1967 to 1969 and organized the International Congress of Chemotherapy in Tokyo. He also organized Japanese Cancer Meeting in 1978. He was appointed to the president of Japan Antibiotics Research Association in 1970.

He was awarded many famed prizes in Japan and in foreign countries. He received the Asahi prize in 1959 by the discovery of kanamycin, the Order of Culture (Bunka-Kunsho), the Japan Academy Prize in 1962 and the First Class of the Rising Sun in 1986. He was often invited by many scientific conferences as the prenary lecturer.

Furthermore he founded three scientific institutes: Episome Institute at Maebashi city in 1960, Institute for Bio-organic Chemistry at Kawasaki city in 1974, and Institute for Chemotherapy at Numazu city in 1985. When these 3 institutes are working in co-operation with the main Institute of Microbial Chemistry, it will be possible to solve many cancer problems in near future.

Friends and colleagues in many countries never enough to be regretted, and pray for the repose of a soul.

Toju HATA
Tokyo, Japan

CONTENTS

xviii

I. SURVEY OF DEVELOPMENT OF ANTITUMOR NATURAL PRODUCTS

NOVEL ANITUMOR ANTIBIOTICS DEVELOPED IN JAPAN

Tomio Takeuchi[*1] and Kazuo Nitta[*2]

Institute of Microbial Chemistry[*1] *and Chiba Cancer Center
Research Institute*[*2]

In 1951 we initiated a screening study for new compounds capable of potent antitumor activity in the culture media of microorganisms and discovered several useful and efficient agents by this systematic screening system. This current study has continued the search for new compounds. We also began preparation of many chemically-derived analogues of antitumor antibiotics with proven activity that may have much greater efficacy and less toxicity than their parent compounds. In this way, new antitumor antibiotics were discovered and introduced as cancer chemotherapeutics: bleomycin, peplomycin, aclacinomycin, 4'-O-tetrahydropyranyladriamycin, and others. Some compounds are now in Phase I studies: liblomycin, 15-deoxyspergualin, neothramycin, and MX2. The immunomodifiers we discovered were bestatin, forphenicinol, and others. Bestatin, put into clinical use in 1987, has been found to prolong the survival of patients with acute non-lymphatic adult leukemia.

Although these antitumor antibiotics are very effective for patients with Hodgkin's disease, malignant lymphoma, acute leukemia, testicular tumor, or skin cancer, they are not efficient for naturally resistant cancers, such as malignant melanoma, gastric cancer, and certain types of pulmonary cancer. In order to find much more efficient antitumor antibiotics or improve the efficacy of cancer chemotherapy, a modification of the screening method or a device of a new method for cancer chemotherapy must be developed.

In addition to our own studies, this review covers new antitumor antibiotics which have been found by others in Japan during the last 10 years: leptomycin, kazusamycin, rhizoxin, FR-900482, FK-973, staurosporin, rebeccamycin, elsamicin, esperamicins, FR-900405, and FR-900406. Most of these have not yet been studied clinically, but esperamicins and their structurally related compounds have been reported to have the strongest antitumor activity. This raises hope for the discovery of even more powerful and effective antitumor antibiotics.

In 1944, Hamao Umezawa initiated his antibiotic research. From 1945 until his death in 1986, we worked with him as co-workers, exchanging opinions and ideas with the mutual goal of furthering studies on antibiotics. In 1951, we decided to open a new area searching for substances of microbial origin that were capable of anticancer activity; at that time no such screening had yet been attempted. Although the project seemed bold and even a "gamble," we felt confident that we would find useful anticancer antibiotics, because of the numberless microorganisms existing in the soil and producing a great

---

[*1] Kamiosaki 3-14-23, Shinagawa-ku, Tokyo 141, Japan (竹内富雄).
[*2] Nitona-cho 666-2, Chiba 280, Japan (新田和男).

number of substances with a variety of structures and different biological activities. Since that time, culture filtrates of every known microorganism have been systematically screened for antitumor antibiotics.

Our confidence was rewarded by the discovery of sarkomycin in 1953, which was reported under the title, "Sarkomycin, an antitumor substance produced by streptomyces" by Umezawa, Takeuchi, Nitta, Yamamoto, and Yamaoka (56). This was the first paper on an antitumor antibiotic discovered by systematic screening. Soon thereafter in 1956, Hata et al. discovered mitomycins A and B (9), from which Wakaki and his colleagues isolated mitomycin C in 1958 (59).

Umezawa and his co-workers first discovered bleomycin in culture filtrates of Streptomyces verticillus in 1962 but did not report it until 1966 (52). It was found to have a marked therapeutic effect against some types of cancer.

In 1964, DiMarco et al. discovered daunorubicin, a compound which was very active against acute leukemia (5). Arcamone and his co-workers isolated doxorubicin in 1969 from Streptomyces peucetius var. caesius, which was very effective against acute leukemia, malignant lymphoma, childhood neuroblastoma, Wilms' tumor, and breast cancer (1).

During the last two decades, progress in combination chemotherapy has produced "cures" of more than 5 years' duration in some cases of acute leukemia, advanced Hodgkin's disease, and malignant lymphomas, and in several types of childhood cancer; however, the majority of these patients has eventually suffered a relapse. One important reason for this was considered to be the inefficacy and toxicity of the cytotoxic drugs used. Therefore, soon after the discovery of bleomycin, we began to improve bleomycins so as to produce more efficient but less toxic ones, at the same time conducting routine screening for more potent antitumor antibiotics. Thus, peplomycin and liblomycin were born from 227 derivatives.

During the last ten years we have isolated numerous new antitumor antibiotics, although most were identified as members of the anthracycline class of antibiotics. Aclacinomycin, discovered in 1975, showed a low cardiac toxicity and no cross-resistance to conventional anthracyclines (30).

In 1981 we found spergualin in a culture medium of a strain of Bacillus laterosporus (40, 51). The structure was entirely different from that of conventional anticancer agents and it had strong antitumor activity, but very low toxicity.

In 1965 we extended our studies to a new area to find specific enzyme inhibitors of microbial origin. Then, bestatin was discovered in 1976 as an aminopeptidase inhibitor (49), and was extensively studied as an immunomodifier for use in cancer treatment.

Recently, various oncogenes have been isolated and their functions studied. Therefore, an attempt was initiated to find inhibitors of oncogene functions for the purpose of obtaining a new type of antitumor drug. Through these studies we learned that herbimycin, originally isolated by Omura et al. in 1979 (34) for its herbicidal activity, and oxanosine, isolated by Shimada et al. in 1981 (37) for its antibacterial activity, had an inhibitory effect on the functions of certain oncogene products. Erbstatin, an inhibitor of the tyrosine kinase of an oncogene (erb B) product, was first isolated by Umezawa et al. in 1986 (50). These inhibitors are expected to be effective against tumors in which cognate oncogenes are activated.

In this review, studies on bleomycin, aclacinomycin, 4'-O-tetrahydropyranyladriamycin (THP), spergualin, bestatin, forphenicinol, and inhibitors of oncogene product function will be only briefly outlined because these agents are separately described later in this monograph. Then some of the new antitumor antibiotics discovered at the Institute of Microbial Chemistry, Tokyo (IMC) during the last ten years will be presented and, finally, mitomycin (9) and neocarzinostatin (26) will be reviewed. Some interesting new antitumor antibiotics recently found by others in Japan will also be described, although no clinical results have yet been reported.

Studies on Useful Antitumor Antibiotics Discovered and Launched by the IMC*

1. Bleomycin

The definite structure of bleomycin was elucidated in 1978 (42), and its total synthesis was completed in 1981 in collaboration with Takita in our institute (43). The pyrimidoblamyl-(β-hydroxyl)histidyl moiety was thought to be the site reactive with DNA. It was assumed that a bleomycin-Fe^{2+}-O_2 complex was formed in the nucleus and cytoplasm and caused DNA double strand scission. The thiazole moiety was considered the DNA binding site, intercalating between bases of double-stranded DNA. The AHM moiety,(2S, 3S, 4R)-4-amino-3-hydroxy-2-methylpentanoic acid, was not only the connective chain between the DNA reaction site and DNA binding site, but was also involved in anticancer activity. Bleomycins with different terminal amines were found to differ in their degree of renal or pulmonary toxicity. When unnatural amines were added to the culture medium of a bleomycin-producing strain, the amines were incorporated into the amine moiety of bleomycins. Therefore, many bleomycin analogues were prepared by fermentation, biosynthesis, or total synthesis.

In this way, many bleomycin analogues were studied for acute and chronic toxicity, therapeutic index, antitumor spectrum, and pulmonary toxicity. As a consequence, peplomycin (57), having phenylethylaminopropylamine as the terminal amine, was chosen as one worthy of clinical study, and was marketed in 1981. After that, liblomycin (57) was selected; it had a bulky lipophilic amine as terminal amine and low or no pulmonary toxicity in animal experiments. It entered Phase I study in 1987.

2. Aclacinomycin A (aclarubicin) and 4′-O-tetrahydropyranyladriamycin (pirarubicin)

Since 1971 we have isolated about 39 new analogues of anthracycline antitumor antibiotics, and aclacinomycin A was found in 1976 (31). Different from daunorubicin and adriamycin, the structure of aclacinomycin A is characterized by an ethyl group at C-9 instead of the acetyl or the hydroxyacetyl group, and the presence of a trisaccharide (rhodosamine, 2-deoxyfucose, and cinerulose) attached *via* a glycosidic linkage at C-7. It is effective against adult myelocytic leukemias, both those sensitive and refractory to daunorubicin or adriamycin, and has thus far caused no congestive heart failure. It was marketed in 1982.

We also discovered baumycins in 1977 (39), which were shown to be 4′-O-(1-alkoxyalkyl) derivatives of daunorubicin, in culture filtrates of daunorubicin-producing strains. Baumycin A showed a strong antitumor activity against L1210 leukemia cells. Thereupon, we synthesized about fifty analogues of 4′-O-acetal derivatives of adriamy-

---

* The chemical structures of the following antibiotics are shown in the papers of the pertinent authors in this monograph: bleomycin, peplomycin, and liblomycin by Takita; aclacinomycin A (aclarubicin) and THP (pirarubicin) by Tone; spergualin by Kunimoto; bestatin (ubenimex) by Ishizuka; oxanosine, herbimycin, and erbstatin by Hori.

cin and daunorubicin, among which THP showed a stronger effect against L1210 than adriamycin and daunorubicin (*55*). THP had significantly lower cardiac toxicity than adriamycin in hamsters. In the Phase I and II studies, THP was found to be effective against lymphatic leukemia, malignant lymphomas, head and neck cancer, ovarian tumor, and uterine cancer (*36*). Such side effects as hair loss, nausea, and vomiting were very slight and no cardiac toxicity has been observed. THP was introduced in 1988.

3. *Spergualin*

Spergualin is a hygroscopic, basic white powder which contains spermidine and guanidine in its structure. It inhibits the focus formation of transformed chicken embryo fibroblasts by Rous sarcoma virus. Moreover, spergualin strongly inhibits the growth of L1210, P-388, C1498, EL-4, RL male I, and especially L1210 (IMC), the latter obtained in 1965 from T. Yamamoto of the University of Tokyo, who brought it from the L1210 strain at the National Cancer Institute (NCI), U.S.A. in 1961 (*28, 40*). Spergualin used at optimum dosage cured mice bearing L1210 (IMC), and the cured mice showed resistance to the cancer when reinoculated with L1210 (10^6 cells). In this case, the effector cells were thought to be T cells (*54*), but the real mechanism of action has not yet been determined.

We carried out total synthesis of spergualin and its analogues; among them, 15-deoxyspergualin was chosen for Phase I study in the U.S.A. and in Japan because it showed the strongest antitumor activity.

4. *Studies on low molecular weight immunomodifiers, bestatin, and forphenicinol*

In 1972 we discovered coriolin B produced by *Coriolus consors* and showed it to enhance the production of antibody in mice. Diketocoriolin B, a derivative of coriolin B, increased the number of antibody-forming cells in the mouse spleen and inhibited Na^+-K^+-ATPase located on the cell membrane. Accordingly, we assumed that the binding of inhibitors to enzymes located on the membrane of immunocompetent cells might give rise to an increase in production of antibody-forming cells. First, in cooperation with Aoyagi in our institue, we looked for enzymes located on the cell surface or on the cell membrane and found that aminopeptidase, alkaline phosphatase, and esterases existed on the cell surface. We then searched for inhibitors of these enzymes and discovered bestatin in 1976, inhibiting aminopeptidase B and leucine aminopeptidase; amastain in 1978, inhibiting aminopeptidase A and leucine aminopeptidase; forphenicine in 1978, inhibiting chicken intestine alkaline phosphatase; and esterastin in 1978, inhibiting esterase.

Bestatin enhanced delayed-type hypersensitivity (DTH) of mice to sheep red blood cells when 1, 10, or 100 μg/mouse was orally given at the time of immunization, whereas 1,000 μg/mouse did not enhance DTH but did increase the number of spleen cells producing antibody to sheep red blood cells. DTH reduced by cyclophosphamide treatment or by Ehrlich carcinoma inoculation was restored to the normal level by oral administration of 10–100 μg/mouse of bestatin. Bestatin showed an inhibitory effect against the growth of solid tumors, as well as enhancing the effect of clinically useful anticancer drugs such as bleomycin, adriamycin, aclacinomycin, and mitomycin. Moreover, bestatin suppressed the spontaneous development of tumors in aged mice. It is noteworthy that bestatin has no or extremely low toxicity in experimental animals.

Bestatin was clinically studied (*2, 35*), and daily doses of 30 or 60 mg were found to restore the low percentage or small number of T cells normally found in cancer patients to the base line level. The reduced activity of natural killer (NK) cells in cancer patients was also restored by oral administration of bestatin. A randomized controlled study of immunotherapy with bestatin was performed in patients with adult non-lymphocytic leukemia, and the result showed a significant prolongation of survival time in the bestatin group compared with that in the control group. Bestatin was marketed in 1987.

Forphenicine, which inhibits chicken intestine alkaline phosphatase, was discovered in 1978 in the culture filtrate of a strain of *Actinomycetes*. Forphenicine enhanced DTH in mice by intraperitoneal administration but not by the oral route. Therefore, forphenicinol, L-(3-hydroxy-4-hydroxymethylphenyl)glycine, was synthesized as an active derivative for oral administration.

Forphenicinol augmented DTH, macrophage phagocytosis, and production of colony-forming units in culture (CFU/c) in bone marrow cell cultures. It exhibited an antitumor effect against slow growing tumors and enhanced the effects of antineoplastic drugs. Forphenicinol also showed a protective effect against *Pseudomonas* infection and, moreover, displayed an extremely low toxicity in experimental animals.

Clinical studies on the effect of forphenicinol on chronic bronchitis with *Pseudomonas* infection (27) and a placebo-controlled randomized trial with forphenicinol on malignant melanoma (10) are now being carried out in Japan.

5. *Inhibitors of oncogene functions*

There is accumulated evidence that oncogenes are involved in the expression of malignant phenotypes, although much remains to be learned about how oncogenes function. In view of such evidence, we initiated the screening of microbial sources for inhibitors of oncogene functions in the hope of finding new types of antitumor drugs which may also be useful in the elucidation of oncogene functions.

A rat kidney cell line (NRK) integrating a temperature-sensitive oncogene, either src^{ts} or ras^{ts}, shows a transformed morphology and a normal morphology at 33°C (the permissive temperature) and 39°C (the nonpermissive temperature), respectively. We found that herbimycin and oxanosine reversed the transformed morphologies of src^{ts} NRK and ras^{ts} NRK, respectively, at 33°C (47). In addition, oxanosine inhibited the *in vitro* growth of these cell lines more strongly at 33°C than at 39°C (13).

Oncogene products of the *src* family are known to have tyrosine kinase activities which are closely correlated with their oncogene functions. An inhibitor of *erb* B-associated tyrosine kinase was newly isolated and named erbstatin.

Other New Antitumor Antibiotics Discovered at IMC

1. *Anthracyclines*

Of the various anthracyclines we obtained, aclarubicin and pirarubicin have been described above. Microbial biosynthetic glycosidation of natural or semisynthetic anthracyclinones with an aglycone-nonproducing mutant of an aclacinomycin A-producing strain produced many hybrid anthracycline antibiotics composed of an exogenous aglycone and aclacinomycin A-sugars, among which 2-hydroxy-aclacinomycin A (Fig. 1) (1981) (32), trisarubicinol (1981) (62) and CG7 had excellent antitumor activity against L1210. CG7 was named betaclamycin A (Fig. 1) from which betaclamycins M, N, S, and T were chemically obtained (1984) (61). All of them were nonmutagenic against

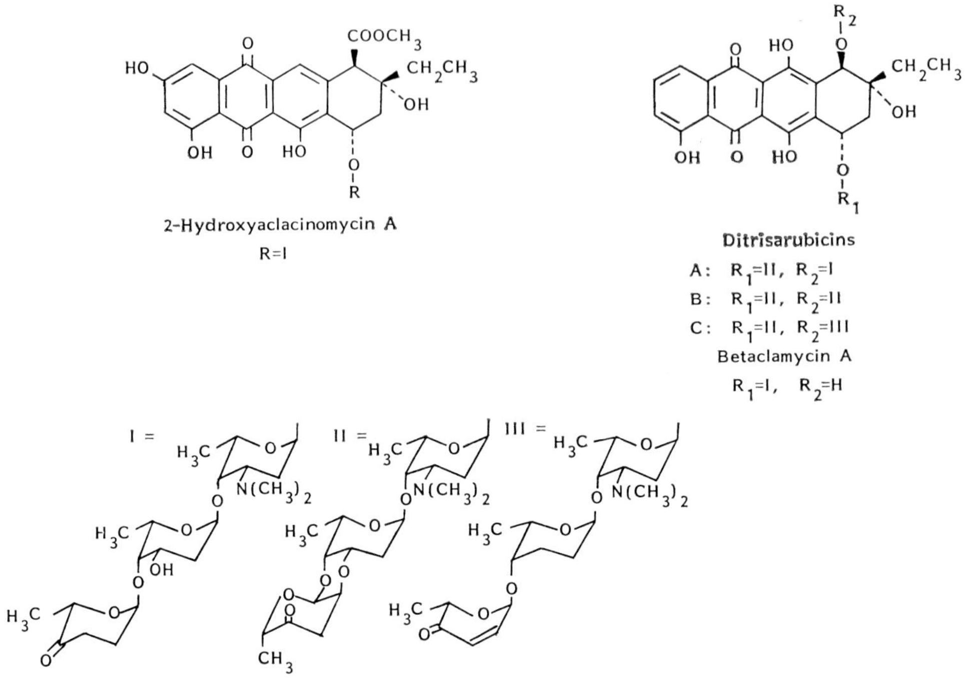

FIG. 1.   2-Hydroxyaclacinomycin A, betaclamycin A, and ditrisarubicins

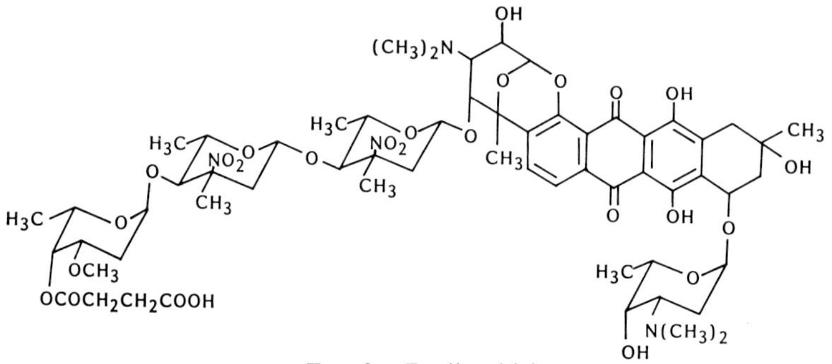

FIG. 2.   Decilorubicin

bacterial mutagenesis tests. 2-Hydroxyaclacinomycin A and betaclamycin A were more resistant than aclacinomycin A to the reductive cleavage at C7 by redox enzymes and inhibited the growth of adriamycin-resistant P388 leukemia cells. The plasma levels of these in dogs were much higher than that of aclacinomycin A.

In a continuation of the screening for cytotoxic antibiotics inhibiting L1210 leukemia, we found ditrisarubicins A, B, and C from the culture filtrate of *Streptomyces cyaneus*. Ditrisarubicins (1983) (*45*) contain trisaccharides at both C-7 and C-10 positions (Fig. 1). These antibiotics strongly inhibit the growth of adriamycin-sensitive and -resistant cells *in vitro*, and their DNA-binding is the strongest of the known anthracyclines.

Decilorubicin (1983) is a new antitumor antibiotic having two nitro sugars (decilonitrose) (Fig. 2) (*12*).

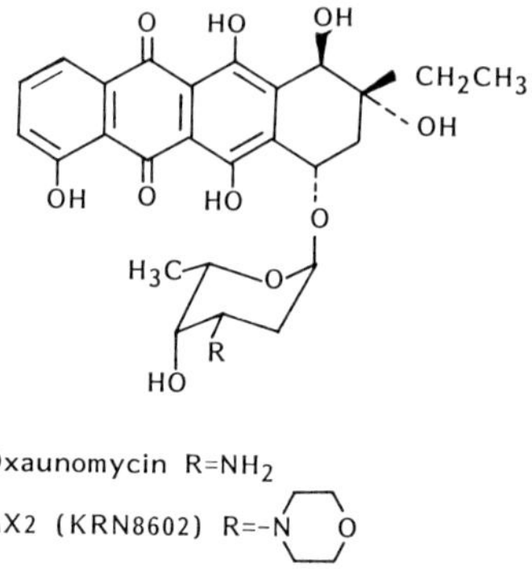

Oxaunomycin R=NH$_2$

MX2 (KRN8602) R=-N

FIG. 3.   Oxaunomycin and MX2

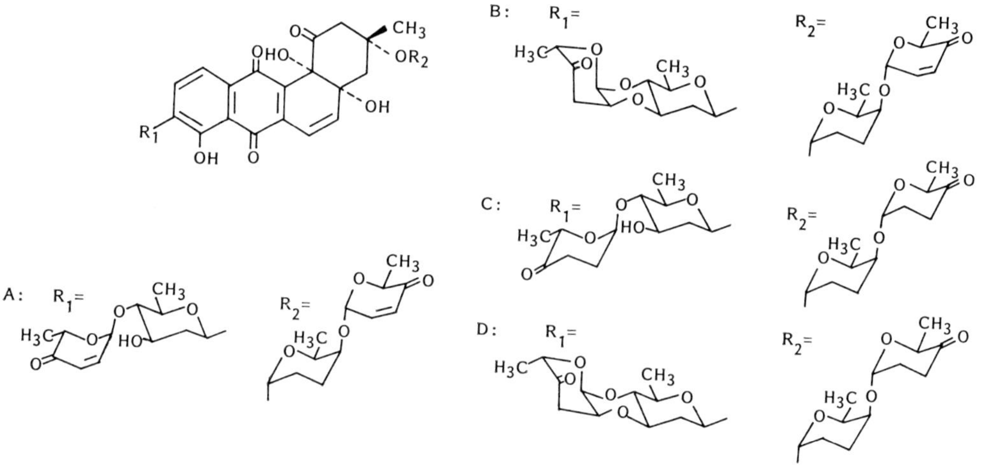

FIG. 4.   Saquayamycins

The new anthracycline oxaunomycin (Fig. 3) (1986) (*60*) has strong cytotoxic action: the concentration giving 50% inhibition of L1210 cell growth was 300 pg/ml. Another characteristic is its stronger inhibiting action on DNA synthesis than on RNA synthesis.

3'-Deamino-3'-morpholino-13-deoxo-10-hydroxycarminomycin hydrochloride (MX2, KRN8602) (Fig. 3) (1987) (*53*) showed strong antitumor activity on adriamycin-sensitive and -resistant P388 leukemias both *in vitro* and *in vivo*. This compound also exhibited strong antitumor activity against P388 leukemia, L1210 leukemia, Lewis lung cancer, and colon 26 cancer in mice (*18*). Subacute toxicity in rats and dogs and cardiac toxicity in hamsters and rabbits were found to be lower than those of adriamycin. The Phase I clinical study is now being carried out in Japan.

2.   *Other new antitumor antibiotics*

From the culture broth of *Streptomyces nodosus*, four new antibiotics were isolated and termed saquayamycins A, B, C, and D (Fig. 4) (1985) (*46*). The compounds are glycosides of aquayamycin and inhibit the growth of adriamycin-sensitive and -resistant p388 leukemia cells.

New 1,4-benzodiazepine antibiotics, neothramycins A and B (1976) (*41*), were found in culture filtrates of *Streptomyces* sp. MC916-C4. They exhibited a marked therapeutic

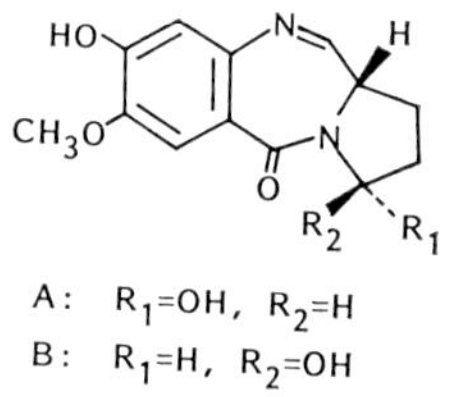

A : R₁=OH, R₂=H
B : R₁=H, R₂=OH

FIG. 5.   Neothramycins

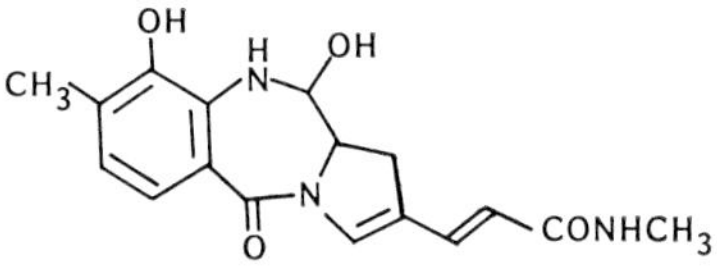

FIG. 6.   Mazethramycin

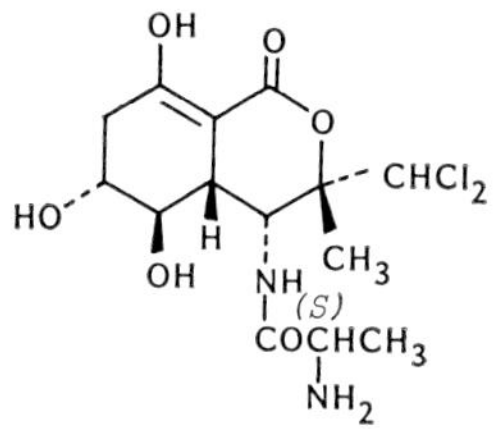

FIG. 7.   Bactobolin

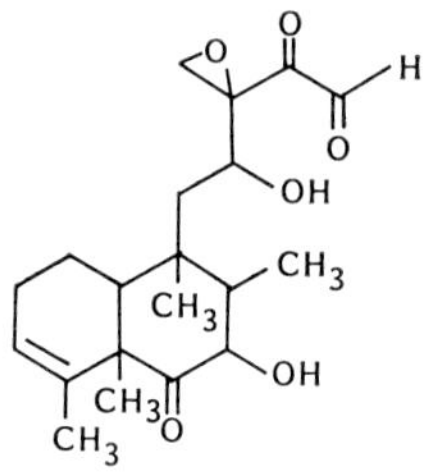

FIG. 8.   Terpentecin

effect on Yoshida rat sarcoma and mouse leukemia L1210. The structures were determined and confirmed by their total synthesis (Fig. 5). There was no myelosuppression nor cardiovascular or central nervous toxicity. The Phase I study is now being conducted in Japan. Another 1,4-benzodiazepine, mazethramycin (Fig. 6) (1980) (22), isolated from a culture of streptomyces, exhibited a marked life span-prolonging action in mice bearing L1210.

A chlorine-containing antibiotic, bactobolin (1979) (19), was found in a culture of *Pseudomonas*. It is structurally related to actinobolin produced by streptomyces (Fig. 7), inhibiting the growth of various bacteria and exhibiting an antitumor action against mouse leukemia L1210.

Terpentecin (Fig. 8) (1985) (44) was isolated from a culture broth of *Kitasatosporia griseola*. This compound has strong antibacterial activity and exhibits strong antitumor activity against L1210, P388, and Ehrlich carcinoma.

Some Interesting Antitumor Antibiotics Discovered by Others in Japan

1. Mitomycin C

Hata *et al.* (1956) isolated a reddish purple antibiotic and a purple-colored one from the culture broth of *Streptomyces caespitosus* (*9*). Both were active against Ehrlich carcinoma and Yoshida sarcoma and were called mitomycins A and B. In 1958, Wakaki *et al.* isolated mitomycin C as dark purple crystals from a culture broth (*59*) and it has been used clinically since that time (Fig. 9). Mitomycins A, B, and C exhibit strong antibacterial activity against gram-positive and gram-negative bacteria and also have considerable toxicity. The aziridine ring is activated by an NADPH-dependent enzyme and binds to the guanine moieties of DNA, forming a cross-linked complex with double-stranded DNA.

Clinically, mitomycin C is used for the treatment of various malignant neoplasms such as sarcoma, leukemia, Hodgkin's disease, malignant lymphoma, choriocarcinoma, and gastrointestinal tract cancers. Side effects consisting of disturbances of the digestive organs, a bleeding tendency (especially bleeding in the intestinal mucosa), leukopenia, thrombocytopenia, and hepatic and renal toxicities have been reported.

Recently, a clinical study of a mitomycin analogue, 7-N-(*p*-hydroxyphenyl)mitomycin C (M-83) (Fig. 9), has been made in Japan (*11*).

2. Neocarzinostatin

Maeda *et al.* (1966) isolated a high molecular weight antitumor antibiotic from the culture broth of *Streptomyces carzinostaticus* and called it neocarzinostatin (*26*). Neocarzinostatin is a peptide preparation which consists of an acidic protein of about 12,100 daltons and a low molecular weight chromophore (Fig. 10) (*6*). This antibiotic possesses antibacterial activity against *Micrococcus luteus* and antitumor activity against ascites type of Ehrlich carcinoma, sarcoma 180, and leukemia L1210.

Clinically, neocarzinostatin has been used for the treatment of acute leukemia, as well as for stomach and pancreatic cancers. Bone marrow suppression and anaphylactic reaction were reported as major side effects.

Neocarzinostatin reacts with the tumor cell membrane and inhibits DNA synthesis and cell mitosis. In a cell-free system, this antibiotic causes DNA single-strand scission non-enzymatically (*25*).

3. Leptomycin and kazusamycin

Hamamoto *et al.* isolated leptomycins A and B in 1983 (Fig. 11) (*8*) from the culture filtrate of a strain of streptomyces. They exhibited a strong inhibitory activity against *Schizosaccharomyces* and *Mucor*.

I. Umezawa *et al.* in 1984 found kazusamycin (*58*) from the culture broth of *Strep-*

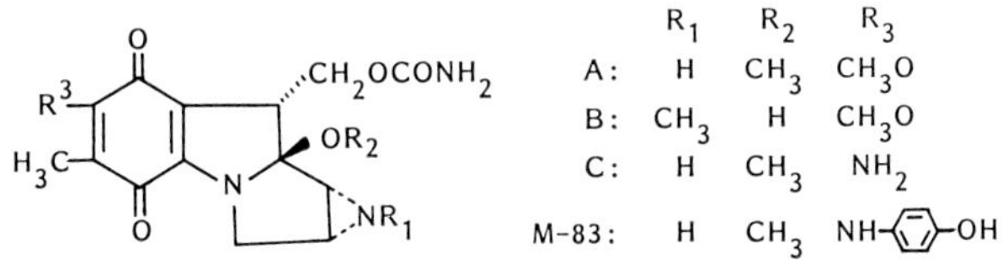

FIG. 9. Mitomycins

A

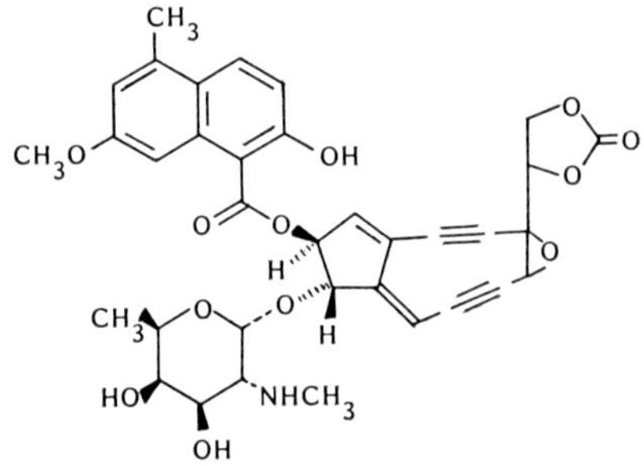

B

10
Ala-Ala-Pro-Thr-Ala-Thr-Val-Thr-Pro-Ser-Ser-Gly-Leu-Ser-Asp-
20   30
Gly-Thr-Val-Val-Lys-Val-Ala-Gly-Ala-Gly-Leu-Gln-Ala-Gly-Thr-
40
Ala-Tyr-Asp-Val-Gly-Gln-Cys-Ala-Trp-Val-Asn-Thr-Gly-Val-Leu-
50   60
Ala-Cys-Asp-Pro-Ala-Asn-Phe-Ser-Ser-Val-Thr-Ala-Asp-Ala-Asp-
70
Gly-Ser-Ala-Ser-Thr-Ser-Leu-Thr-Val-Arg-Arg-Ser-Phe-Glu-Gly-
80   90
Phe-Leu-Phe-Asp-Gly-Thr-Arg-Trp-Gly-Thr-Val-Asn-Cys-Thr-Thr-
100
Ala-Ala-Cys-Gln-Val-Gly-Leu-Ser-Asp-Ala-Ala-Gly-Asp-Gly-Glu-
110
Pro-Gly-Val-Ala-Ile-Ser-Phe-Asn

FIG. 10.   Neocarzinostatin

A: chromophore structure.   B: structure of the protein portion.

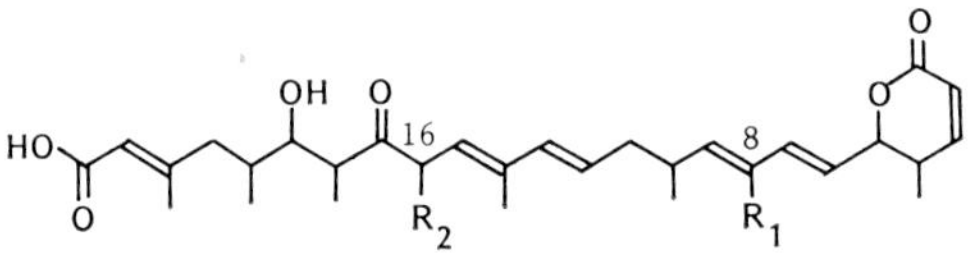

Kazusamycin B: $R_1=CH_3$ $R_2=CH_2OH$
Kazusamycin A: $R_1=CH_2CH_3$ $R_2=CH_2OH$
Leptomycin A : $R_1=CH_3$ $R_2=CH_3$
Leptomycin B : $R_1=CH_2CH_3$ $R_2=CH_3$

FIG. 11.   Kazusamycins and leptomycins

tomyces sp. No. 81-484. Kazusamycin B was isolated as one of the major products, together with kazusamycin A and already known congeners leptomycins A and B. Their structures were shown to have an unsaturated branched-chain fatty acid with a terminal δ-lactam ring (Fig. 11). Kazusamycin B showed potent cytocidal activity against L1210 and P388 leukemia cells *in vitro*.

4. Rhizoxin

In 1982 Iwasaki *et al.* isolated rhizoxin (*16*), a new 16-membered macrocyclic lactone, from the culture broth of a plant pathogenic fungus, *Rhizopus chinensis* Rh-2 (Fig. 12). Rhizoxin is one of the ansamacrolides.

Rhizoxin inhibited mitosis of tumor cells just like vinca alkaloids, as evidenced by morphological and flow cytometry analysis, and it was found to have considerably strong activity against L1210 and P388 leukemia cells and B16 melanoma. Rhizoxin was also found to be effective against vincristine- and adriamycin-resistant tumor cells *in vitro* and *in vivo*.

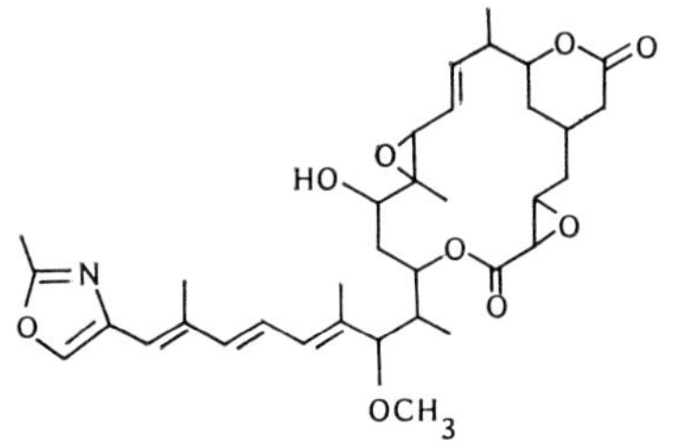

FIG. 12. Rhizoxin

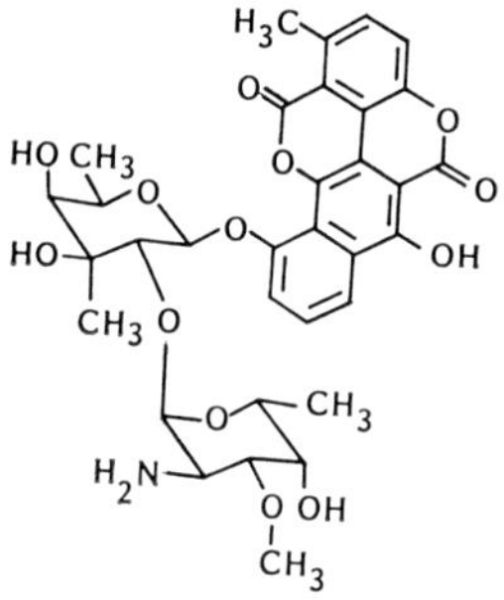

FIG. 13. Elsamicin A

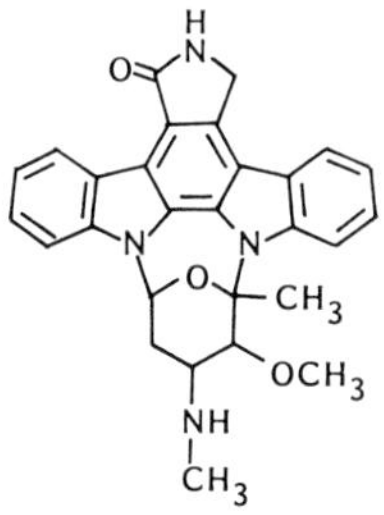

FIG. 14. Staurosporine

5. *Elsamicin*

The new antitumor antibiotic elsamicin A was found by Konishi *et al.* in 1986 (*21*) in the culture broth of an unidentified actinomycetes strain isolated from a soil sample from El Salvador. It is structurally similar to chartreusin, containing chartarin as the aglycone (Fig. 13). Elsamicin A showed a strong effect in prolonging the life span of mice bearing P388 leukemia, L1210 leukemia, or B16 melanoma.

6. *Staurosporine*

Omura *et al.* isolated a new alkaloid, AM-2282 (*33*), from cultures of *Streptomyces staurosporeus* in 1977. It showed an antimicrobial activity against fungi and yeasts. In 1981, Oka *et al.* found a potent platelet aggregation inhibitor from the culture broth of streptomyces strain M-193 (*29*), and it was identified as AM-2282. The structure was determined in 1983 by X-ray crystallographic analysis (*7*) and it was called staurosporine (Fig. 14). Staurosporine was shown to have an indolocarbazole structure. Staurosporine has many interesting characteristics, *e.g.*, it inhibits protein kinase and shows strong cytotoxic activity against the growth of some tumor lines.

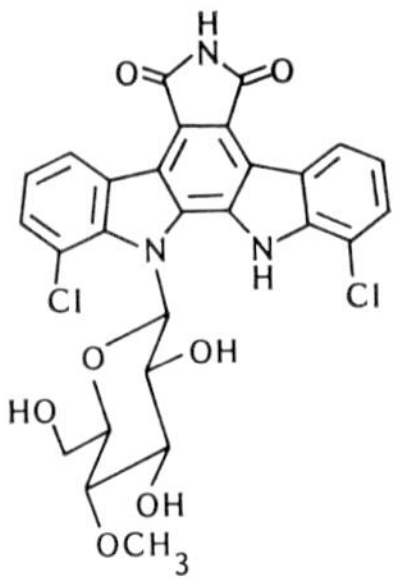

Fig. 15.   Rebeccamycin

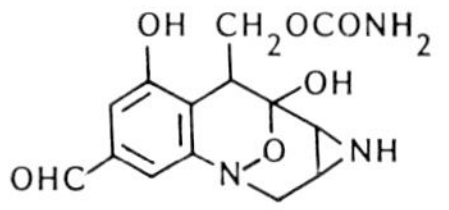

Fig. 16.   FR-900482

Rebeccamycin (*4*), a novel antitumor agent developed by Bristol-Myers Co., is structurally related to staurosporine (Fig. 15). As rebeccamycin has an antitumor activity
against P388 leukemia, L1210 leukemia, and B16 melanoma in mice, staurosporine and
rebeccamycin may be promising agents for cancer treatment.

7.   FR-900482 and FK973

Iwami *et al.* discovered in 1987 a new antitumor antibiotic, FR-900482 (*15, 38*) from
the fermentation broth of *Streptomyces sandaensis*. Its structure was determined as 4-
formyl-6,9-dihydroxy-14-oxa-1,11-diazatetracyclo-tetradeca-2,4,6-triene-8-ylmethyl car-
bamate (Fig. 16).

The antitumor activity of FR-900482 was stronger than that of mitomycin C *in vitro*.
It prolonged the life span of mice bearing ascitic P388, L1210, B16, MM46, Ehrlich, or
EL 4 tumors. FR-900482 was also effective against mitomycin C- or vincristine-resistant
P388, but not against cyclophosphamide-resistant P388.

The 6,9-O-11-N-triacetyl derivative (FK973) of FR-900482 showed a stronger antitumor activity than the mother compound and is now undergoing clinical trial.

8.   Esperamicins, FR-900405, and FR-900406

Konishi *et al.* isolated potent esperamicin antitumor antibiotics in 1984 from the
culture of *Actinomadura verrucosospora* (*20*). Esperamicins contain principal components,
A_1 and A_2, and minor congeners, A_{1b}, A_3, B_1, and B_2 (Fig. 17). Esperamicins A_1 and A_2
exhibit antimicrobial activity against gram-positive and gram-negative bacteria and
fungi, and display the strongest antitumor activity among anticancer drugs so far discovered: the growth of various tumor strains is inhibited at the extremely low concentration of 1–3 pg/ml. These drugs exhibit strong antitumor activity against mice bearing
P388 leukemia, B16 melanoma, or Lewis lung cancer.

Iwami *et al.* found new antitumor antibiotics, FR-900405 and FR-900406, in 1985
(*14, 17*) in the culture broth of a strain of *Actinomadura pulveracea*. FR-900405 exhibited
very strong antitumor activity and was found to be identical with esperamicin A_{1b}.

In this connection, PD-114759 and PD-115028 (*3*) were isolated by Warner-

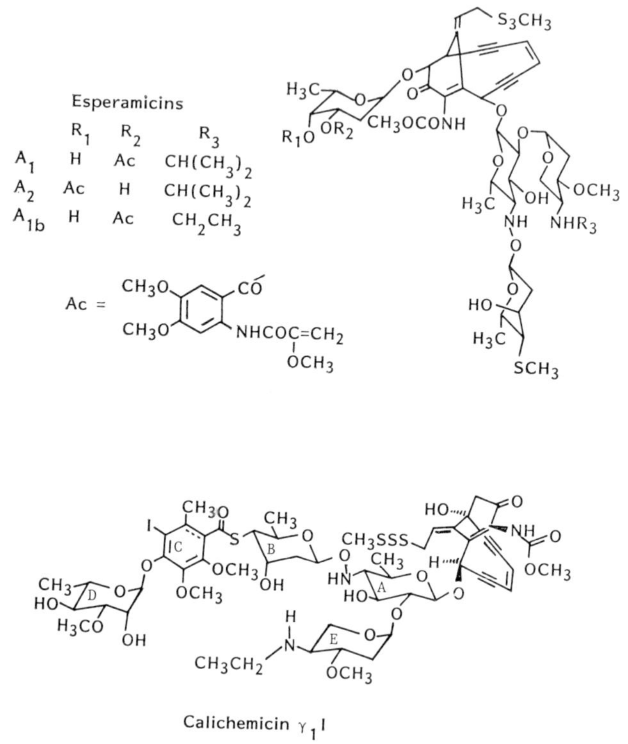

FIG. 17. Esperamicins and calichemicin γ_1 I

Lambert / Parke-Davis Pharmaceutical Research from a fermentation broth of *A. pulveracea*. These compounds exhibited excellent activity *in vivo* against P388 leukemia and a variety of solid tumors. PD-114759 was found to be identical with esperamicin A_1, and PD-115028 with esperamicin A_2.

Calichemicins, the products of a strain of *Micromonospora echinospora*, were found by Lederle Laboratories. They showed extraordinary potency against murine tumors and were approximately 4,000-fold more active than adriamycin, with the optimal dose at 0.5–1.5 µg/kg (*23, 24*). Calichemicins have a novel structure related to esperamicins, FR-900406, PD-114759, and PD-115028 (Fig. 17).

Esperamicin-calichemicin antibiotics with extraordinarily potent antitumor activity appear promising for use in cancer chemotherapy.

REFERENCES

1. Arcamone, F., Cassinelli, G., Fantini, G., Grein, A., Orezzi, P., Pol, C., and Spalla, C. Adriamycin, 14-hydroxydaunomycin, a new antitumor antibiotic from *S. peucetius* var. *caesius*. *Biotechnol. Bioenz.*, **11**, 1101–1110 (1969).
2. Blomgren, H., Näslund, I., Esposti, P-L., Johansen, L., and Aaskoven, O. Adjuvant bestatin immunotherapy in patients with transitional cell carcinoma of the bladder; clinical results of a randomized trial. *Cancer Immunol. Immunother.*, **25**, 41–46 (1987).
3. Bunge, R. H., Hurley, T. R., Smitka, T. A., Willmer, N. E., Brankiewicz, A. J., Steinman, C. E., and French, J. C. PD 114,759 and PD 115,028, novel antitumor antibiotics

with phenomenal potency. I. Isolation and characterization. *J. Antibiot.*, **37**, 1566–1571 (1984).

4. Bush, J. A., Long, B. H., Catino, J. J., Bradner, W. T., and Tomita, K. Production and biological activity of rebeccamycin, a novel antitumor agent. *J. Antibiot.*, **40**, 668–678 (1987).

5. DiMarco, H., Silvestrini, R., Gaetani, M., Soldati, M., Orezzi, P., Dasdia, T., Scarpinato, B. M., and Valentini, L. 'Daunomycin,' a new antibiotic of the rhodomycin group. *Nature*, **201**, 706–707 (1964).

6. Edo, K., Mizugaki, M., Koide, Y., and Ishida, N. The structure of neocarzinostatin chromophore possessing a novel bicyclo-[7, 3, 0]-dodecadiyne system. *Tetrahedron Lett.*, **26**, 331–334 (1985).

7. Furusaki, A., Hashiba, N., Matsumoto, T., Hirano, A., Iwai, Y., and Omura, S. X-ray crystal structure of staurosporine: A new alkaloid from a *Streptomyces* strain. *J. Chem. Soc. Chem. Commun.*, 800–801 (1978).

8. Hamamoto, T., Gunji, S., Tsuji, H., and Beppu, T. Leptomycins A and B, new antifungal antibiotics. I. Taxonomy of the producing strain and their fermentation, purification and characterization. *J. Antibiot.*, **36**, 639–645 (1983).

9. Hata, T., Sano, Y., Sugawara, R., Matsumae, A., Kanamori, K., Shima, T., and Hoshi, T. Mitomycin, a new antibiotic from *Streptomyces*. I. *J. Antibiot.*, **A9**, 141–146 (1956).

10. Ikeda, S., Ishihara, K., and Ogawa, N. Double blind study of forphenicinol in malignant melanoma and squamous cell carcinoma of the skin. *Biotherapy*, **1**, 114–122 (1978) (in Japanese).

11. Imai, R., Ashigawa, T., Urakawa, C., Morimoto, M., and Nakamura, N. Antitumor activity of 7-*N*-phenyl derivatives of mitomycin C in the leukemia P338 system. *Jpn. J. Cancer Res.* (*Gann*), **71**, 560–562 (1980).

12. Ishii, K., Kondo, S., Nishimura, Y., Hamada, M., Takeuchi, T., and Umezawa, H. Decilorubicin, a new anthracycline antibiotic. *J. Antibiot.*, **36**, 451–453 (1983).

13. Itoh, O., Kuroiwa, S., Atsumi, S., Umezawa, K., Takeuchi, T., and Hori, M. Induction by the guanosine analogue oxanosine of reversion toward the normal phenotype of *K-ras*-transformed rat kidney cells. *Cancer Res.*, **49**, 996–1000 (1989).

14. Iwami, M., Kiyoto, S., Nishikawa, M., Terano, H., Kohsaka, M., Aoki, H., and Imanaka, H. New antitumor antibiotics, FR-900405 and FR-900406. I. Taxonomy of the producing strain. *J. Antibiot.*, **38**, 835–839 (1985).

15. Iwami, M., Kiyoto, S., Terano, H., Kohsaka, M., Aoki, H., and Imanaka, H. A new antitumor antibiotic, FR-900482. I. Taxonomic studies on the producing strain: A new species of the genus streptomyces. *J. Antibiot.*, **40**, 589–593 (1987).

16. Iwasaki, S., Kobayashi, H., Furukawa, J., Namikoshi, M., Okuda, S., Sato, Z., Matsuda, I., and Noda, T. Studies on macrocyclic lactone antibiotics. VII. Structure of a phytotoxin "rhizoxin" produced by *Rhizopus chinensis*. *J. Antibiot.*, **37**, 354–362 (1984).

17. Kiyoto, S., Nishikawa, M., Terano, H., Kohsaka, M., Aoki, H., Imanaka, H., Kawai, Y., Uchida, I., and Hashimoto, M. New antitumor antibiotics, FR-900405 and FR-900406. II. Production, isolation, characterization and antitumor activity. *J. Antibiot.*, **38**, 840–848 (1985).

18. Komeshima, N., Tsuruo, T., and Umezawa, H. Antitumor activity of new morpholino anthracyclines. *J. Antibiot.*, **41**, 548–553 (1988).

19. Kondo, S., Horiuchi, Y., Hamada, M., Takeuchi, T., and Umezawa, H. A new antitumor antibiotic, bactobolin produced by *Pseudomonas*. *J. Antibiot.*, **32**, 1069–1071 (1979).

20. Konishi, M., Ohkuma, H., Saitoh, K., Kawaguchi, H., Golik, J., Dubay, G., Groenewold, G., Krishnan, B., and Doyle, T. W. Esperamicins, a novel class of potent antitumor antibiotics. I. Physicochemical data and partial structure. *J. Antibiot.*, **38**, 1605–1609 (1985).

21. Konishi, M., Sugawara, K., Kofu, F., Nishiyama, Y., Tomita, K., Miyaki, T., and

Kawaguchi, H. Elsamicins, new antitumor antibiotics related to chartreusin. I. Production, isolation, characterization and antitumor activity. *J. Antibiot.*, **39**, 784–791 (1986).

22. Kunimoto, S., Masuda, T., Kanbayashi, N., Hamada, M., Naganawa, H., Miyamoto, M., Takeuchi, T., and Umezawa, H. Mazethramycin, a new member of anthramycin group antibiotics. *J. Antibiot.*, **33**, 665–667 (1980).

23. Lee, M. D., Dunne, T. S., Siegel, M. M., Chang, C. C., Morton, G. O., and Borders, D. B. Calichemicins, a novel family of antitumor antibiotics. 1. Chemistry and partial structure of calichemicin γ_1^1. *J. Am. Chem. Soc.*, **109**, 3464–3466 (1987).

24. Lee, M. D., Dunne, T. S., Chang, C. C., Ellstad, G. A., Siegel, M. M., Morton, G. O., McGahren, W. J., and Borders, D. B. Calichemicins, a novel family of antitumor antibiotics. 2. Chemistry and structure of calichemicin γ_1^1. *J. Am. Chem. Soc.*, **109**, 3466–3468 (1987).

25. Maeda, H., Aikawa, S., and Yamashita, A. Subcellular fate of protein antibiotic neocarzinostatin in culture of lymphoid cell line from Burkitt's lymphoma. *Cancer Res.*, **35**, 554–559 (1975).

26. Maeda, H., Kumagai, K., and Ishida, N. Characterization of neocarzinostatin. *J. Antibiot.*, **A19**, 253–259 (1966).

27. Matsumoto, K., Nagatake, T., Rikitomi, N., Uzuka, Y., and Harada, T. Clinical trial of a new immunomodulator, forphenicinol, against severe respiratory infections. 13th International Congress of Chemotherapy, Vienna (1983).

28. Nishikawa, K., Shibasaki, C., Takahashi, K., Nakamura, T., Takeuchi, T., and Umezawa, H. Antitumor activity of spergualin, a novel antitumor antibiotic. *J. Antibiot.*, **39**, 1461–1466 (1986).

29. Oka, S., Kodama, M., Takeda, H., Tomizuka, N., and Suzuki, H. Staurosporine, a potent platelet aggregation inhibitor from a *Streptomyces* species. *Agric. Biol. Chem.*, **50**, 2723–2727 (1986).

30. Oki, T., Matsuzawa, Y., Yoshimoto, A., Numata, K., Kitamura, I., Hori, S., Takamatsu, A., Umezawa, H., Ishizuka, M., Naganawa, H., Suda, H., Hamada, M., and Takeuchi, T. New antitumor antibiotics, aclacinomycins A and B. *J. Antibiot.*, **28**, 830–834 (1975).

31. Oki, T., Takeuchi, T., Oka, S., and Umezawa, H. New anthracycline antibiotic aclacinomycin A: Experimental studies and correlations with clinical trials. *Recent Results Cancer Res.*, **76**, 21–40 (1981).

32. Oki, T., Yoshimoto, A., Matsuzawa, Y., Takeuchi, T., and Umezawa, H. New anthracycline antibiotic, 2-hydroxyaclacinomycin A. *J. Antibiot.*, **34**, 916–918 (1981).

33. Omura, S., Iwai, Y., Hirano, A., Nakagawa, A., Awaya, J., Tsuchiya, H., Takahashi, Y., and Masuma, R. A new alkaloid AM-2282 of *Streptomyces* origin. Taxonomy, fermentation, isolation and preliminary characterization. *J. Antibiot.*, **30**, 275–282 (1977).

34. Omura, S., Iwai, Y., Takahashi, Y., Sadakane, N., Nakagawa, A., Oiwa, H., Hasegawa, Y., and Ikai, T. Herbimycin, a new antibiotic produced by a strain of streptomyces. *J. Antibiot.*, **32**, 255–261 (1979).

35. Ota, K., Kurita, S., Yamada, K., Masaoka, T., Uzuka, Y., and Ogawa, N. Immunotherapy with bestatin for acute nonlymphocytic leukemia in adults. *Cancer Immunol. Immunother.*, **23**, 5–10 (1986).

36. Saito, T. and other 19 authors. Phase II study of (2''R)-4'-O-tetrahydropyranyladriamycin (THP) in patients with solid tumors. *Jpn. J. Cancer Chemother.*, **13**, 1060–1069 (1986) (in Japanese).

37. Shimada, N., Yagisawa, N., Naganawa, H., Takita, T., Hamada, M., Takeuchi, T., and Umezawa, H. Oxanosine, a novel nucleoside from actinomycetes. *J. Antibiot.*, **34**, 1216–1218 (1981).

38. Shimomura, K., Hirai, O., Mizota, T., Matsumoto, S., Mori, J., Shibayama, F., and Kikuchi, H. A new antitumor antibiotic, FR-900482. III. Antitumor activity in trans-

plantable experimental tumors. *J. Antibiot.*, **40**, 600–606 (1987).

39. Takahashi, Y., Naganawa, H., Takeuchi, T., Umezawa, H., Komiyama, T., Oki, T., and Inui, T. The structure of baumycins A1, A2, B1, B2, C1 and C2. *J. Antibiot.*, **30**, 622–624 (1977).

40. Takeuchi, T., Iinuma, H., Kunimoto, S., Masuda, T., Ishizuka, M., Takeuchi, M., Hamada, M., Naganawa, H., Kondo, S., and Umezawa, H. A new antitumor antibiotic, spergualin: Isolation and antitumor activity. *J. Antibiot.*, **34**, 1619–1621 (1981).

41. Takeuchi, T., Miyamoto, M., Ishizuka, M., Naganawa, H., Kondo, S., Hamada, M., and Umezawa, H. Neothramycins A and B, new antitumor antibiotics. *J. Antibiot.*, **29**, 93–96 (1976).

42. Takita, T., Muraoka, Y., Nakatani, T., Fujii, A., Umezawa, Y., Naganawa, H., and Umezawa, H. Chemistry of bleomycin. XIX. Revised structures of bleomycin and phleomycin. *J. Antibiot.*, **31**, 801–804 (1978).

43. Takita, T., Umezawa, Y., Saito, S., Morishima, H., Umezawa, H., Muraoka, Y., Suzuki, M., Ohtsuka, M., Kobayashi, S., Ohno, M., Tsuchiya, T., Miyake, T., and Umezawa, S. Total synthesis of bleomycin A2. *In* "Peptides: Synthesis-Structure-Function. Proc. of the 7th American Peptide Symposium," ed. H. Rich and E. Gross, pp. 29–39 (1981). Pierce Chemical Company.

44. Tamamura, T., Sawa, T., Isshiki, K., Masuda, T., Homma, Y., Iinuma, H., Naganawa, H., Hamada, M., Takeuchi, T., and Umezawa, H. Isolation and characterization of terpentecin, a new antitumor antibiotic. *J. Antibiot.*, **38**, 1664–1669 (1985).

45. Uchida, T., Imoto, M., Masuda, T., Imamura, K., Hatori, Y., Sawa, T., Naganawa, H., Hamada, M., Takeuchi, T., and Umezawa, H. New antitumor antibiotics, ditrisarubicins A, B and C. *J. Antibiot.*, **36**, 1080–1083 (1983).

46. Uchida, T., Imoto, M., Watanabe, Y., Miura, K., Dobashi, T., Matsuda, N., Sawa, T., Naganawa, H., Hamada, M., Takeuchi, T., and Umezawa, H. Saquayamycins, new aquayamycin-group antibiotics. *J. Antibiot.*, **38**, 1171–1181 (1985).

47. Uehara, Y., Hori, M., Takeuchi, T., and Umezawa, H. Screening of agents which convert 'transformed morphology' of Rous sarcoma virus-infected rat kidney cells to 'normal morphology': Identification of an active agent as herbimycin and its inhibition of intracellular *src* kinase. *Jpn. J. Cancer Res. (Gann)*, **76**, 672–675 (1985).

48. Umezawa, H. Studies on antibiotics and enzyme inhibitors. *Rev. Infect. Dis.*, **9**, 147–164 (1987).

49. Umezawa, H., Aoyagi, T., Suda, H., Hamada, M., and Takeuchi, T. Bestatin, an inhibitor of aminopeptidase B, produced by actinomycetes. *J. Antibiot.*, **29**, 97–99 (1976).

50. Umezawa, H., Imoto, M., Sawa, T., Isshiki, K., Matsuda, N., Uchida, T., Iinuma, H., Hamada, M., and Takeuchi, T. Studies on a new epidermal growth factor-receptor kinase inhibitor, erbstatin, produced by MH435-hF3. *J. Antibiot.*, **39**, 170–173 (1986).

51. Umezawa, H., Kondo, S., Iinuma, H., Kunimoto, S., Ikeda, Y., Iwasawa, H., Ikeda, D., and Takeuchi, T. Structure of an antitumor antibiotic, spergualin. *J. Antibiot.*, **34**, 1622–1624 (1981).

52. Umezawa, H., Maeda, K., Takeuchi, T., and Okami, Y. New antibiotics, bleomycin A and B. *J. Antibiot.*, **A19**, 200–209 (1966).

53. Umezawa, H., Nakajima, S., Kawai, H., Komeshima, N., Yoshimoto, H., Urata, T., Odagawa, A., Otsuki, N., Tatsuta, K., Otake, N., and Takeuchi, T. New morpholino anthracyclines, MX, MX2, and MY5. *J. Antibiot.*, **40**, 1058–1061 (1987).

54. Umezawa, H., Nishikawa, K., Shibasaki, C., Takahashi, K., Nakamura, T., and Takeuchi, T. Involvement of cytotoxic T-lymphocytes in the antitumor activity of spergualin against L1210 cells. *Cancer Res.*, **47**, 3062–3065 (1987).

55. Umezawa, H., Takahashi, Y., Kinoshita, M., Naganawa, H., Masuda, T., Ishizuka, M., Tatsuta, K., and Takeuchi, T. Tetrahydropyranyl derivatives of daunomycin and adria-

mycin. *J. Antibiot.*, **32**, 1082–1084 (1979).

56. Umezawa, H., Takeuchi, T., Nitta, K., Yamamoto, T., and Yamaoka, S. Sarkomycin, an antitumor substance produced by streptomyces. *J. Antibiot.*, **A6**, 101 (1953).
57. Umezawa, H., Takita, T., Saito, S., Muraoka, Y., Takahashi, K., Ekimoto, H., Minamide, S., Nishikawa, K., Fukuoka, T., Nakatani, T., Fujii, A., and Matsuda, A. New analogs and derivatives of bleomycin. *In* "Bleomycin Chemotherapy," ed. B. I. Sikic, M. Rozencweig, and S. K. Carter, pp. 289–301 (1985). Academic Press, Inc., New York.
58. Umezawa, I., Komiyama, K., Oka, H., Okada, K., Tomisaka, S., Miyano, T., and Takano, S. A new antitumor antibiotic, kazusamycin. *J. Antibiot.*, **37**, 706–711 (1984).
59. Wakaki, S., Marumo, H., Tomioka, K., Shimizu, G., Kato, E., Kamada, H., Kudo, S., and Fujimoto, Y. Isolation of new fractions of antitumor mitomycins. *Antibiot. Chemother.*, **8**, 228–240 (1958).
60. Yoshimoto, A., Fujii, S., Johdo, O., Kubo, K., Ishikura, T., Naganawa, H., Sawa, T., Takeuchi, T., and Umezawa, H. Intensely potent anthracycline antibiotic oxaunomycin produced by a blocked mutant of the daunorubicin-producing microorganism. *J. Antibiot.*, **39**, 902–909 (1986).
61. Yoshimoto, A., Matsuzawa, Y., Ishikura, T., Sawa, T., Takeuchi, T., and Umezawa, H. New anthracycline derivatives from betaclamycin A. *J. Antibiot.*, **37**, 920–922 (1984).
62. Yoshimoto, A., Matsuzawa, Y., Matsushita, Y., Oki, T., Takeuchi, T., and Umezawa, H. Trisarubicinol, new antitumor anthracycline antibiotic. *J. Antibiot.*, **34**, 1492–1494 (1981).

DEVELOPMENT OF ANTITUMOR NATURAL PRODUCTS AT THE NATIONAL CANCER INSTITUTE

Matthew SUFFNESS

Developmental Therapeutics Program, Division of Cancer Treatment, National Cancer Institute, NIH*

The National Cancer Institute's (NCI) drug development program in natural products was begun in 1957 to increase the rate at which new drugs were brought to clinical studies. Its purpose was to compliment the activities of pharmaceutical companies and academic researchers and to provide a National resource for developing anticancer drugs with special attention to those which did not have strong economic potential. Depending on the needs of the public and the level of activity in the pharmaceutical industry, the NCI program has emphasized development of improved analogs of clinical agents or novel mechanistic and structural types. Four examples of compounds in current clinical trials in which the NCI played a strong role are acivicin, echinomycin, taxol, and 2'-deoxycoformycin (DCF). These represent novel chemotypes with different biochemical mechanisms and are respectively, an amino acid derivative with glutamine antagonist activity, a quinoxaline antibiotic which is a bifunctional intercalator, an unusual diterpene which stabilizes microtubules, and a potent inhibitor of adenosine deaminase. Clinical data to date are promising for DCF in hairy cell leukemia and T-cell malignancies and for taxol in ovarian cancer.

The intention of this paper is to provide an overview of the activities of the National Cancer Institute (NCI) in drug development of natural products from the beginnings of the drug development program to the present, to review some of the program's accomplishments and to discuss briefly several drugs of current interest.

There have been previous reviews of various aspects of the NCI program in natural products including plant products (*105, 106*), fermentation products (*19*), marine products (*5, 107*), the screening programs (*5, 31, 113*) the organization of preclinical new drug research (*20*) and the clinical trials program (*16, 124*). It seemed appropriate to bring some of that material together here to use as a basis for understanding the NCI's efforts in natural products drug development. The relationship in drug development of the NCI to the pharmaceutical industry and to researchers in academic settings has undergone changes over the years. Many of these changes transcend the science and development of natural products and therefore cannot be viewed in isolation from the overall philosophies of the NCI and the U.S. Congress.

Origins of Natural Products Drug Development Program

The NCI was established in 1937 with the mission "to provide for, foster and aid

---

* Bethesda, MD 20892, U.S.A.

in coordinating research related to cancer." It was not until the early 1950's however that serious consideration began to be given to establishment at NCI of a program for drug development. This was based on the clinical responses with nitrogen mustard in Hodgkin's disease (32), aminopterin in childhood leukemia (25) and 6-mercaptopurine in leukemia (7).

The first broadly based drug development programs were initiated at the Sloan-Kettering Institute for Cancer Research, the Chester Beatty Institute in Great Britain and the University of Tokyo. The Sloan-Kettering program grew out of a reorientation of the war effort with nitrogen mustards so that the Chemical Warfare Service became the nucleus of the Sloan-Kettering chemotherapy program (125). Both synthetic compounds and fermentation broths were tested at Sloan-Kettering, and in the early 1950's that program accounted for approximately 75% of the total chemotherapy screening capacity in the United States.

Insufficient capacity was available for researchers to have their new materials tested at Sloan-Kettering and this led to pressure from industrial and academic sources for a place to have their compounds tested as well as pressure from clinicians who wanted to follow up the leads that would be discovered. A meeting in 1952 of the National Advisory Cancer Council (the NCI's chief advisory board) considered the area of chemotherapy to justify increased support, but also felt that the state of knowledge was insufficient to warrant developing an engineered program. This group recommended increased support for chemotherapy in both the laboratory and clinical areas through increased grant funding. Despite the success of wartime programs, such as the antimalarial program and the penicillin production program, they were regarded unfavorably by many scientists who felt that they were dominated by a very few people, they were too secretive and they were too costly.

Pressure for a major program continued to mount and in 1954 Congress asked NCI to consider establishing a directed program of research in cancer chemotherapy. An *ad hoc* review committee concluded that such a program directed by the NCI was not appropriate and recommended increased funding of existing centers and that the NCI play a larger role on a voluntary basis by means of organizing meetings and symposia and producing newsletters for information exchange. These steps to improve communication were taken and also a series of large research grants were made to research institutions and medical schools to establish or expand integrated (preclinical and clinical) chemotherapy research programs.

In 1955, only a year later, Congress mandated that a program be organized on a national basis at the NCI. This led to formation of the Cancer Chemotherapy National Service Center (CCNSC) as the unit within NCI for coordination and operation of a national chemotherapy program to support research in the area and provide services to investigators in the field. The establishment of the CCNSC was by a joint committee including other involved Government agencies (the Atomic Energy Commission, the Veterans Administration and the Food and Drug Administration) and private foundations (American Cancer Society and the Damon Runyon Memorial Fund for Cancer Research). The CCNSC developed quickly and in 1956 the first contracts were awarded for screening, mouse breeding, screening methods development, pharmacology, and clinical studies. The first fermentation broths were tested in 1957 and that date can be said to mark the beginnings of natural product drug development at the NCI. Although Hartwell and collaborators had done some screening of plant extracts on a research basis before the

TABLE I. Examples of *In Vitro* Prescreens Used by NCI Fermentation Contractors

Cytotoxicity	Enzyme inhibition
KB cells	DNA polymerase
P388 cells	RNA polymerase
L1210 cells	Reverse transcriptase
Human colon lines	Cell surface enzymes
Human lung lines	Alkaline phosphatase
Leukemias *vs.* solid tumors	Esterase
Murine *vs.* human lines	Leucine aminopeptidase
Sensitive *vs.* resistant lines	Phospholipase
Antimetabolites	Others
Folic acid	Tubulin binding
Amino acids	DNA damage
Purines	Membrane changes
Pyrimidines	Metabolic activation

establishment of the CCNSC, the first major collection, extraction and screening of plants began in 1960. In 1962 14,200 fermentation broths and 5,200 plant extracts were screened (*94*, *98*) and over the next 20 years a similar level of screening was maintained.

Following the foundation of a contract program in microbial sources of antitumor agents in 1957, the first four years were mainly spent in the evaluation of fungi; this was a direct result of the success of the wartime penicillin production program and the consequent hope for other breakthrough drugs from this class of organism (*19*). From about 1961 through 1985 the NCI program mainly examined streptomycetes as sources of new agents. The main reason for this was that the NCI contractors who were performing the work were mainly pharmaceutical companies whose antitumor programs were offshoots of their antimicrobial programs and streptomycetes were extremely good sources of anti-infectives. The main contractors for the drug discovery aspect of the fermentation program were the Upjohn Company, Parke-Davis Co. (later Warner-Lambert / Parke-Davis), Bristol-Myers Company, the Institute of Microbial Chemistry and the Michigan Department of Public Health.

It is not possible to discuss in detail the screening methods used due to the proprietary nature of some of the information and the large number of different approaches employed over the years, but it can be summarized by stating that the universal pattern was to find *in vitro* activity in the broth and then subsequently concentrate the active principle and perform *in vivo* evaluation. That is, no primary *in vivo* testing was done in the microbial program in contrast to the NCI protocols for synthetic samples or plant extracts where the initial evaluation was always *in vivo*. The *in vitro* prescreens used by the contractors sought a wide spectrum of different end points directed towards cytotoxic phenomena as well as enzyme inhibition screens (Institute of Microbial Chemistry) and antimetabolite screens (Upjohn). Some of the assays used are listed in Table I.

Selection of Drugs for Development

The types of drugs selected for development by the NCI have varied considerably over the years and must be understood in the context of the Institute's mission and the perceived role of drug development in the economy. The presence of a drug development program in the NCI is somewhat unusual as a part of NIH and as a part of any Government agency for the following reasons: (1) the heart of the mission of NIH is to conduct and promote basic biomedical research leading to improved understanding and treatment of human disease. The large, highly targeted screening and drug development program at NCI is unique within the NIH: (2) in the U.S. economic system, drug development and marketing are considered to be a function of the Pharmaceutical industry and it is generally considered inappropriate for the Government to compete with industry or to supplement industrial efforts in drug development.

Drug discovery and development efforts by the Government have been largely confined to: national emergencies, such as pencillin production during World War II; tropical diseases, where the victims lack ability to pay for drugs and hence there is no profit for the Pharmaceutical industry; and rare diseases where the sales volume is inadequate to make production commercially justifiable. A major step forward with regards to drugs for rare diseases was the Orphan Drug Act of 1983 which permitted a guarantee of exclusive marketing rights in the U.S. for a period of seven years, even if there was no patent status. This Act also reduced the requirements for licensure of "orphan" drugs to correspond with the projected market size and the potential risk to the patients involved. Certain types of cancer with relatively low incidence would qualify as "rare diseases" under the terms of the Orphan Drug Act so the possibility of development of drugs discovered for rare cancer types is enhanced.

The changes in attitudes in the pharmaceutical industry and the developments of new concepts of therapy for cancer have been reflected in what the NCI has done in drug development. The first breakthroughs in chemotherapy were the nitrogen mustads, and antimetabolites of purines, pyrimidines, and folates in the 1940's and 1950's. At that time mortality from leukemia and lymphoma was exceedingly high and there was essentially no hope for cure or significant remission. These new drugs gave hope and there was a short burst of interest in the cancer drug market by a few companies. The next development in chemotherapy was the advent of combination chemotherapy where several drugs with different mechanisms of action and toxicities were combined to give additive effects. Some of these therapies were MOPP (mechlorethamine, Oncovin, procarbazine, prednisone), COPP (cytoxan, Oncovin, and prednisone), and VAMP (vincristine, 6-mercaptopurine, methotrexate, prednisone). These pioneering combinations again gave encouragement to the pharmaceutical industry as multiple drugs and multiple courses of therapy were involved making the prospective market larger. However, the lack of effectiveness of such combinations against solid tumors was a discouraging factor for industry and several major pharmaceutical companies ceased or decreased their efforts. During the 1970's there was less emphasis on new drug discovery for cancer in the pharmaceutical industry in the U.S. Several good new drugs had been discovered which were not antimetabolities and which had activity beyond the leukemia and lymphoma area. These included bleomycin, doxorubicin, cisplatin, and etoposide. NCI management felt at this time that the greatest probability for rapid success in new therapies was through improved analogs of these, and other, drugs. Since many companies and private researchers in universities around the world were working on analogs of the same structures it was apparent that a large number of similar analogs would be brought forward for clinical trials. This would cause tremendous problems in judging between them and also the high cost of clinical studies, the limited population of patients willing to enter clinical trials, and the limited number of highly qualified clinical investigators made it necessary to try to set up committees to review data and select those compounds in each group which were most worthy of NCI support. These groups were called Analog Committees and they were created for anthracyclines, platinums, bleomycin, antifolates, nucleosides, actinomycins, amino acid antimetabolites and enzymes, mitotic inhibitors, and alkylating agents. These committees included tumor biologists, biochemists, medicinal chemists, pharmacologists, and clinicians and they discussed in detail the problems in development of each class of analogs and determined what criteria should be sought for improvement of the class. Thus for the anthracyclines a major goal was reduced cardiotoxicity, while for the platinums the goals were stability in solution, reduced renal toxicity and activity against the platinum resistant L1210 leukemia subline.

With the exception of the antimetabolite groups (nucleosides, antifolates, amino acid derivatives) which had fairly narrow spectra of activity against mouse tumor models, the other analog classes generally had broad spectrum activity, and the limiting factors in selection of improved analogs were decreased toxicities along with enough confidence in the toxicity models to believe that they were predictive. The NCI played an important role in development and standardization of toxicity models during this period.

The fermentation program in natural products was also very active in analog development by starting new projects in two areas, directed biosynthesis and microbial transformation. The program in directed biosynthesis produced some quite interesting analogs of actinomycin D, while the microbial transformation project gave rise to interesting analogs of compounds such as anguidine, daunomycin, quadrone, and bruceantin. None of these ultimately became development candidates however.

Later on, in the 1980's, as the best of the second and third generation analogs entered clinical trials in the U.S., Europe, and Japan, it seemed that further major therapeutic advances among analogs of standard agents were less likely than formerly, and the emphasis in the NCI's drug discovery and drug development area shifted more towards novel structure types and novel mechanistic types of compounds. The 1980's also have brought an increased sophistication in tumor biology, in understanding of newer targets of drug action, such as toposisomerases and protein kinases, and furthermore in the capabilities to design and engineer screening systems with relatively low cost and high capacity to look for target specific leads. Thus the emphasis in selection of compounds to be developed at the NCI has moved very heavily towards novel chemotypes. Another major change in the 1980's has been the increased availability of highly purified biologicals and the NCI established a separate drug discovery and development program, the Biological Response Modifiers Program, to exploit this area (80).

Compounds in Development

At present there are a substantial number of natural product derived compounds in various stages of preclinical or clinical study at the NCI but only four will be covered in this chapter as examples. Others which are very interesting but are not included are didemnin B, menogaril, bryostatin, homoharringtonine, and 15-deoxyspergualin. The last of these, 15-deoxyspergualin, a derivative of spergualin which was discovered by Umezawa and co-workers has shown outstanding activity against murine L1210 leukemia and is also of considerable interest as an immunosuppressive agent. It is not discussed here since other chapters in this memorial volume describe it in detail.

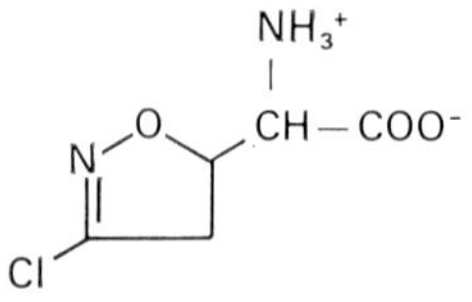

Acivicin

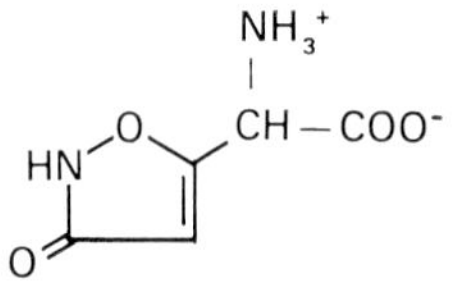

Ibotenic Acid

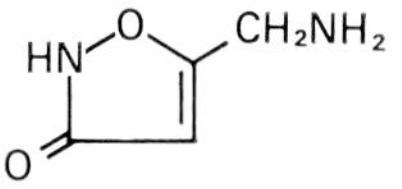

Muscimol

FIG. 1.   Acivicin and structurally related neurotoxins

1. *Acivicin*

The discovery of acivicin (AT-125; L-(αS, 5S)-α-amino-3-chloro-4,5-dihydro-5-isoxazoleacetic acid), Fig. 1, came as a result of a program at the Upjohn Company to seek analogs of amino acids as antimetabolites which might be useful in cancer chemotherapy (*36, 38*). The basis for the origins of an amino acid antimetabolite screen were 2-fold, the depletion of amino acids which are necessary for growth and development of tumor cells (*e.g.*, asparagine depletion by asparaginases) and the inhibition of biosynthesis of purines and pyrimidines resulting in decreased *de novo* synthesis of nucleotides. The screen used in detection of antimetabolite activities as devised by Hanka *et al.* (*36*) utilized a microbial disc assay with test organisms grown on both fully supplmented, complex media and limited, chemically defined media which were deficient in specific purines, pyrimidines, or amino acids. A large variety of fermentation broths were screened and those which showed enhanced inhibition of microbial growth on the restricted media were considered as leads. Acivicin was a very minor component in the lyophilized crude broth of *Streptomyces sviceus* (*38*) but could be isolated by following the antimetabolite activity (*37, 39*). The structure elucidation and complete relative and absolute stereochemistry were determined (*68*) and acivicin was subsequently synthesized (*51*).

The antitumor activity of acvicin in mice was greatest against leukemias (*44*) as might be expected for an antimetabolite. The standard schedule of daily intraperitoneal (i.p.) injections for 9 days against the i.p. implanted L1210 leukemia gave an increase in life span (ILS) of 65%. Almost equivalent activity was found with subcutaneous (s.c.) treatment against the i.p. L1210 but oral activity was only marginal. Activity was also seen with i.p. treatment of intracranial L1210 and s.c. treatment of s.c. implanted L1210 tumor (*44*). A schedule dependency study found that the best schedule for activity against L1210 was injection every 3 hr on days 1, 5, and 9 which gave an ILS of 104%.

TABLE II.   Summary of Single Agent Phase II Trials of Acivicin[a]

Disease site	Schedule	Evaluable patients	CR	PR	Response rate (%)
Breast	d×5	37	0	0	0
	72 hr CI	25	0	1	4
CNS	d×5	27	1	3	15
Colorectal	d×5	50	0	1	2
	72 hr CI	67	1	3	6
Leukemia	d×7	6	0	—	—
Pancreas	d×5	4	0	0	—
NSCL	d×5	106	0	5	5
SCLC	d×5	7	0	0	—
NHL	d×5	11	1	0	—
Melanoma	72 hr CI	38	0	1	3
Mesothelioma	72 hr CI	21	0	0	0
Ovarian	d×5	23	0	1	4
	72 hr CI	31	0	0	0
Renal	d×5	10	0	0	—
	72 hr CI	29	0	1	3

[a] From NCI annual report to the FDA, 1987.
NSCL, non-small cell lung; SCLC, small cell lung cancer; NHL, non-Hodgkin's lymphoma.

Good activity was seen against the P388 leukemia, the M5076 sarcoma and the MX-1 human mammary xenograft, while B16 melanoma, Lewis lung carcinoma, and three human colon xenografts were not responsive (44).

Acivicin was initially found to be an inhibitor of L-asparagine synthetase (12) and subsequently to be an irreversible inhibitor of a number of enzymes catalyzing transfer of amido groups from L-glutamine (46). Key enzymes involved in purine synthesis (e.g., phosphoribosylpyrophosphate (PRPP) aminotransferase and GMP synthetase) and in pyrimidine synthesis (carbamoylphosphate synthetase and CTP synthetase) are strongly inhibited by acivicin. A variety of experiments in P388 leukemia cells, hepatoma cells and other models have shown synergy with 5-fluorouracil, 6-thioguanine, PALA, actinomycin D, and dipyridamole (21, 22, 75).

Several other glutamine antagonists have been studied in man and azaserine, 6-diazo-5-oxo-L-norleucine (DON), and azotomycin all have shown limited but definite clinical activity (8). Thus there was clinical interest in studies with acivicin.

Phase I studies were conducted on a variety of schedules and central nervous system (CNS) toxicity was found to be dose limiting on most schedules including single daily bolus, 24-hr infusion and 72-hr infusion schedules (22, 75). The CNS toxicity may relate to the structural similarity of acivicin with known neurotoxins such as ibotenic acid (Fig. 1) and muscimol (Fig. 1; 53). Rats, mice, and rabbits did not exhibit behavioral changes but a dose related ataxia was seen in cats (71, 73). The concomitant administration of an amino acid infusion was shown to prevent this toxicity while retaining antitumor activity (72).

In a related study, growth of methylcholanthrene-induced sarcomas in rats was inhibited approximately equally whether they were fed rat chow or maintained on total parenteral nutrition (9).

Two schedules of administration for acivicin, daily for 5 days and a 72-hr continuous

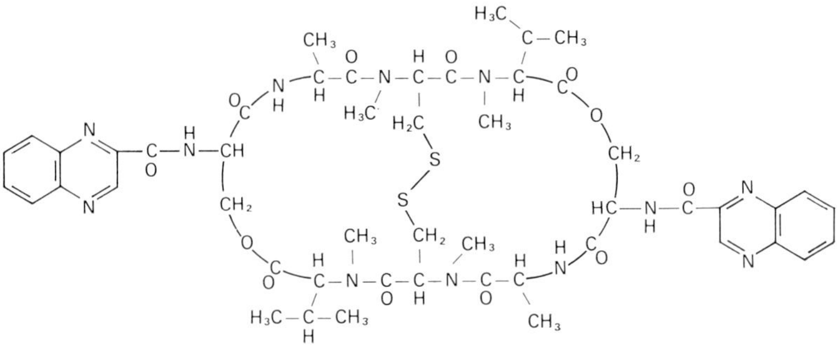

Triostin A

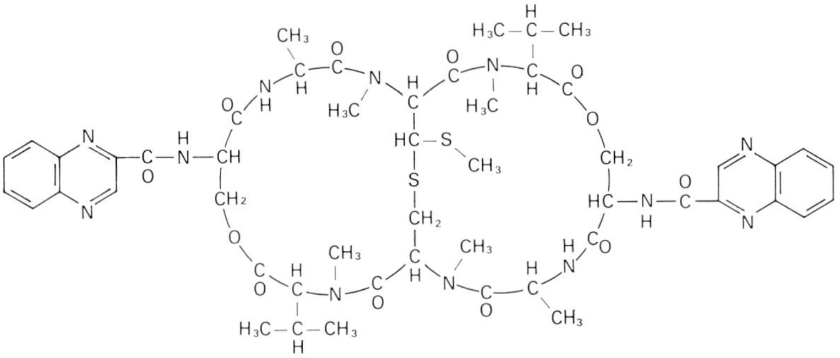

Echinomycin (quinomycin A)

FIG. 2.   Typical quinoxaline antibiotics

infusion, have been utilized in Phase II studies. Results are summarized in Table II. The most promising study to date has been in recurrent glioma where one complete remission and three partial remissions were seen in 27 evaluable patients (109). The observation that CNS toxicity in the cat model could be prevented by amino acid infusion has led to a Phase I trial now underway combining aminosyn with acivicin to determine whether higher blood levels of acivicin can be achieved without CNS toxicity.

2. Echinomycin

Echinomycin (also known as quinomycin A) has been studied forr over 30 years dating from its isolation from *Streptomyces echinatus* and the discovery of its activity against gram positive bacteria in 1957 (13). The correct chemical structure was determined in 1975 (Fig. 2) (14, 69). Echinomycin is characterized as a quinoxaline antibiotic and this class is named for the two aromatic quinoxaline rings on either end of the molecule. The quinoxaline antibiotics are further subdivided into two series, the triostins and the quinomycins which differ only in the organization of the sulfide crosslinks in the peptidyl portion of the molecule (Fig. 2) (50). Extensive biological studies in Japan in the 1960's found that the quinoxalines, in addition to antibacterial activity, had anti-mycoplasma (50), antitumor (48, 49, 70), antiviral (111), and anti-bacteriophage (91) activities. The antiviral activity was modest against polio virus whereas the antimycoplasma activity was quite strong (50). The effects of echinomycin and other quinoxalines were studied against more than thirty tumor models in mice, rats, and hamsters and echinomycin showed

TABLE III.   Summary of Antitumor Evaluation of Echinomycin at the NCI[a]

System	Treatment schedule	Activity
Murine tumors		
i.p. B16 melanoma	i.p. Q1D, days 1– 9	++
s.c. CD8F$_1$ mammary tumor	i.p. Q7D, days 1–29	–
s.c. Colon 38 tumor	i.p. Q7D, days 2–16	–
i.p. L1210 leukemia	i.p. Q1D, days 1– 9	–
i.v. Lewis lung carcinoma	i.p. Q1D, days 1– 9	–
i.p. P388 leukemia	i.p. Q1D, days 1– 9	++
Human tumor xenografts		
s.r.c. CX-1 colon tumor	s.c. Q1D, days 1–10	–
s.r.c. LX-1 lung tumor	s.c. Q1D, days 1–10	–
s.r.c. MX-1 mammary tumor	s.c. Q1D, days 1–10	–
s.c. CX-1 colon tumor	i.p. Q4D, days 19–27	–
s.c. LX-1 lung tumor	i.p. Q4D, days 21–29	–
s.c. MX-1 mammary tumor	i.p. Q4D, days 18–25	–

[a] After Foster et al. (26).

positive activity against only the Sarcoma 180 (ascitic type), Ehrlich carcinoma, and Jensen sarcoma models (49). In these studies quinomycin C was more active than either echinomycin or quinomycin B. Detailed studies in the Ehrlich ascites carcinoma in mice and the AH-130 hepatoma in rats found that triostin C was more active than echinomycin in both systems and had a broader therapeutic index (70), however none of the quinoxalines was brought to clinical trials at that time. It was not until echinomycin was restudied by the NCI in the late 1970's that enough interest was generated to consider it as a clinical candidate.

Echinomycin is a very potent compound *in vivo*, and in antitumor evaluations in mice active doses were typically from 50 to 250 μg/kg/dose depending on the schedule and route of administration and the strain of the host animals. The spectrum of activity for echinomycin in the studies of Katagiri and Sugiura was narrow (49) and in testing at the NCI against a panel of murine tumors and human tumor xenografts in athymic mice, activity was noted only in the P388 leukemia and B16 melanoma systems (26) (Table III). Schedule dependency studies in the B16 melanoma model against i.p. implanted tumor with i.p. drug administration showed the greatest ILS of 91% on a daily schedule for 9 days. A single dose or five daily doses were less effective. Oral administration on the same three schedules showed only marginal activity on the daily×nine schedule and inactivity on the single and daily×five schedules indicating that the oral route was not promising. The intravenous route gave moderate activity on the single and daily×five schedules establishing that echinomycin was active when the site of tumor and the site of administration of drug were distant (26).

Somewhat encouraging results were found by Cobb et al. using a 6-day subrenal capsule xenograft assay with fresh surgical explants of human tumors. They studied 69 tumors of a variety of histologies including breast, lung, colon, ovarian, and cervical. Echinomycin met their activity standard of tumor graft regression greater than 20% against 15 of 69 tumors with the greatest response rate seen in ovarian cancers (11).

Early studies on the mechanism of action of quinoxaline antibiotics found considerable effects on nucleic acid synthesis. Gauze et al. noted selective suppression of RNA synthesis in Ehrlich ascites carcinoma cells (30), while Sato et al. found that RNA synthesis in *Staphylococcus aureus* was completely blocked by echinomycin which also had a lesser effect on DNA and protein synthesis (*92*). Ward *et al.* found inhibition of synthesis of both DNA and RNA in studies with bacterial and mammalian cells (*117*). They were able to conclude through studies of ultraviolet absorption spectral shifts and inhibition of DNA-primed RNA synthesis that the effects on RNA synthesis were secondary to echinomycin-DNA binding and that there was base specificity in the binding to DNA (*117*). Studies by Waring's group found that at low ionic strength echinomycin created an unwinding angle on duplex bacteriophage DNA that was almost twice that of ethidium indicating that echinomycin was a bifunctional intercalating agent, the first such agent to be recognized (*119*). Not only was echinomycin specific for double helical DNA but it also showed specificity for particular base sequences, especially those rich in guanine and cytosine nucleotides (*114, 118*). "Footprinting" of echinomycin found that there was a binding site of the size of four base pairs. The strong binding sites have a central two-base pair sequence of 5'-CG-3'. The key recognition elements for echinomycin are in the sequences 5'-ACGT-3' and 5'-TCGT-3' (*112*). The closely related triostin A has been crystallized as a complex with a DNA duplex, 5'-CGTACG-3', and has been solved crystallographically. There is direct evidence that triostin A is a bis-intercalator that brackets a 5'-CG-3' sequence (*115*).

Although the biologically active quinomycins and triostins all exhibit properties of bifunctional intercalation, they vary in base sequence specificity. This has been ascribed to differences in their conformations in solution (*57*). The natural quinoxalines differ only in the peptidal portion and all have the same quinoxaline nucleus. Lee and Waring studied analogs having opened lactones and cleaved sulfide bridges and found these inactive, and also prepared an analog with benzyl ethers replacing the quinoxaline ring which still possessed some DNA binding. They concluded that the structure and conformation of the sulfur-containing bridge was important to sequence specificity (*57, 58*). Other analogs have been prepared by directed biosynthesis (*29, 63*) especially with modifications of the quinoxaline rings (*27*). It was found that when quinoxaline was replaced by quinoline there were considerable differences in unwinding angle and sequence specificity leading to the conclusion that the chromophore as well as the peptide play an important role (*27*).

Based on the *in vivo* antitumor data and the unique mechanism of interaction with DNA, echinomycin was advanced to toxicology studies (*26*). Two schedules were evaluated in both mice and dogs, a single bolus and a single daily dose for five consecutive days. Major toxicities were found with the gastrointestinal, hepatic, and lymphoreticular systems (*26*).

Phase I trials were carried out on four different schedules:
1) single bolus every 28 days (*3, 40, 41*)
2) 24-hr infusion every 28 days (*54*)
3) daily for five consecutive days every 28 days (*110*)
4) once weekly for 4 weeks (*35, 82*)

The dose limiting toxicity in all studies was gastrointestinal with nausea and vomiting predominating. The two schedules selected for Phase II trials are once weekly for 4 weeks and once every 4 weeks. Results of Phase II trials have not yet been published but the NCI's Phase II trials objective is to study echinomycin in all of the major tumor types.

Useful reviews of the early biological and mechanistic studies (*50*), the detailed mechanism (*118*), and the preclinical development (*26*) can be consulted for further details.

3. *Taxol*

The cytotoxic and antitumor activities in extracts of *Taxus brevifolia* were discovered in the NCI program for collection and screening of plants (*106*), and isolation and structure elucidation of taxol was done by Wall's group at the Research Triangle Institute (*116*). Taxol (Fig. 3) is a member of the taxane group of diterpenes, a small and rare structure type found only in the genus *Taxus* in the family Taxaceae. *Taxus* species, known by the common name of yew, include the western yew, (*T. brevifolia*), the European yew (*Taxus baccata*) and the Japanese yew (*Taxus cuspidata*). The yews are all very slow growing trees or shrubs which have very dense strong and yet flexible wood and were in older times highly valued for production of bows. Taxol is concentrated in the bark and, to a lesser extent, in the needles of the yew.

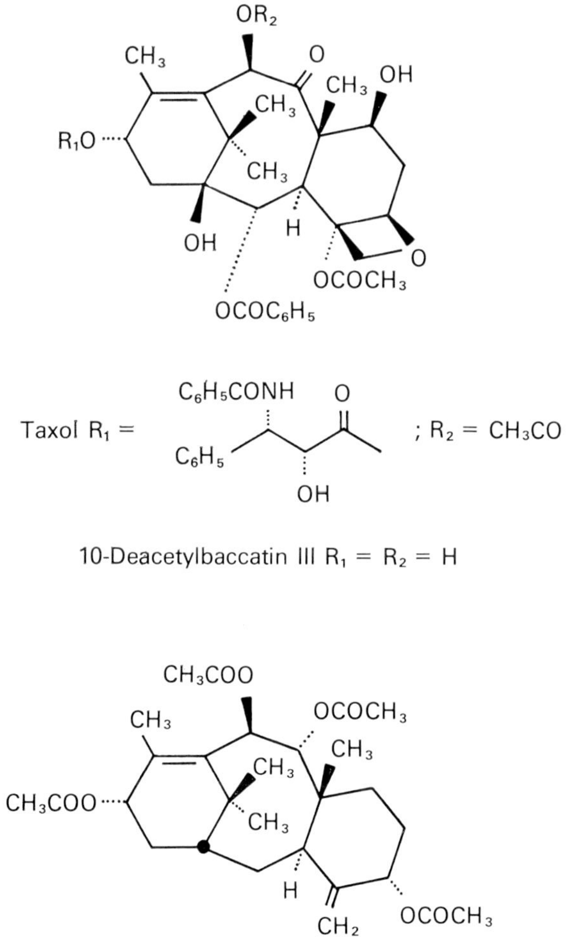

Taxol $R_1 = $ [structure] ; $R_2 = CH_3CO$

10-Deacetylbaccatin III $R_1 = R_2 = H$

Taxusin

FIG. 3. Taxol and related compounds

The synthesis of taxol is a most formidable task which to date has not been achieved although recently Holton's group have completed the synthesis of taxusin (Fig. 3), a highly functionalized taxane (42, 126). Also very recently, a chemical conversion of 10-deacetyl baccatin III (Fig. 3) to taxol has been described. This is important since 10-deacetyl baccatin can be extracted and isolated from the leaves (needles) of T. baccata which, in contrast to bark of T. brevifolia, are a rapidly renewable resource (15).

The relationship of structure to activity among taxol and related compounds is not well defined since all the compounds available are either naturally-occurring close analogs, such as cephalomannine, baccatin III, cinnamoyltaxinine, xylosyl taxol, and their derivatives or simple derivatives of taxol, including 7-epi isomers and 2' and/or 7-acetates (97, 108). Many points of the structure of taxol have not been probed because they are not readily accessible from taxol, and compounds similar enough to taxol to be useful in a structure-activity sense have not been prepared by total synthesis. The points that are fairly clear are that an ester at position 13 is needed for activity, esterification or epimerization at C-7 retains activity but decreases potency, and deacetylation at C-10 doesn't alter activity much (56, 81, 108). Esterification at C-2' of the ester side chain does not result in loss of activity (64) and indeed the esters here are readily hydrolyzed to taxol. This is important for the attempted preparation of more water soluble pro-drugs of taxol designed to release taxol under physiological conditions (64, 108).

Taxol has a fascinating and wholly unique mechanism of action in that it binds to microtubules and stabilizes them (67, 95, 96) thus shifting the equilibrium between the soluble protein, tubulin, and microtubules, the polymerized form of tubulin. Since microtubules form the mitotic spindle, taxol blocks cell division in mitosis (28). Other natural products which are antimitotics including colchicine, vincristine, podophyllotoxin, and maytansine, all bind to tublin and inhibit polymerization rather than promoting it as taxol does. Taxol has thus become a new probe for studying microtubules (43) and microtubule associated processes such as mitosis, flagellar motion, cellular secretion, the cytoskeleton, and muscle contraction (108). In the last five years more than 300 studies

TABLE IV. Antitumor Activity of Taxol in Murine Tumors and Human
Tumor Xenografts at the NCI

System	Treatment schedule	Activity
Murine tumors		
i.p. B16 melanoma	i.p. Q1D, days 1– 9	++
s.c. CD8F$_1$ mammary tumor	i.p. Q7D, days 1–29	−
s.c. Colon 38 tumor	i.p. Q7D, days 2– 9	−
i.p. L1210 leukemia	i.p. Q1D, days 1–15	+
i.v. Lewis lung carcinoma	i.p. Q1D, days 1– 9	−
i.p. P388 leukemia	i.p. Q1D, days 1– 5	+
i.p. P1534 leukemia	i.p. Q1D, days 1–10	++
Human tumor xenografts		
s.r.c. CX-1 colon tumor	s.c. Q1D, days 1–10	+
s.r.c. LX-1 lung tumor	s.c. Q1D, days 1–10	+
s.r.c. MX-1 mammary tumor	s.c. Q1D, days 1–10	++

Activity: ++ reproduced activity; ≥50% ILS for i.p. and i.v. implanted tumors (≥75% ILS for i.p. P388), ≥90% inhibition of tumor growth for s.c. and s.r.c. implanted tumors. + reproduced activity; 25–49% ILS for B16 and L1210, 20–74% ILS for P388, 40–49% ILS for Lewis lung. 58–89% and 80–99% inhibition of tumor growth for colon 38 and the xenografts, respectively. − inactive.

have been published which utilized taxol as a reagent to isolate microtubules or to study their role in biological processes.

Taxol was selected for development towards clinical trials based on its strong activity against the B16 melanoma and the MX-1 human mammary tumor xenograft. It is also highly active against the P1534 leukemia and moderately active against the L1210 and P388 murine leukemias and colon and lung xenografts in testing at the NCI (see Table IV) (108). Jacrot *et al.* (45) have reported good activity of taxol against 3 of 4 human tumor xenografts in nude mice. These were a hepatic metastasis of a breast tumor, a tumor of the base of the tongue and a cutaneous meta tasis of bronchial cancer. Additional studies found activity against human breast, endometrial, ovarian, brain, lung, and tongue tumors (87) and against another ovarian xenograft (86). A study against two pancreatic xenografts however, found taxol to be inactive (103).

Toxicology studies of taxol were conducted in rats and dogs using both single dose and five daily dose protocols. The major toxicity in both species was found to be tissues with rapid turnover including hematopoietic, lymphatic, and gastrointestinal systems. The dose limiting toxicity in both species was dose related myelosuppression. In dogs, on the single dose schedule, unpredictable and lethal toxicity was seen with the vehicle alone. The key component of the vehicle believed responsible for the toxicity is Cremophor EL, a surfactant known to cause histamine release (55, 74). The formulation of taxol has been a major problem because its solubility in water is very poor and the optimal antitumor dose of typically 5–20 mg/kg/dose. While not large, this dosage is several times larger than other very insoluble natural products such as echinomycin or didemnin B which also require surfactant formulations (see Table V) (55, 74). The amount of Cremophor administered in a dose of taxol is high and has led to problems in clinical studies (discussed below). Prodrug approaches thus far have not been entirely satisfactory because the solubility of taxol in aqueous solutions is so poor that even a small amount of hydrolysis of prodrug in the administration fluid will result in a cloudy appearance. Further efforts on prodrugs are continuing and other solubilization and surfactant studies are ongoing. Work on water soluble derivatives and prodrugs has also been hampered by the limited supply of taxol available as a starting material.

Taxol entered clinical trials in 1983 under NCI sponsorship and is now in Phase II trials. A summary of published Phase I trials is found in Table VI. All of the early trials using bolus or short (1 to 3 hr) infusions experienced anaphylactoid reactions or other hypersensitivity responses, but premedication with steroids (dexamethasone), antihistamines (diphenhydramine), and H-2 antagonists (cimetidine or ranitidine) coupled with extension of the infusion time to 24 hr virtually eliminated serious hypersensitivity reactions. The hypersensitivity reactions observed in Phase I trials (104) are generally

TABLE V. Cremophor EL Concentration in Investigational Drugs

Drug	Cremophor EL (ml)/ unit of drug	Phase II dose	
		Drug/m²	Cremophor EL/m²
Teniposide	0.05/mg	165 mg	8.25 ml
Echinomycin	0.00000025/μg	2 mg	0.5 ml
Taxol	0.08/mg	200 mg	16.0 ml
Didemnin B	0.03/mg	3.47 mg	0.10 ml
Miconazole	0.01/mg	200–1,200 mg/infusion (total dose)	2–12 ml/infusion

TABLE VI. Phase I Studies with Taxol

Investigator and reference	Schedule	Patients	DLT	Recommended for Phase II
Kris *et al.* (*52*)	3-hr infusion Q3W	17	Hypersensitivity reaction	NO
Donehower *et al.* (*18*)	1-hr or 6-hr infusion Q3W	30	Leukopenia	NO
Wiernik *et al.* (*121*)	1-hr to 6-hr infusion Q3W	34	Leukopenia; neurotoxicity	NO
Legha *et al.* (*59*)	1-hr infusion daily ×5	20	Leukopenia	NO
Grem *et al.* (*33*)	1-hr or 6-hr infusion daily ×5	16	Leukopenia	NO
Wiernik *et al.* (*120*)	24-hr CI Q3W	26	Peripheral neuropathy	YES
Ohnuma *et al.* (*79*)	24-hr CI Q3W	42	Leukopenia	YES
Rowinsky *et al.* (*88*)	24-hr CI Q3W	12	Mucositis; pharyngitis	YES

typical for cremophor-induced histaminic reactions (*55*). Minor responses and some partial remissions were seen in several of the Phase I trials, and in particular a Phase I trial reported by Wiernik *et al.* (*120*) noted 4 partial responses among 12 melanoma patients.

Phase II trials of taxol have been restricted by drug supply and only three trials have been reported thus far. A trial with 18 renal cell carcinoma patients on a 24-hr continuous infusion schedule had no responders (*23*), but a trial on the same schedule in advanced, refractory ovarian cancer found 5 partial responses in 15 evaluable patients (33% response rate) (*89*). The latter is a very encouraging result in this population. *In vitro* studies of the cytotoxicity of taxol to human ovarian cell lines found that there was a correlation between microtubule bundling and cytotoxicity which related to duration of exposure to taxol. It was suggested that indirect immunofluorescence with antitubulin may predict the taxol sensitivity of ovarian tumors (*90*). A Phase II study in melanoma was less promising than the results reported for Phase I but nonetheless two complete remissions were observed and this trial had an overall response rate complete response (CR) plus partial response (PR) of 18% (*24*). Further trials in ovarian cancer and melanoma are underway and other disease sites will be studied as more drug becomes available. Important cancer types including lung, colon, and breast have not yet been studied in clinical trials.

4. 2'-Deoxycoformycin

One of the most promising compounds currently in clinical trials is 2'-deoxycoformycin (DCF; pentostatin). It was discovered at the Warner-Lambert Company as a result of its prolongation of the activity of vidarabine (adenosine arabinoside; Ara-A) in a fermentation broth of *Streptomyces antibioticus* (*17, 122*). It has also been subsequently prepared by total synthesis (*4*). Adenosine deaminase (ADA) is a particularly important enzyme as part of the salvage pathway that converts ATP-derived adenosine to hypoxanthine in cells which lack *de novo* purine biosynthesis (*2*). Inhibition of ADA leads to increased levels of adenosine and 2'-deoxyadenosine which are toxic to some cell types even at low concentrations. Among various cell types studied, T-lymphocytes are particularly sensitive to increased levels of 2' deoxyadenosine. Thus DCF which is a very tight-binding inhibitor of ADA can be expected to have selective cytotoxicity towards T-cells and may be expected to have activity against T-cell leukemias and lymphomas. It has also been found that B-lymphocytes are quite sensitive to the cytotoxic effects of

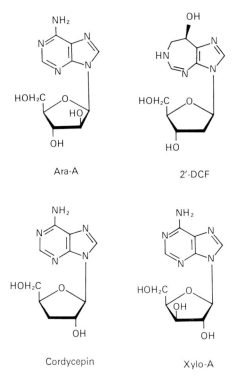

Ara-A

2'-DCF

Cordycepin

Xylo-A

Fig. 4.   2'-Deoxycoformycin and compounds whose activity it potentiates

adenosine leading to the exploration of DCF in B-cell leukemias and lymphomas. The selective toxicity of ADA inhibitors towards lymphocytes also suggests that they might be immunosuppressive agents and indeed these compounds represent a new class of immunomodulating drugs. In the case of severe combined immunodeficiency syndrome, a hereditary defect in which ADA is absent, the normal immune function is absent.

There are, however, other biochemical changes which may occur after DCF administration including inhibition of S-adenosyl homocysteine hydrolase (with secondary effects on S-adenosyl methionine pools and the ability to methylate DNA and RNA), DNA strand breaks or incorporation of DCF triphosphates into DNA, effects mediated through immunomodulation, and changes in cell membranes and transport. Therefore the mechanism of action of DCF is complex and requires further clarification.

DCF has no activity as an antitumor agent in traditional models. Two standard leukemia models were tested for response, the P388 and L1210 murine leukemias. DCF was inactive in the P388 model on a daily×9 schedules at doses of 4 mg/kg/inj. and below, while higher doses were toxic. Even at doses which could be shown to inhibit the deaminase activity of L1210 cells, DCF had no effect against the i.p. implanted L1210 leukemia on either a daily schedule for 9 days or an intermittent schedule (61). Testing against the standard models in the NCI panel of *in vivo* tumors including the B16 melanoma, colon 26 and colon 38, ependymoblastoma, Lewis lung, and human lung, colon, and mammary xenografts revealed no activity.

The ADA-inhibiting activity of 2'-DCF does clearly, and in some cases dramatically, enhance the antitumor activity of compounds which are metabolically inactivated by ADA (*1, 47, 61, 83, 84*). The compounds whose activity is potentiated include Ara-A,

(61) cordycepin (3'-deoxyadenosine) (47), and adenosine xyloside (Xylo-A) (83) (see Fig. 4). Because Ara-A was known to have good antiviral activity (93) and weak antitumor activity and because it was known to be rapidly deaminated and inactivated by ADA it was considered that an inhibitor of ADA might be combined with Ara-A to convert it into a longer lived, more potent and hopefully highly active antitumor agent. While the activity of Ara-A was clearly potentiated by DCF, bringing such a combination forward to clinical trials was extremely difficult because there were many ways to study such a combination. In principle, one could vary the dose of Ara-A while holding the DCF dose constant or conversely the Ara-A dose could be fixed while varying the dose of DCF. There are sound arguments on both sides of this question and despite large numbers of combination studies in mice with Ara-A and DCF it was impossible to predict in advance which combination of doses of the two agents would be best. Thus the preliminary preclinical toxicology plan for the combination which was discussed with the FDA (Food and Drug Administration) used multiple dose levels of each agent in combination with the other. This was equivalent to at least six to eight single agent studies. Serious questions were raised about whether the DCF-Ara-A combination had sufficient potential value to justify the great expense involved in toxicology. The political climate at the FDA was also unfavorable towards selecting only one or two combinations for toxicology studies since at this time the FDA was removing a number of fixed combinations of antibiotics from the market. This was based on the idea that a fixed combination would not necessarily provide optimum therapy, and better treatment would result from each agent being prescribed separately as was appropriate to the individual case. Because DCF had no antitumor activity *in vivo* as a single agent there did not seem to be any possibility to have an Investigational New Drug Application approved by the FDA for single agent Phase I studies and the further development of DCF seemed blocked. NCI staff did not believe that the potential of DCF was high enough to warrant the huge expense of the combination toxicology studies with Ara-A and furthermore even if such studies were done, there would then arise the questions of how many combinations should be taken to Phase I trials and the source of the large patient resource which would be needed to evaluate the combinations.

Fortunately, Dr. John Smyth in England had been involved in preclinical studies with DCF and was quite interested in its lymphotoxic activities. He was able to conduct a single agent trial at the Institute of Cancer Research based on the biochemical and pharmacological data. This trial entered 18 patients with a variety of advanced cancers refractory to prior chemotherapy. The dose of DCF administered was from 0.1 to 0.25 mg/kg daily for one to 5 days. The major toxicity was a marked decrease in circulating lymphoblasts with little effect on neutrophil or platelet counts or hemoglobin level.

Hyperuricemia was seen and one patient developed life-threatening renal failure. Subsequently all patients were given allopurinol and no further renal dysfunction was encountered. Three of seven patients with acute lymphocytic leukemia (ALL) responded to DCF (99). This was judged sufficient to pursue the drug further and toxicology studies were performed in the U.S. using DCF as a single agent. Based on this data and the responses seen in Smyth's trial in England, Phase I trials in the U.S. were approved and began in 1979. It is not possible to individually review the many clinical trials performed with DCF in this paper so only a brief overall summary will be given. Several reviews available have summarized various aspects of the preclinical and clinical trials with DCF (62, 76, 78, 101, 102). In Phase I clinical trials there were a significant number of serious toxicities noted, depending on dose and schedule, including CNS, renal, nausea and vomiting, and lymphoid depletion. The best tolerated schedule recommended for Phase II trials is a dose of 4 mg/m² every other week. This is a dose which gives good inhibition of ADA. Higher or more frequent dosing seems to add toxicity without particular benefit. The clinical pharmacology and pharmacokinetics of DCF have been studied in detail (65, 66, 100). A significant number of responses were seen in Phase I trials including some complete remissions. Responsive diseases in Phase I were ALL (adult and pediatric), Hodgkin's disease, non-Hodgkin's lymphoma, diffuse histiocytic lymphoma, and mycosis fungoides. Early Phase II trials found an extremely high response rate with DCF in hairy cell leukemia which has held up through a number of trials (10, 60, 76). There is about a 90% response rate with about 60% complete remissions including some cases refractory or intolerant to alpha interferon (aIFN). Several studies are underway in hairy cell leukemia patients who have failed on aIFN in order to obtain good statistics on response rate in this population. Two Phase III trials are underway which are conducting a randomized comparison of DCF and aIFN in hairy cell leukemia. Although DCF has not yet been approved for marketing for hairy cell leukemia, the NCI has applied for special status (Group C) which will allow distribution to all patients needing the drug without them having to be on a particular protocol. Other diseases where DCF is clearly active in Phase II trials are chronic lymphocytic leukemia (CLL) and mycosis fungoides (78, 101, 103). Adult T-cell leukemia / lymphoma may be responsive but insufficient patients are available in the U.S. Trials are underway in Japan and preliminary data have been reported (123). Further studies will be undertaken as more drug becomes available. The immunosuppression due to DCF can have serious consequences (77) but DCF could also be beneficial in studies of transplantation if the neurotoxicity of the drug is not limiting. The original reason for development of DCF, its potentiation of Ara-A, has now largely been abandoned. There were several reports of patient treatment with the combination (34, 85) but the need for the combination has been obviated by the discovery of 2-fluoro-Ara-A, a derivative of Ara-A which is resistant to deamination (6). This drug is now in clinical trials as its more soluble monophosphate (FAMP; 2-fluoro-ara-A monophosphate).

CONCLUSIONS

While it is too early to know whether acivicin or echinomycin will be clinically active, the results with taxol are quite encouraging and DCF appears to have an excellent prospect for becoming a marketed drug. It is reasonable to say that none of these drugs would probably have reached clinical trials without strong NCI support; the NCI's philosophy of being willing to take on drugs which have unusual properties and would not otherwise be supported has been successful enough that it should clearly be continued. The strong cooperation of NCI and industry was abolutely critical for acivicin (Upjohn Company) and DCF (Warner-Lambert / Parke-Davis Co.) and it is hoped that such cooperation will continue in the future.

The Institute of Microbial Chemistry has been a very strong collaborator with the NCI. Professor Umezawa's studies were always dedicated to the health of all mankind and he helped the NCI many times in working with colleagues in Japan. One of the most interesting drugs now in early clinical development at the NCI is 15-deoxyspergualin, discovered in Professor Umezawa's laboratories and provided by the cooperation of the Institute of Microbial Chemistry, the Takara Shuzo Company and Nippon Kayaku Company. The close collaboration between the NCI in the United States and cancer researchers in Japan is a tribute to Professor Umezawa's efforts towards international cooperation in discovery and development of new antibiotic and antitumor drugs.

Acknowledgments

I wish to thank Dr. D. Dale Shoemaker, Drug Regulatory Affairs Branch, NCI for reports and references on the drugs discussed and Ms. Brenda Lee for typing the Manuscript.

REFERENCES

1. Adamson, R. H., Zaharevitz, D. W., and Johns, D. G. Enhancement of the biological activity of adenosine analogs by the adenosine deaminase inhibitor 2'-deoxycoformycin. *Pharmacology*, **15**, 84–89 (1977).

2. Agarwal, R. P., Spector, T., and Parks, R. E., Jr. Tight-binding inhibitors. IV. Inhibition of adenosine deaminase by various inhibitors. *Biochem. Pharmacol.*, **26**, 359–367 (1977).

3. Andrews, W. G., Harvey, J. H., McFadden, M., Byrne, P. J., Ahlgren, J. D., and Woolley, P. V. A Phase I study of echinomycin administered on an intermittent bolus schedule. *Proc. Am. Soc. Clin. Oncol.*, **4**, 42 (C-159) (1985).

4. Baker, D. C. and Putt, S. R. A total synthesis of pentostatin, the potent inhibitor of adenosine deaminase. *J. Am. Chem. Soc.*, **101**, 6127–6128 (1979).

5. Boyd, M. R., Shoemaker, R. H., Cragg, G. M., and Suffness, M. New avenues of investigation of marine biologicals in the anticancer drug discovery program of the National Cancer Institute. *In* "Pharmaceuticals and the Sea," ed. C. W. Jefford, K. L. Rinehart, and L. S. Shield, pp. 27–43 (1988). Technomic Publishing Co., Lancaster, Pennsylvania.

6. Brockman, R. W., Schabel, F. M., Jr., and Montgomery, J. A. Biological activity of 9-B-D-arabinofuranosyl-2-fluoroadenine, a metabolically stable analog of 9-B-D-arabinofuranosyladenine. *Biochem. Pharmacol.*, **26**, 2193–2196 (1977).

7. Burchenal, J. H., Murphy, M. L., Ellison, R. R., Sykes, M. P., Tan, T. C., Leone, L. A., Karnofsky, D. A., Craver, L. F., Dargeon, H. W., and Rhoads, C. P. Clinical evaluation of a new antimetabolite, 6-mercaptopurine, in the treatment of leukemia and allied diseases. *Blood*, **8**, 965–999 (1953).

8. Catane, R., von Hoff, D. D., Glaubiger, D. L., and Muggia, F. M. Azaserine, DON, and Azotomycin: three diazo analogs of L-glutamine with clinical antitumor activity. *Cancer Chemother. Rep.*, **63**, 1033–1038 (1979).

9. Chance, W. T., Cao, L., Nelson, J. L., Foley-Nelson, T., and Fischer, J. E. Acivicin reduces tumor growth during total parenteral nutrition. *Surgery*, **102**, 386–394 (1987).

10. Cheson, B. D. and Martin, A. Clinical trials in hairy cell leukemia. *Ann. Intern. Med.*, **1106**, 871–878 (1987).

11. Cobb, W. R., Bogden, A. E., Reich, S. D., Griffin, T. W., Kelton, D. E., and LePage, D. J. Activity of two phase I drugs N-methylformamide (NSC-3051) and Echinomycin (NSC-526417) against fresh surgical explants of human tumors in the 6-day subrenal capsule (SRC) assay. *Invest. New Drugs*, **1**, 5–9 (1983).

12. Cooney, D. A., Jayaram, H. N., Ryan, J. A., and Bono, V. H. Inhibition of L-asparagine synthetase by a new amino acid antibiotic with antitumor activity: L-αS, 5S-α-amino-3-chloro-4,5-dihydro-5-isoxazoleacetic acid (NSC-163501). *Cancer Chemother. Rep.*, **58**, 793–802 (1974).

13. Corbaz, R., Ettlinger, L., Gäumann, E., Keller-Schierlein, W., Kradolfer, F., Neipp, L.,

Prelog, V., Reusser, P., and Zähner, H. Stoffwechselprodukte von actinomyceten. Echino-mycin. *Helv. Chim. Acta*, **40**, 199–204 (1957).

14. Dell, A., Williams, D. H., Morris, H. R., Smith, G. A., Feeney, J., and Roberts, G. C. Structure revision of the antibiotic echinomycin. *J. Am. Chem. Soc.*, **97**, 2495–2502 (1975).

15. Denis, J. N., Greene, A. E., Guenard, D., Gueritte-Voegelein, F., Mangatal, L., and Potier, P. A highly efficient, practical approach to natural taxol. *J. Am. Chem. Soc.*, **110**, 5917–5919 (1988).

16. DeVita, V. T., Oliverio, V. T., Muggia, F. M., Wiernik, P. W., Ziegler, J., Goldin, A., Rubin, D., Henney, J., and Schepartz, S. The drug development and clinical trials pro-grams of the Division of Cancer Treatment, National Cancer Institute. *Cancer Clin. Trials*, **2**, 195–216 (1979).

17. Dion, H. W., Woo, P.W.K., and Ryder, A. Isolation and properties of a vidarabine de-aminase inhibitor, co-vidarabine. *Ann. N. Y. Acad. Sci.*, **284**, 21–29 (1977).

18. Donehower, R. C., Rowinsky, E. K., Grochow, L. B., Longnecker, S. M., and Ettinger, D. S. Phase I trial of taxol in patients with advanced cancer. *Cancer Treat. Rep.*, **71**, 1171–1177 (1987).

19. Douros, J. D. National Cancer Institute's Fermentation Development Program. *Recent Results Cancer Res.*, **63**, 33–48 (1978).

20. Driscoll, J. S. The preclinical new drug research program of the National Cancer In-stitute. *Cancer Treat. Rep.*, **68**, 63–76 (1984).

21. Earhart, R. H. Acivicin: A new antimetabolite. *Cancer Treat. Rev.*, **36**, 161–181 (1987).

22. Earhart, R. H. and Neil, G. L. Acivicin in 1985. *Adv. Enzyme Regul.*, **24**, 179–205 (1986).

23. Einzig, A. I., Gorowski, E., Sasloff, J., and Wiernik, P. H. Phase II trial of taxol in pa-tients with renal cell carcinoma. *Proc. Am. Assoc. Cancer Res.*, **29**, A884 (1988).

24. Einzig, A. I., Trump, D. L., Sasloff, J., Gorowski, E., Dutcher, J., and Wiernik, P. H. Phase II pilot study of taxol in patients with malignant melanoma. *Proc. Am. Soc. Clin. Oncol.*, **7**, 249 (A963) (1988).

25. Farber, S., Diamond, L. K., Mercer, R. D., Sylvester, R. F., Jr., and Wolff, J. A. Tem-porary remissions in acute leukemia in children produced by folic acid antagonist 4-amino-pteroylglutamic acid (aminopterin). *N. Engl. J. Med.*, **238**, 787–793 (1948).

26. Foster, B. J., Clagett-Carr, K., Shoemaker, D. D., Suffness, M., Plowman, J., Trissel, L. A., Grieshaber, C. K., and Leyland-Jones, B. Echinomycin: the first bifunctional intercalating agent in clinical trials. *Invest. New Drugs*, **3**, 403–410 (1986).

27. Fox, K. R., Gauvreau, D., Goodwin, D. C., and Waring, M. J. Binding of quinoline analogues of echinomycin to deoxyribonucleic acid: role of the chromophores. *Biochem. J.*, **191**, 729–742 (1980).

28. Fuchs, D. A. and Johnson, R. K. Cytologic evidence that taxol, an antineoplastic agent from *Taxus brevifolia*, acts as a mitotic spindle poison. *Cancer Treat. Rep.*, **62**, 1219–1222 (1978).

29. Gauvreau, D. and Waring, M. J. Directed biosynthesis of novel derivatives of echino-mycin by *Streptomyces echinatus*. I. Effect of exogenous analogues of quinoxaline-2-car-boxylic acid on the fermentation. *Can. J. Microbiol.*, **30**, 439–450 (1984).

30. Gauze, G. G., Dudnik, Y. V., Loshgareva, N. P., and Zbarsky, I. B. Inhibition of RNA synthesis by antibiotic 6270 from echinomycin group in bacterial and tissue cells. *Anti-biotiki*, **11**, 426–429 (1966).

31. Goldin, A., Schepartz, S. A., Venditti, J. M., and DeVita, V. T., Jr. Historical develop-ment and current strategy of the National Cancer Institute drug development program. *In* "Methods in Cancer Research," ed. V. T. DeVita, Jr. and H. Busch, Vol. 16A, pp. 165–245 (1979). Academic Press, New York.

32. Goodman, L. S., Wintrobe, M. M., Dameshek, W., Goodman, M. J., Gilman, A., and McLennan, M. T. Nitrogen mustard therapy. Use of methyl-bis(beta-chloroethyl)amine

hydrochloride and tris(beta-chloroethyl)amine hydrochloride for Hodgkin's disease, lymphosarcoma, leukemia, and certain allied and miscellaneous disorders. *J. Am. Med. Assoc.*, **132**, 126–132 (1946).

33. Grem, J. L., Tutsch, K. D., Simon, K. J., Alberti, D. B., Willson, J.K.V., Tormey, D. C., Swaminathan, S., and Trump, D. L. Phase I study of taxol administered as a short i.v. infusion daily for 5 days. *Cancer Treat Rep.*, **71**, 1179–1184 (1987).

34. Grever, M. R., Malspeis, L., Kraut, E. H., Wilson, H. E., Staubus, A. E., Coleman, M. S., and Balcerzak, S. P. Combination of 2′-deoxycoformycin and vidarabine in advanced malignancy: Clinical and biochemical observations. *Cancer Treat. Symp.*, **2**, 97–104 (1984).

35. Haas, C., Baker, L., Leichman, L., and Decker, D. Phase I evaluation of echinomycin administered on a weekly×4 schedule. *Proc. Am. Soc. Clin. Oncol.*, **3**, 29 (C-112) (1984).

36. Hanka, L. J. *In vitro* system for detection of antimetabolites of specific amino acids. *Cancer Treat Rep.*, **63**, 1133–1136 (1979).

37. Hanka, L. J. and Dietz, A. U-42126, a new antimetabolite antibiotic. Production, biological activity and taxonomy of the producing organism. *Antimicrob. Agents. Chemother.*, **3**, 425–431 (1973).

38. Hanka, L. J., Kuentzel, S. L., Martin, D. G., Wiley, P. F., and Neil, G. L. Detection and assay of antitumor antibiotics. *Recent Results Cancer Res.*, **63**, 69–76 (1978).

39. Hanka, L. J., Martin, D. G., and Neil, G. L. A new antitumor antimetabolite, (αS, 5S)-α-amino-3-chloro-4,5-dihydro-5-isoxazoleacetic acid (NSC-163501): Antimicrobial reversal studies and preliminary evaluation against L1210 mouse leukemia *in vivo*. *Cancer Chemother. Rep.*, **57**, 141–147 (1973).

40. Harvey, J. H., McFadden, M., Andrews, W. G., Byrne, P. J., Ahlgren, J. D., and Woolley, P. V. Phase I study of echinomycin administered on an intermittent bolus schedule. *Cancer Treat. Rep.*, **69**, 1365–1368 (1985).

41. Harvey, J., Priego, V., Binder, R., Byrne, P., Smith, F., and Woolley, P. A Phase I study of echinomycin (quinomycin A), NSC-526417 administered on an intermittent bolus schedule. *Proc. Am. Soc. Clin. Oncol.*, **3**, 35 (C-137) (1984).

42. Holton, R. A., Juo, R. R., Kim, H. B., Williams, A. D., Harusawa, S., Lowenthal, R. E., and Yogai, S. A synthesis of taxusin. *J. Am. Chem. Soc.*, **110**, 6558–6560 (1988).

43. Horwitz, S. B., Parness, J., Schiff, P. B., and Manfredi, J. J. Taxol: a new probe for studying the structure and function of microtubules. *Cold Spring Harbor Symp. Quant. Biol.*, **46**, 219–226 (1982).

44. Houchens, D. P., Ovejera, A. A., Sheridan, M. A., Johnson, R. K., Bogden, A. E., and Neil, G. L. Therapy for mouse tumors and human tumor xenografts with the antitumor antibiotic AT-125. *Cancer Treat. Rep.*, **63**, 473–476 (1979).

45. Jacrot, M., Riondel, J., Picot, F., Leroux, D., Mouriquand, C., Beriel, H., and Potier, P. Action du taxol vis-a-vis de tumeurs humaines transplantees sur des souris athymiques. *C. R. Seances Acad. Sci. Ser. 3*, **297**, 597–600 (1983).

46. Jayaram, H. N., Cooney, D. A., Ryan, J. A., *et al.* L-(αS, 5S)-α-amino-3-chloro-4,5-dihydro-5-isoxazoleacetic acid (NSC-163501): a new amino acid antibiotic with the properties of an antagonist of L-glutamine. *Cancer Treat. Rep.*, **59**, 481–491 (1975).

47. Johns, D. G. and Adamson, R. H. Enhancement of the biological activity of cordycepin (3′-deoxyadenosine) by the adenosine deaminase inhibitor 2′-deoxycoformycin. *Biochem. Pharmacol.*, **25**, 1441–1444 (1977).

48. Katagiri, K. and Matsuura, S. Studies on the antitumor activity of quinoxaline antibiotics. *J. Antibiot. Ser. B*, **16**, 122–125 (1963).

49. Katagiri, K. and Sugiura, K. Antitumor action of the quinoxaline antibiotics. *Antimicrob. Agents Chemother.*, **1961**, 162–168 (1961).

50. Katagiri, K., Yoshida, T., and Sato, K. Quinoxaline antibiotics. *In* "Antibiotics Vol. III.

Mechanism of Action of Antimicrobial and Antitumor Agents," ed. J. W. Corcoran and F. E. Hahn, pp. 234–251 (1974). Springer-Verlag, Berlin.

51. Kelly, R. C., Schletter, I., Stein, S. J., and Wierenga, W. Total synthesis of α-amino-3-chloro-4,5-dihydro-5-isoxazoleacetic acid (AT-125), an antitumor antibiotic. *J. Am. Chem. Soc.*, **101**, 1054–1055 (1979).

52. Kris, M. G., O'Connell, J. P., Gralla, R. J., Wertheim, M. S., Parente, R. M., Schiff, P. B., and Young, C. W. Phase I trial of taxol given as a 3-hour infusion every 21 days. *Cancer Treat. Rep.*, **70**, 605–607 (1986).

53. Krogsgaard-Larsen, P., Honore, T., and Hansen, J. J. New class of glutamate antagonists structurally related to ibotenic acid. *Nature*, **284**, 64–66 (1980).

54. Kuhn, J., von Hoff, D., Schick, M., Clark, G., Kisner, D., Weiss, G., Melnik, T., and Coltman, C., Jr. Phase I trial of echinomycin (NSC-526417). *Proc. Am. Soc. Clin. Oncol.*, **3**, 24 (C-91) (1984).

55. Lassus, M., Scott, D., and Leyland-Jones, B. Allergic reactions associated with Cremophor containing antineoplastics. *Proc. Am. Soc. Clin. Oncol.*, **4**, 268 (1985).

56. Lataste, H., Senilh, V., Wright, M., Guenard, D., and Potier, P. Relationships between the structures of taxol and baccatine III derivatives and their *in vitro* action on the disassembly of mammalian brain and *Physarum* amoebal tubulins. *Proc. Natl. Acad. Sci. U.S.A.*, **81**, 4090–4094 (1984).

57. Lee, J. S. and Waring, M. J. Bifunctional intercalation and sequence specificity in the binding of quinomycin and triostin antibiotics to deoxyribonucleic acid. *Biochem J.*, **173**, 115–128 (1978).

58. Lee, J. S. and Waring, M. J. Interaction between synthetic analogues of quinoxaline antibiotics and nucleic acids: changes in mechanism and specificity related to structural alterations. *Biochem J.*, **173**, 129–144 (1978).

59. Legha, S. S., Tenney, D. M., and Krakoff, I. R. Phase I study of taxol using a 5-day intermittent schedule. *J. Clin. Oncol.*, **4**, 762–766 (1986).

60. Lembersky, B. C., Ratain, M. J., Westbrook, C., and Golomb, H. M. Rapid response to 2'-deoxycoformycin in advanced hairy cell leukemia after failure of interferons alpha and gamma. *Am. J. Hematol.*, **27**, 60–62 (1988).

61. LePage, G. A., Worth, L. S., and Kimball, A. P. Enhancement of the antitumor activity of arabinofuranosyladenine by 2'-deoxycoformycin. *Cancer Res.*, **36**, 1481–1485 (1976).

62. Lofters, W., Campbell, M., Gibbs, W. N., and Cheson, B. 2'-deoxycoformycin therapy in adult T-cell leukemia / lymphoma. *Cancer*, **60**, 2605–2608 (1987).

63. Low, C. M., Fox, K. R., and Waring, M. J. DNA sequence selectivity of three biosynthetic analogues of the quinoxaline antibiotics. *Anticancer Drug Des.*, **1**, 149–160 (1986).

64. Magri, N. F. and Kingston, D. G. Modified taxols. 4. Synthesis and biological activity of taxols modified in the side chain. *J. Natl. Prod.*, **51**, 298–306 (1988).

65. Major, P. P., Agarwal, R. P., and Kufe, D. W. Clinical pharmacology of deoxycoformycin. *Blood*, **58**, 91–96 (1981).

66. Malspeis, L., Weinrib, A. B., Staubus, A. E., Grever, M. R., Balcerzak, S. P., and Neidhart, J. A. Clinical pharmacokinetics of 2'-deoxycoformycin. *Cancer Treat. Symp.*, **2**, 7–15 (1984).

67. Manfredi, J. J., Parness, J., and Horwitz, S. B. Taxol binds to cellular microtubules. *J. Cell Biol.*, **94**, 688–696 (1982).

68. Martin, D. G., Duchamp, D. J., and Chidester, C. G. The isolation, structure and absolute configuration of U-42126, a novel antitumor antibiotic. *Tetrahedron Lett.*, **1973**, 2549–2552 (1973).

69. Martin, D. G., Mizsak, S. A., Biles, C., Stewart, J. C., Baczynskyj, L., and Meulman, P. A. Structure of quinomycin antibiotics. *J. Antibiot.*, **28**, 332–336 (1975).

70. Matsuura, S. Studies on quinoxaline antibiotics. IV. Selective antitumor activity of each

quinoxaline antibiotic. *J. Antibiot. Ser A*, **18**, 43–46 (1965).

71. McGovren, J. P., Piercey, M. J., Einspahr, F. J., Tang, A. H., Schreur, P.J.K.D., Williams, M. G., and Curtis, D. R. Studies on the central nervous system (CNS) toxicity of acivicin (NSC-163501). *Proc. Am. Assoc. Cancer Res.*, **26**, 370 (1985).

72. McGovren, J. P. and Williams, M. G. Prevention of acivicin-induced CNS toxicity by concomitant amino acid infusion. *Proc. Am. Assoc. Cancer Res.*, **27**, 421 (1986).

73. McGovren, J. P., Williams, M. G., and Stewart, J. C. Interspecies comparison of acivicin pharmacokinetics. *Drug Metab. Dispos.*, **16**, 18–22 (1988).

74. National Cancer Institute Clinical Brochure, Taxol (NSC-125973) (1983). Drug Regulatory Affairs Branch. Div. of Cancer Treatment, NCI, Bethesda, MD.

75. O'Dwyer, P. J., Alonso, M. T., and Leyland-Jones, B. Acivicin: a new glutamine antagonist in clinical trials. *J. Clin. Oncol.*, **2**, 1064–1071 (1984).

76. O'Dwyer, P. J., Marsoni, S., Alonso, M. T., and Wittes, R. E. 2'-Deoxycoformycin: summary and future directions. *Cancer Treat. Symp.*, **2**, 1–5 (1984).

77. O'Dwyer, P. J., Spiers, A.S.D., and Marsoni, S. Association of severe and fatal infections and treatment with pentostatin. *Cancer Treat. Rep.*, **70**, 1117–1120 (1986).

78. O'Dwyer, P. J., Wagner, B., Leyland-Jones, B., Wittes, R. E., Cheson, B. D., and Hoth, D. F. 2'-Deoxycoformycin (pentostatin) for lymphoid malignancies: Rational development of an active new drug. *Ann. Intern. Med.*, **108**, 733–743 (1988).

79. Ohnuma, T., Zimet, A. S., Coffey, V. A., Holland, J. F., and Greenspan, E. M. Phase I study of taxol in a 24-hr infusion schedule. *Proc. Am. Assoc. Cancer Res.*, **26**, 167 (1985).

80. Oldham, R. K. Biological Response Modifiers Program. *J. Biol. Resp. Modif.*, **1**, 81–100 (1982).

81. Parness, J., Kingston, D.G.I., Powell, R. G., Harracksingh, C., and Horwitz, S. B. Structure-activity study of cytotoxicity and microtubule assembly *in vitro* by taxol and related taxanes. *Biochem. Biophys. Res. Commun.*, **105**, 1082–1089 (1982).

82. Pazdur, R., Haas, C. D., Baker, L. H., Leichman, C. G., and Decker, D. Phase I study of echinomycin. *Cancer Treat. Rep.*, **71**, 1217–1219 (1987).

83. Peale, A. L. and Glazer, R. I. Potentiation by 2'-deoxycoformycin of the inhibitory effect of xylosyladenine on nuclear RNA synthesis in L1210 cells *in vitro. Biochem. Pharmacol.*, **27**, 2543–2547 (1978).

84. Plunkett, W. Inhibition of adenosine deaminase to increase the antitumor activity of adenine nucleoside analogs. *Ann. N. Y. Acad. Sci.*, **451**, 150–159 (1985).

85. Plunkett, W., Feun, L. G., Benjamin, R. S., Keating, M., and Freireich, E. J. Modulation of vidarabine metabolism by 2'-deoxycoformycin for therapy of acute leukemia. *Cancer Treat. Symp.*, **2**, 23–27 (1984).

86. Riondel, J., Jacrot, M., Nissou, M. F., Picot, F., Beriel, H., Mouriquand, C., and Potier, P. Antineoplastic activity of two taxol derivatives on an ovarian tumor xenografted into nude mice. *Anticancer Res.*, **8**, 387–390 (1988).

87. Riondel, J., Jacrot, M., Picot, F., Beriel, H., Mouriquand, C., and Potier, P. Therapeutic response to taxol of six human tumors xenografted into nude mice. *Cancer Chemother. Pharmacol.*, **17**, 137–142 (1986).

88. Rowinsky, E. K., Burke, P. J., Karp, J. E., Ettinger, D. S., Tucker, R. W., and Donehower, R. C. Phase I study of taxol in refractory adult acute leukemia. *Proc. Am. Assoc. Cancer Res.*, **29**, 215 (A855) (1988).

89. Rowinsky, E. K., Donehower, R. C., Rosenshein, N. B., Ettinger, D. S., and McGuire, W. P. Phase II study of taxol in advanced ovarian epithelial malignancies. *Proc. Am. Soc. Clin. Oncol.*, **7**, A523 (1988).

90. Rowinsky, E. K., Donehower, R. C., and Tucker, R. W. Microtubule changes and cytotoxicity produced by taxol in human ovarian cell lines. *Proc. Am. Assoc. Cancer Res.*, **28**, 423 (1987).

91. Sato, K., Niinomi, Y., Katagiri, K., Matsukage, A., and Minagawa, T. Prevention of phage multiplication by quinomycin A. *Biochim. Biophys. Acta*, **174**, 230–238 (1969).

92. Sato, K., Shiratori, O., and Katagiri, K. The mode of action of quinoxaline antibiotics: Interaction of quinomycin A with DNA. *J. Antibiot. Ser. A*, **20**, 270–276 (1967).

93. Schabel, F. M. The antiviral activity of 9-B-D-arabinofuranosyladenine. *Chemotherapy*, **13**, 321–338 (1968).

94. Schepartz, S. A. History of the National Cancer Institute and the plant screening program. *Cancer Treat. Rep.*, **60**, 975–977 (1976).

95. Schiff, P. B., Fant, J., and Horwitz, S. B. Promotion of microtubule assembly *in vitro* by taxol. *Nature*, **277**, 665–667 (1979).

96. Schiff, P. B. and Horwitz, S. B. Taxol stabilizes microtubules in mouse fibroblast cells. *Proc. Natl. Acad. Sci. U.S.A.*, **77**, 1561–1565 (1980).

97. Senilh, V., Blechert, S., Colin, M., Guenard, D., Picot, F., Potier, P., and Varenne, P. Mise en evidence de nouveaux analogues du taxol extraits de *Taxus baccata*. *J. Natl. Prod.*, **47**, 131–137 (1984).

98. Sessoms, S. M., Coghill, R. D., and Waalkes, T. P. Review of the Cancer Chemotherapy National Service Center program. *Cancer Chemother. Rep.*, **7**, 25–46 (1960).

99. Smyth, J. F., Chassin, M. M., Harrap, K. R., Adamson, R. H., and Johns, D. G. 2'-Deoxycoformycin (DCF): Phase I trial and clinical pharmacology. *Proc. Am. Assoc. Cancer Res.*, **20**, 47 (A-187) (1979).

100. Smyth, J. F., Paine, R. M., Jackman, A. L., Harrap, K. R., Chassin, M. M., Adamson, R. H., and Johns, D. G. The clinical pharmacology of the adenosine deaminase inhibitor 2'-deoxycoformycin. *Cancer Chemother. Pharmacol.*, **5**, 93–101 (1980).

101. Smyth, J. F., Prentice, H. G., Proctor, S., and Hoffbrand, A. V. Deoxycoformycin in the treatment of leukemias and lymphomas. *Ann. N. Y. Acad. Sci.*, **451**, 123–127 (1985).

102. Spiers, A.S.D. The activity of deoxycoformycin (pentostatin) in refractory leukemias and lymphomas. *Ann. N. Y. Acad. Sci.*, **451**, 138–141 (1985).

103. Sternberg, C. N., Sordillo, P. P., Cheng, E., Chuang, Y. J., and Niedzwiecki, D. Evaluation of new anticancer agents against human pancreatic carcinomas in nude mice. *Am. J. Clin. Oncol.*, **10**, 219–221 (1987).

104. Strauman, J. J. Symptom distress in patients receiving Phase I chemotherapy with taxol. *Oncol. Nurs. Forum*, **13**, 40–43 (1986).

105. Suffness, M. The discovery and development of antitumor drugs from natural products. *In* "Advances in Medicinal Plant Research," ed. A. J. Vlietinck and R. A. Dommisse, pp. 101–133 (1985). Wissenschaftliche Verlagsgesellschaft mbH, Stuttgart.

106. Suffness, M. and Douros, J. Drugs of plant origin. *In* "Methods in Cancer Research" ed. V. T. DeVita and H. Busch, Vol. 16, Part A, pp. 73–126 (1979). Academic Press, New York.

107. Suffness, M. and Douros, J. Current status of the NCI plant and animal products program. *J. Natl. Prod.*, **45**, 1–14 (1982).

108. Suffness, M. and Cordell, G. A. Antitumor alkaloids. *In* "The Alkaloids," ed. A. Brossi, Vol. 25, pp. 6–18 and 280–288 (1985). Academic Press, New York.

109. Taylor, S. and Eyre, H. J. Randomized Phase II trials of acivicin (AT-125, NSC-163501) and fludarabine in recurrent malignant gliomas: A SWOG study. *Proc. Am. Soc. Clin. Oncol.*, **6**, 71 (#275) (1987).

110. Taylor, S., Slavik, M., Stephens, R., and Sayre, R. Phase I trial of echinomycin (NSC-526417) daily ×5 schedule. *Invest. New Drugs*, **2**, 106 (1984).

111. Tsunoda, A. Chemoprophylaxis of poliomyelitis in mice with quinomycin. *J. Antibiot. Ser. A*, **15**, 60–66 (1962).

112. Van Dyke, M. M. and Dervan, P. B. Echinomycin binding sites on DNA. *Science*, **225**, 1122–1127 (1984).

113. Venditti, J. M., Wesley, R. A., and Plowman, J. Current NCI preclinical antitumor screening *in vivo*. Results of tumor panel screening 1976–1982 and future directions. *Adv. Pharmacol. Chemother.*, **20**, 1–20 (1984).

114. Wakelin, L.P.G. and Waring, M. J. The binding of echinomycin to deoxyribonucleic acid. *Biochem. J.*, **157**, 721–740 (1976).

115. Wang, A.H.J., Ughetto, G., Quigley, G. J., Hakoshima, T., Van der Marel, G. A., Van Bloom, J. H., and Rich, A. The molecular structure of a DNA-triostin A complex. *Science*, **225**, 1115–1121 (1984).

116. Wani, M. C., Taylor, H. L., Wall, M. E., Coggon, P., and McPhail, A. T. Plant antitumor agents. VI. The isolation and structure of taxol, a novel antileukemic and antitumor agent from *Taxus brevifolia*. *J. Am. Chem. Soc.*, **93**, 2325–2327 (1971).

117. Ward, D. C., Reich, E., and Goldberg, I. H. Base specificity in the interaction of polynucleotides with antibiotic drug. *Science*, **149**, 1259–1263 (1965).

118. Waring, M. J. and Fox, K. R. Molecular aspects of the interaction between quinoxaline antibiotics and nucleic acids. *In* "Molecular Aspects of Anticancer Drug Action," ed. S. Neidle and M. J. Waring, pp. 127–156 (1983). Verlag Chemie, Basel.

119. Waring, M. J. and Wakelin, L.P.G. Echinomycin. A bifunctional intercalating antibiotic. *Nature*, **252**, 653–657 (1974).

120. Wiernik, P. H., Schwartz, E. L., Einzig, A., Strauman, J. J., Lipton, R. B., and Dutcher, J. P. Phase I trial of taxol given as a 24 hour infusion every 21 days: responses observed in metastatic melanoma. *J. Clin. Oncol.*, **5**, 1232–1239 (1987).

121. Wiernik, P. H., Schwartz, E. L., Strauman, J. J., Dutcher, J. P., Lipton, R. B., and Paietta, E. Phase I clinical and pharmacokinetic study of taxol. *Cancer Res.*, **47**, 2486–2493 (1987).

122. Woo, P.K.W., Dion, H. W., Lange, S. M., Dahl, L. F., and Durham, L. J. Novel adenosine and ara-A deaminase inhibitor, (R)-3-(2-deoxy-B-D-erythropentofuranosyl)-3, 6, 7, 8-tetrahydroimidazol-[4, 5-d] [1, 3] diazepin-8-01. *J. Heterocycl. Chem.*, **11**, 641–643 (1974).

123. Yamaguchi, K., Yul, L. S., Oda, T., Maeda, Y., Ishii, M., Fujita, K., Kagiyama, S., Nagai, K., Suzuki, H., and Takatsuki, K. Clinical consequences of 2′-deoxycoformycin treatment in patients with refractory adult T-cell leukaemia. *Leukemia Res.*, **10**, 989–993 (1986).

124. Zubrod, C. G. Origins and development of chemotherapy research at the National Cancer Institute. *Cancer Treat. Rep.*, **68**, 9–19 (1984).

125. Zubrod, C. G., Schepartz, S., Leiter, J., Endicott, K. M., Carrese, L. M., and Baker, C. G. The chemotherapy program of the National Cancer Institute: History, analysis and plans. *Cancer Chemother. Rep.*, **50**, 349–540 (1966).

126. Zurer, P. Chemists closing in on synthesis of scarce anticancer agent taxol. *Chem. Engin. News*, **10**, 22–23 (1988).

ANTITUMOR NATURAL PRODUCTS OTHER THAN ANTIBIOTICS UNDER DEVELOPMENT IN JAPAN

Shigeru TSUKAGOSHI

*Cancer Chemotherapy Center, Japanese Foundation for Cancer Research**

Clinically active drugs with novel structures are sought, and antitumor natural products can be a good source for such new structures. Antitumor antibiotics and plant products such as various anthracyclines, mitomycins, bleomycins and other antibiotics, and vinca alkaloids like etoposide and others are excellent anticancer drugs in clinical use. This article reviews antitumor natural products other than antibiotics under clinical or experimental study in Japan. A derivative of camptothecin, a cyclic hexapeptide preparation and a derivative of ellipticine are now being clinically tested, and an effort to discover antitumor substances from marine organisms and plants has also been undertaken. Several novel compounds such as peptides, polyether, alkaloids, prostanoid, *etc.* with antitumor activity have been isolated from marine sponges, octocorals, bryozoans, and plants, and these may be good candidates for further testing.

Antitumor natural products have been surveyed as possible anticancer drugs for clinical use, and in the past, antitumor antibiotics, marine and plant products have provided the main candidate compounds. Currently many antibiotics including the derivatives of doxorubicin and daunorubicin, and plant products such as vinca alkaloids are being used clinically for the treatment of human neoplasms. We need, however, anticancer drugs with greater tumor-selective activity and less toxicity than those known at present. Many natural antitumor products have been investigated in Japan, and in this paper, recent studies on candidate compounds from natural origins other than the antitumor antibiotics under clinical and pre-clinical investigation are reviewed. A camptothecin (CPT) derivative, a cyclic hexapeptide preparation and an ellipticine derivative are examples of substances under clinical trials in Japan.

In addition to antitumor antibiotics, there are many antitumor compounds originating from natural products in various stages of preclinical and clinical investigation in Japan. Some examples these of compounds follow.

Antitumor Compounds Originating from Natural Products under Clinical Study

1. A camptothecin derivative, CTP-11, under Phase II study

Camptothecin (Fig. 1) is an antitumor alkaloid isolated from *Camptotheca acuminata*, a Chinese plant (*41*), and has been evaluated to have clinical usefulness. In the initial screening test in the National Cancer Institute (NCI) of the United States, the compound was found to possess a significant activity to mouse leukemia L1210 and rat Walker 256

---

* Kami-Ikebukuro 1-37-1, Toshima-ku, Tokyo 170, Japan (塚越　茂).

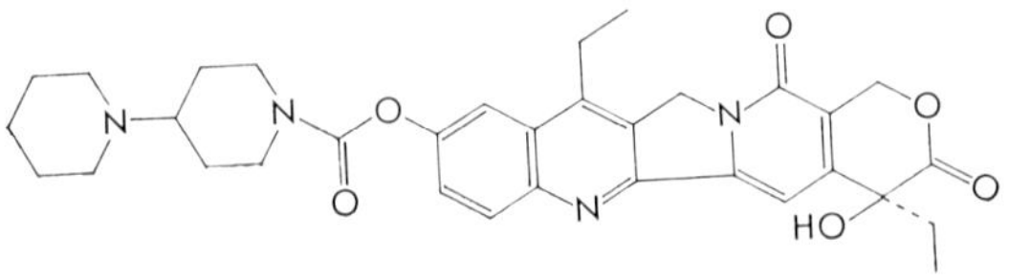

46 S. TSUKAGOSHI

FIG. 1. Structure of CPT-11

TABLE I. Antitumor Activity of CPT-11 against Mouse L1210
Leukemia Implanted Intraperitoneally[a]

Table dose (mg/kg)	CPT-11		Doxorubicin	
	T/C (%)	40 day-survivors	T/C (%)	40 day-survivors
Control	100	0		
1.56	129	0	138	0
6.25	160	0	167	0
12.5	198	0	229	0
25.0	226	0	214	1/6
50.0	269	0	143	0
100.0	414	5/6	90	0
200.0		6/6	71	0

[a] Data from Kunimoto *et al.* (*30*). L1210 cells (5×10^5/mouse) were inoculated i.p. into CDF_1 mice and drugs were given i.p. on days 1–9. Tumor-free survivors were excluded from T/C (%).

carcinosarcoma. Since this compound produced specific toxicity to the intestinal mucosa of monkeys and beagles, the possibility was raised of its clinical usefulness against human gastrointestinal carcinoma. In the Phase II study of camptothecin by patients with gastrointestinal adenocarcinoma, however, various toxic symptoms such as nausea, vomiting, diarrhea, stomatitis, dermatitis, alopecia, hemorrhagic cystitis, and bone marrow suppression were noted and the clinical response was minimal (*34*). In other clinical trials, unpredictable toxicities were also reported (*3, 5, 35*).

To find new derivatives having less toxicity and potent antitumor efficacy, an attempt was made to synthesize several derivatives of camptothecin in Japan (*29*). Among them, 7-ethyl-10-[4-(1-piperidino)-1-piperidino]carbonyloxycamptothecin (CPT-11) (Fig. 1) was found to be a stable and water-soluble compound and active against various murine tumors such as mouse L1210 and P388 leukemias, mouse sarcoma-180, Meth-A, B16 melanoma, Lewis lung carcinoma, and others (*30, 36*). Table I indicates the antitumor activity of CPT-11 against mouse L1210 leukemia (*30*). Inhibition of spontaneous and experimental metastases and antitumor effects of CPT-11 against multi-drug resistant tumor lines were also reported (*33, 40*). The acute toxicities (LD_{50}) of CPT-11 by intraperitoneal (i.p.) and oral (p.o.) administration were 117.5 and 765.3 mg/kg, respectively, much less than those of camptothecin (*30*). CPT-11 has so far been found mainly to inhibit DNA synthesis and to be a topoisomerase 1 inhibitor (*1*) like the mother compound. CPT-11 is now under Phase II study in Japan.

The Phase I study (*4*) was carried out by intravenous (i.v.) infusion starting from 50 mg/m²; the maximum tolerated dose (MTD) was found to be more than 250 mg/m² and the dose-limiting factor was leukopenia. The main side effects observed were transient leukopenia, gastro-intestinal disturbance and alopecia, none of which was serious

---

and there were no other serious side effects. This compound is under Phase II study in Japan.

2. An antitumor cyclic hexapeptide, RA-700, under Phase I study

In 1983, Itokawa *et al.* (*16*) isolated several compounds having potent antitumor activities from methanol extracts of dried roots of *Rubia cordifolia* and *Rubia akane*, which are common grasses in the Japanese islands and were used as dye sources many years ago. Itokawa *et al.* reported the basic chemical structure of the compound to be a cyclic structure consisting of six amino acids (*16–18*). This original structure was found to be almost identical to that of bouvardin or deoxybouvardin isolated from *Bouvardia ternifolia* (Rubiaceae) by Jolad *et al.* (*23*). From the preliminary tests on the antitumor activities (*19, 20*), one of the compounds, RA-700 (Fig. 2), was selected for further testing as an antitumor compound. It has been reported that bouvardin was markedly effective against mouse p388 leukemia, moderately so against mouse L1210 leukemia and B16 melanoma, but not as effective against murine solid tumors (*2, 23*). RA-700 was found effective against mouse P388 leukemia and colon 38, and moderately so against Lewis lung carcinoma and B16 melanoma (*6*). Table II indicates the antitumor activity of RA-700 to mouse colon 38 in comparison with mitomycin C (*6*). Inoue *et al.* (*11*) reported

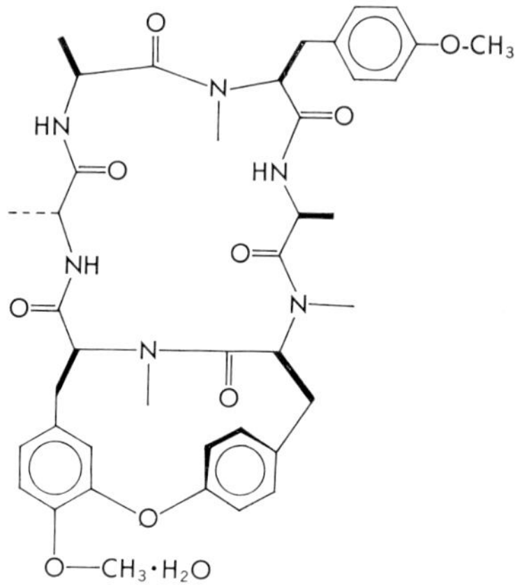

FIG. 2. Structure of RA-700

TABLE II. Antitumor Activity of RA-700 against Mouse Colon 38[a]

Drug	Dose (mg/kg/day)	Growth inhibition (%)		
		Day 22	Day 37	Cured mice
None (saline)		0	0	0/17
RA-700	0.25	40.7	16.9	0/8
	1.0	62.7	58.7	1/8
	2.5	95.5	66.1	5/8
	4.0	—	—	8/8
Mitomycin C	0.5	88.9	85.4	1/8
	1.0	toxic	—	—

[a] Reported by Hamanaka *et al.* (*6*). Mouse colon 38 tumor brei was inoculated s.c. to BDF$_1$ mice, and drugs were given i.v. on days 1–11.

48   S. TSUKAGOSHI

that RA-700 was sensitive to human ovarian, non-small cell lung, breast, and colorectal carcinomas in a human tumor clonogenic assay. Marked antitumor activity of RA-700 was also reported against mouse MM2 mammary carcinoma and rat Yoshida sarcoma. Acute toxicities of RA-700 (LD_{50}) were 32.1 mg/kg in male and 33.5 mg/kg in female mice, respectively, by single i.v. administration and by five consecutive-day 14.1 mg/kg/ day injections to ICR or BDF_1 mice (6). In the preliminary experiments with mouse P388 leukemia cells, a marked inhibition of the incroporation of [³H]leucine into protein was observed, suggesting that the mechanism of action of RA-700 is mainly the inhibition of protein synthesis (15). In the study of treatment schedules of RA-700 using mouse P388 leukemia, the compound was most effective when given daily in small doses. RA-700 also showed a time-dependent feature like vincristine (11, 39). Inhibition of the experimental lymph node metastasis of P388 cells and pulmonary metastasis of B16-BL6 cells was also reported (6). RA-700 is currently under Phase I study by i.v. infusion, and no details have yet been disclosed.

3. *Antitumor ellipticine glycoside preparation, SUN 4599, under Phase I study*

Ellipticine (Fig. 3) and 9-methoxyellipticine are uleine alkaloids originally isolated from *Ochorosia elliptica* Labill (*Apocynacease*), and their potent antitumor activities against murine tumors have been documented (31). Drugs of this group are reportedly strong inhibitors of the synthesis of biopolymers such as DNA, RNA, and protein. In clinical trials of ellipticine, a lactate formulation of 9-methoxyellipticine and 9-hydroxy-2-methylellipticinium acetate were water-soluble and found to be effective against human myeloblastic leukemia and breast cancer, respectively (24, 32). Ellipticine derivatives, however, are usually water-insoluble and development of the formulation for the clinical trials was difficult. To improve water-solubility, sugar moieties were attached to the ellipticine structure by Honda *et al.* in 1987. A study on the structure-activity relationship of about 50 such ellipticine derivatives revealed that, SUN4599 (Fig. 4), an L-arabino-pyranoside derivative of ellipticine, was highly active to mouse leukemia L1210 and less toxic than other derivatives (9, 10). The acute toxicity (LD_{59}) of SUN4599 against *ddY* mice was 17.8 mg/kg and against ICR mice was 28.0 mg/kg, and the LD_{50} against beagles

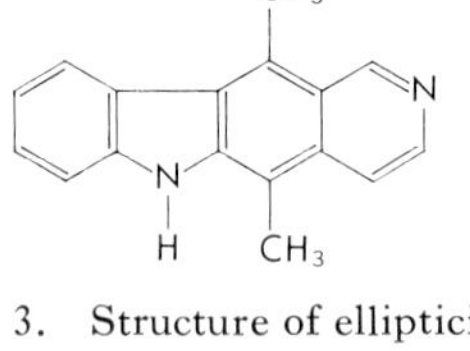

FIG. 3. Structure of ellipticine

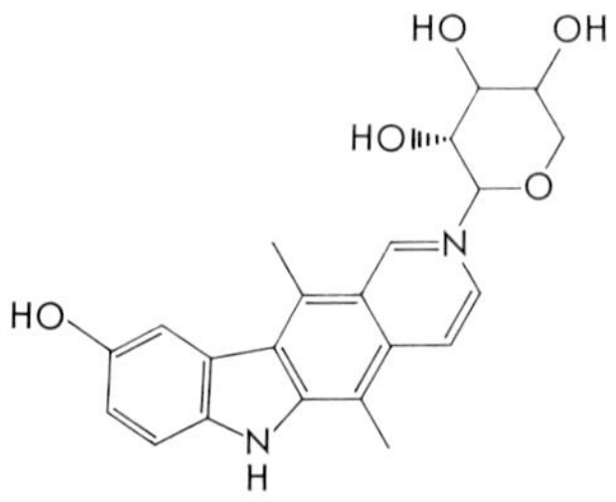

FIG. 4. Structure of SUN 4599

TABLE III.   Antitumor Effects of SUN4599 and Related Compounds
against Mouse L1210 Leukemia[a]

Drug	Dose (mg/kg)	ILS (%)
Control	0	0
SUN4599	1.25	37
	5.0	57
	10.0	113
	20.0	1/6[b]
	40.0	4/6[b]
	80.0	Toxic
Ellipticine	120.0	128
Elliptinium	5.0	48
Doxorubicin	2.5	90
Cisplatin	2.0	120

[a] Reported by T. Honda et al. (10). L1210 (10^5) cells were inoculated i.p. to BDF_1 mice and the drugs were given i.p. daily for 5 days.

[b] 80-day survivors/test mice.

TABLE IV.   Antitumor Effects of SUN4599 and Related Compounds
against Mouse L1210 Leukemia by i.v. Injection[a]

Drug	Dose (mg/kg)	ILS (%)
Control	0	0
SUN4599	10.0	82
	20.0	198
	30.0	2/6[b]
Ellipticine	2.5	10
Doxorubicin	2.5	30

[a] Reported by T. Honda et al. (10). Treatment schedules were the same as in Table III.

[b] 80-day survivors/test mice.

was more than 20 mg/kg. Tables II and IV indicate the antitumor activities of SUN-4599 and related compounds in comparison with doxorubicin and cisplatin against mouse L1210 leukemia. SUN4599 was active against a variety of murine tumors including mouse leukemias L1210 and P388, B16 melanoma, colon 38, Ehrlich carcinoma, and sarcoma 180. This compound was also effective to vincristine-resistant mouse P388 leukemia and various human tumor xenografts, and significantly inhibited experimental tumor metastases to various organs. Experimental tumor metastases to various organs were also inhibited significantly by SUN4599. DNA, RNA, and protein syntheses of mouse L1210 leukemia cells were inhibited by SUN4599 with dose- and time-dependent patterns. The Phase I study of SUN4599 by i.v. infusion is in progress in Japan.

New Antitumor Natural Products under Investigation

1.   Experimentally active marine products

a)   Kitagawa et al. (28) recently reported the isolation of new antitumor prostanoids from Okinawan soft coral (stolonifer), *Clavularia viridis* Quoy and Gaimard (*Stolonifera, Clavalariidae*), and elucidated their structures. That of claviridenone-a, is shown in Fig. 5. These prostanoids are reported to have a growth-inhibiting effect on cultured mouse

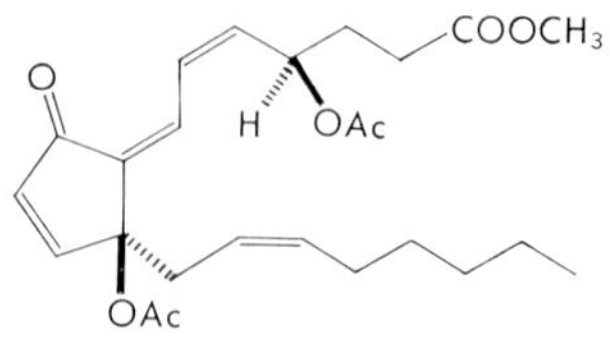

FIG. 5.   Structure of claviridenone-a

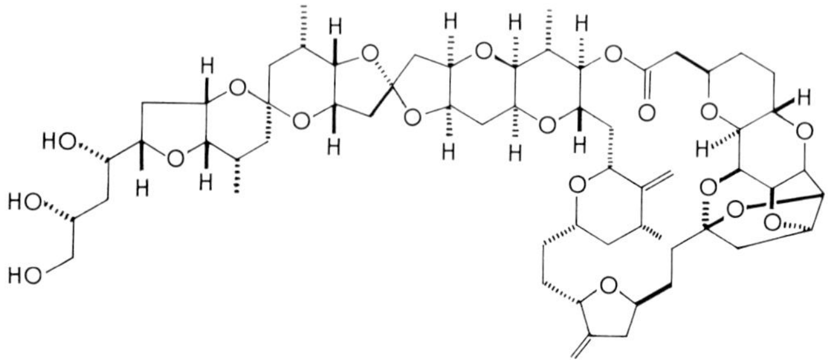

FIG. 6.   Structure of halichondrin B

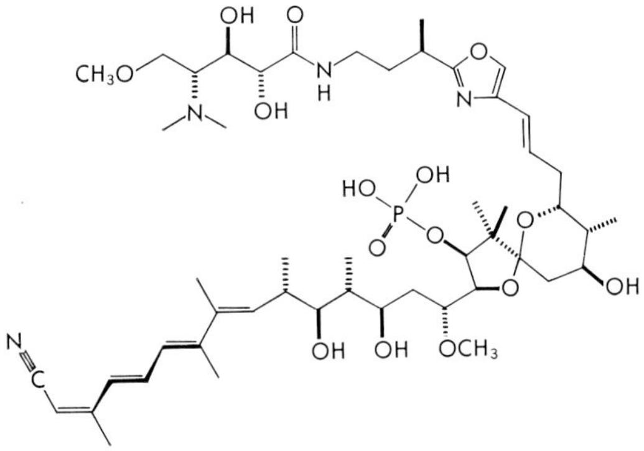

FIG. 7.   Structure of calyculin A

L1210 leukemia cells; other antitumor activities have not yet been studied in detail.

b)   In 1986, Hirata and Uemura (8) reported isolation of eight poly-ether macrolides, halichondrins, from a sponge, *Halichondria okadai*; halichondrin B (Fig. 6) was found to have strongest antitumor effect and an *in vitro* test against mouse B16 melanoma cells showed an IC_{50} of 0.093 ng/ml. T/C% by i.p. injection of 5 µg/kg was 244%; there was no acute toxicity. Calyculin A (Fig. 7) was also isolated by Kato *et al.* (25) from the sponge, *Discodermia calyx*. Against cultured mouse L1210 leukemia cells, this compound showed growth-inhibiting activity (IC_{50}: 1.75 ng/ml).

c)   Suzuki *et al.* (38) recently isolated cytotoxic compounds from a marine red alga, *Laurencia obtusa* (Hudson) Lamouroux. This tri-terpen compound, thyrsiferyl 23-acetate (Fig. 8), showed cytotoxic activity against cultured mouse P388 leukemia cells *in vitro* (ED_{50}: 0.3 ng/ml.) Amphidinolide-B (Fig. 9) was also isolated by Ishibashi *et al.* (12) from a marine dinoflagellate *Amphidinium* species.

d)   An interesting alkaloid, manzamine A hydrochloride (Fig. 10) was recently discovered from a sponge of *Halclona* species by Sakai *et al.* (37) IC_{50} of this alkaloid against

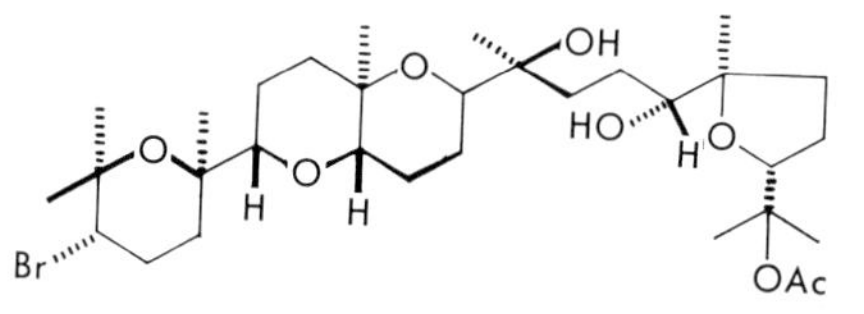

FIG. 8.   Structure of thyrsiferyl 23-acetate

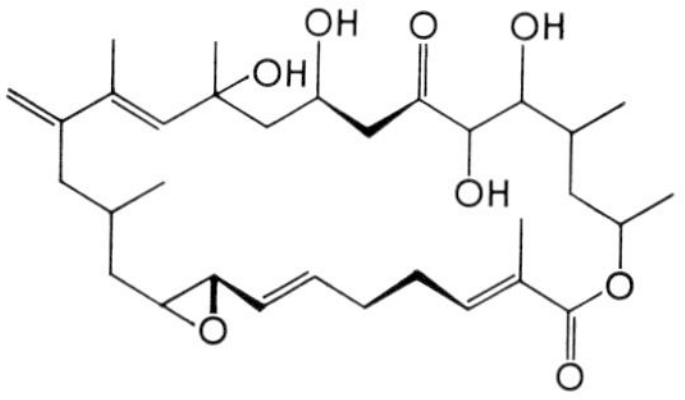

FIG. 9.   Structure of amphidinolide B

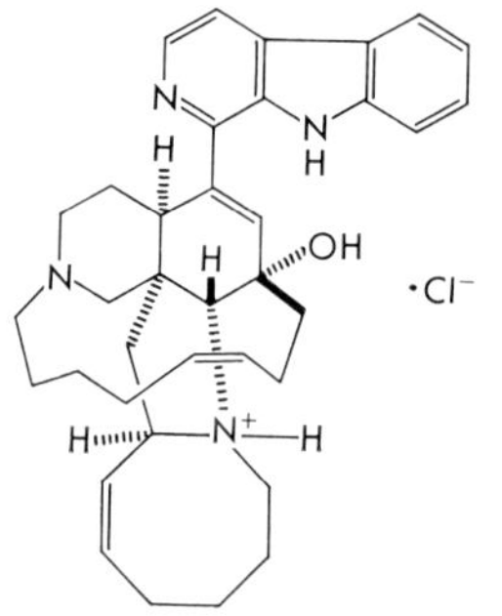

FIG. 10.   Structure of manzamine A hydrochloride

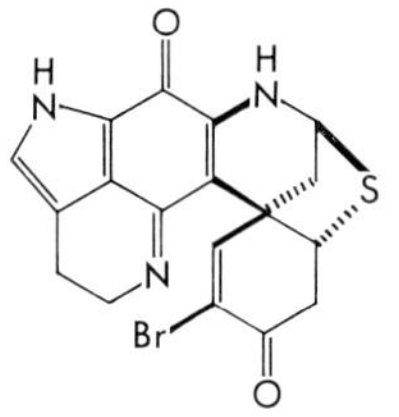

FIG. 11.   Structure of prianosin A

cultured mouse P388 leukemia cells was 0.07 μg/ml. Another *in vitro* active alkaloid, prianosin A (Fig. 11), was found the from Okinawan sponge, *Prianos melanos*, by Koba-yashi *et al.* (*26*). Prianosin A exhibited a growth-inhibiting effect against cultured mouse L1210 (IC$_{50}$: 37 ng/ml) and L5178Y (IC$_{50}$: 14 ng/ml) leukemia cells.

2.   *Some new antitumor compounds of plant origin*

Plants are a primary source of new candidate antitumor drugs expected to have clinical use. The following are examples of such antitumor compounds of plant origin under investigation in Japan.

a)   Cytotoxic diterpens: Four new labdane-type diterpenes, coronarin A, B, C, and D (Fig. 12) were isolated as the cytotoxic constituents from the rhizomes of *Hedychium coronarium* Zingiberaceae by Itokawa *et al.* (*13*). The Fig. 12, IC$_{50}$ values in parentheses in Fig. 12 indicate their cytotoxic activities against cultured V-79 cells.

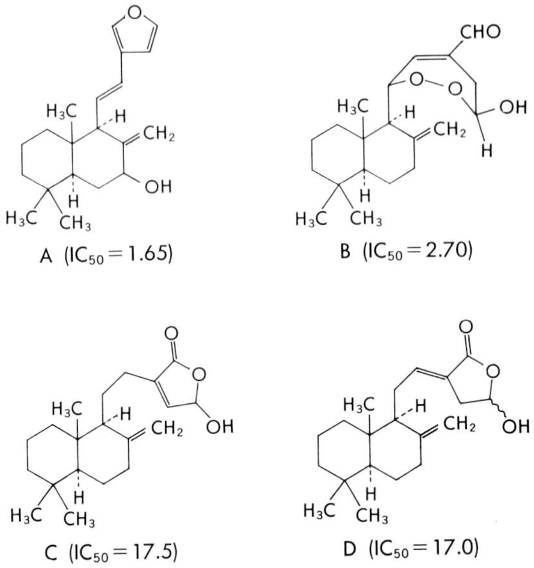

A (IC$_{50}$ = 1.65)   B (IC$_{50}$ = 2.70)

C (IC$_{50}$ = 17.5)   D (IC$_{50}$ = 17.0)

(IC$_{50}$ indicates μg/ml against V-79 cells)

FIG. 12.   Structures of coronarin A, B, C, and D

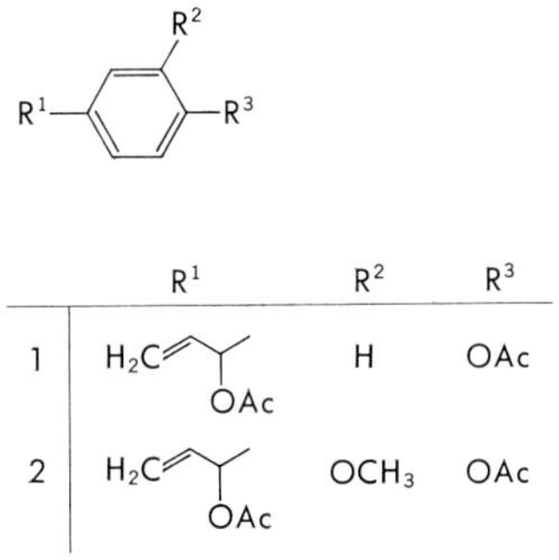

	R^1	R^2	R^3
1	H$_2$C⟍⟋⟍ OAc	H	OAc
2	H$_2$C⟍⟋⟍ OAc	OCH$_3$	OAc

FIG. 13.   Structures of 1′-acetoxychavicol acetate (1) and 1′-acetoxyeugenol acetate (2)

TABLE V.   Antitumor Activity of Sinococuline against Mouse P388 Leukemia[a]

Dose (mg/kg)	T/C (%)	Body weight change
10	154.6	+0.9
25	167.0	+0.6
50	177.0	−0.6
100	200.0	−4.7

[a] Data reported by Itokawa et al. (22). Mouse P388 leukemia (10^6 cells) was inoculated i.p. to CDF$_1$ mice and the drug was given i.p. on days 1–5.

b)   In antitumor screening tests on the alcoholic extracts of 60 species of Indonesian medicinal plants, Itokawa et al. (14) recently isolated 1′-acetoxychavicol acetate and 1′-acetoxyeugenol acetate (Fig. 13). These compounds showed a significant growth-inhibitory activity against mouse sarcoma 180 in vivo.

c) Antitumor activities against mouse sarcoma 180 of the compounds isolated from *Ginkgo biloba* L. were recently identified as anacardic acid, bilobol and cardanol also by Itokawa *et al.* (*21*).

d) Sinococuline was isolated as an antitumor morphinane alkaloid from *Cocclus triolbus* (Menispermaceae) recently by Itokawa *et al.* (*22*). This compound showed a significant antitumor activity against mouse P388 leukemia *in vivo* (Table V).

CONCLUSION

Antitumor compounds of natural origin other than the antitumor antibiotics already under experimental and clinical investigation were reviewed. It is hoped that at least some of these new compounds may prove clinically useful as antitumor drugs, and an active survey of antitumor marine and plant products is, therefore, on-going in Japan.

REFERENCES

1. Andoh, T., Okada, K., and Ogura, M. Biological function of DNA topoisomerase and its implication in cancer chemotherapy. *Jpn. J. Cancer Chemother.*, **15**, 1–14 (1988) (in Japanese).
2. Chitnis, M. P., Alate, A. D., and Menon, R. S. Effect of bouvardin on the growth characteristics and nucleic acid and protein syntheses profiles of P388 leukemia cells. *Chemotherapy*, **27**, 126–130 (1981).
3. Creaven, P. J., Allen, L. M., and Muggia, F. M. Plasma camptothecin (NSC-100880) levels during a 5-day course of treatment: relation to dose and toxicity. *Cancer Chemother. Rep.*, **56**, 573–580 (1972).
4. Furue, H., Suminaga, M., Wakui, A., Kanbe, M., Hasegawa, K., Niitani, H., Kawachi, S., Ota, K., Ariyoshi, H., Taguchi, T., Ota, J., Hattori, T., and Saheki, T. Phase I study of a new anticancer agent, CPT-11. *J. Jpn. Soc. Cancer Ther.*, **28**(9), 120 (1988) (in Japanese).
5. Gottieb, J. A. and Luce, J. K. Treatment of malignant melanoma with camptothecin (NSC-100880). *Cancer Chemother. Rep.*, **56**, 103–109 (1972).
6. Hamanaka, T., Ohgoshi, M., Kawahara, K., Yamakawa, K., Tsuruo, T., and Tsukagoshi, S. A novel antitumor cyclic hexapeptide (RA-700) obtained from *Rubiae radix*. *J. Pharmacobio-Dyn.*, **10**, 616–623 (1987).
7. Higa, T., Okuda, R. K., and Severns, R. M. Unprecedented constituents of a new species of acron worm. *Tetrahedron*, **43**, 1063–1070 (1987).
8. Hirata, Y. and Uemura, D. Halichondrins-antitumor polyether macrolides from a marine sponge. *Pure Appl. Chem.*, **58**, 701–710 (1986).
9. Honda, T., Inoue, M., Kato, M., Shima, K., and Shimamoto, T. Stereoselective synthesis of 9-hydroxyellipticine glycosides; novel and highly active antitumor agents. *Chem. Pharm. Bull.*, **35**, 3975–3978 (1987).
10. Honda, T., Kato, M., Inoue, M., Shimamoto, T., Shima, K., Nakanishi, T., Yoshida, T., and Noguchi, T. Synthesis and antitumor activity of quaternary ellipticine glycoside, a series of novel and highly active antitumor agents. *J. Med. Chem.*, **31**, 1295–1305 (1988).
11. Inoue, K., Mukaiyama, T., Kobayashi, T., and Ogawa, M. Activity of RA-700, a cyclic hexapeptide from *Rubia radix* in the human tumor clonogenic assay. *Invest. New Drugs*, **4**, 231–236 (1986).
12. Ishibashi, M., Ohizumi, Y., and Hamashima, M. Amphidinolide-B, a novel macrolide with potent antineoplastic activity from the marine dinoflagellate *Amphidinium* sp. *J. Chem. Soc. Chem. Commun*, 1127–1129 (1987).

13. Itokawa, H., Morita, H., Katou, I., Takeya, K., Cavalheiro, A. de Pliveira, R.C.B., Ishige, M., and Motidome, M. Cytotoxic diterpenes from the rhizomes of *Hedychium coronarium*. *Planta Med.*, **4**, 311–315 (1988).

14. Itokawa, H., Morita, H., Sumitomo, T., Totsuka, N., and Takeya, K. Antitumor principles from *Alpinia galanoga*. *Planta Med.*, **1**, 32–33 (1987).

15. Itokawa, H., Takeya, K., Hamanaka, T., Takanashi, M., Mori, N., and Tsukagoshi, S. Studies on the antineoplastic cyclic hexapeptides obtained from *Rubiae radix*. III. Antineoplastic activity of RA-700 on animal tumors and cultured cell lines. *In* "Recent Advances in Chemotherapy. Anticancer Section. 1," ed. J. Ishigami, p. 163 (1985). Univ. Tokyo Press, Tokyo.

16. Itokawa, H., Takeya, K., Mihara, K., Mori, N., Hamanaka, T., Sonobe, T., and Iitaka, Y. Studies on the antitumor cyclic hexapeptides obtained from *Rubiae radix*. *Chem. Pharm. Bull.*, **31**, 1424–1427 (1983).

17. Itokawa, H., Takeya, K., Mori, N., Hamanaka, T., Sonobe, T., and Mihara, K. Isolation and antitumor activity of cyclic hexapeptides isolated from *Rubiae radix*. *Chem. Pharm. Bull.*, **32**, 284–290 (1984).

18. Itokawa, H., Takeya, K., Mori, N., Kidokoro, S., and Yamamoto, H. Studies on antitumor cyclic hexapeptides RA obtained from *Rubiae radix*, Rubiaceae (IV); Quantitative determination of RA-VII and RA-V in commercial *Rubiae radix* and collected plants. *Planta Medica*, **51**, 313–316 (1984).

19. Itokawa, H., Takeya, K., Mori, N., Sonobe, T., Serisawa, N., Hamanaka, T., and Mihashi, S. Studies on antitumor cyclic hexapeptides RA obtained from *Rubiae radix*, Rubiaceae. III. On derivatives of RA-V and their *in vivo* activities. *Chem. Pharm. Bull.*, **32**, 3216–3226 (1984).

20. Itokawa, H., Takeya, K., Mori, N., Takahashi, M., Yamamoto, H., Sonobe, T., and Kidokoro, S. Cell growth-inhibitory effects of derivatives of antitumor cyclic hexapeptide RA-V obtained from *Rubia radix* (V). *Jpn. J. Cancer Res. (Gann)*, **75**, 929–936 (1984).

21. Itokawa, H., Totsuka, N., Nakahara, K., Takeya, K., Lepoittevin, J. P., and Asakawa, Y. Antitumor principles from *Ginkgo biloba* L. *Chem. Pharm. Bull.*, **35**, 3016–3020 (1987).

22. Itokawa, H., Tsuruoka, S., Takeya, K., Mori, N., Sonobe, T., Kosemura, S., and Hamanaka, T. An antitumor morphinane alkaloid, Sinococuline, from *Cocculus trilobus*. *Chem. Pharm. Bull.*, **35**, 1660–1662 (1987).

23. Jolad, S. D., Hoffman, J. J., Torrance, R. M., Wiedhopf, J. R., Cole, S. K., Arora, S. K., Bates, R. B., Gargiulo, R. I., and Kriek, G. R. Bouvardin and deoxybouvardin, antitumor cyclic hexapeptides from *Bouvardia ternifolia* (Rubiaceae). *J. Am. Chem. Soc.*, **99**, 8040–8044 (1977).

24. Juret, P., Heron, J. F., Covettle, J. E. *et al.* Hydroxy-9-methyl-2-ellipticinium for osseus metastases from breast cancer: 5-year experience. *Cancer Treat. Rep.*, **66**, 1909–1916 (1982).

25. Kato, Y., Fusetani, N., and Matsunaga, S. Calyculin A, a novel antitumor metabolite from the marine sponge *Discodermia calyx*. *J. Am. Chem. Soc.*, **108**, 2780–2781 (1986).

26. Kobayashi, J., Cheng, J., and Ishibashi, M. Prianosin A, a novel antileukemic alkaloid from the Okinawan marine sponge *Prianos melanos*. *Tetrahedron Lett.*, **28**, 4939–4942 (1987).

27. Kitagawa, I., Cui, Z., and Son, B. W. Nephtheoxydiol, a new cytotoxic hydroperoxygermacrane sesquiterpene, and related sesquiterpenoids from an Okinawan soft coral of *Nephthea* sp. *Chem. Pharm. Bull.*, **35**, 124–135 (1987).

28. Kitagawa, I., Kobayashi, M., Yasuzawa, T., Son, B. W., and Yoshihara, M. New prostanoids from soft coral. *Tetrahedron*, **41**, 995–1005 (1985).

29. Kunimoto, T., Nitta, K., Tanaka, T., Uehara, N., Baba, H., Takeuchi, M., Yokokura, T., Sawada, S., Miyasaka, T., and Mutai, M. Antitumor activity of a new camptothecin

derivative, SN-22, against various murine tumors. *J. Pharmacobio-Dyn.*, **10**, 148–151 (1987).

30. Kunimoto, T., Nitta, K., Tanaka, T., Uehara, N., Baba, H., Takeuchi, M., Yokokura, T., Sawada, S., Miyasaka, T., and Mutai, M. Antitumor activity of 7-ethyl-10[4-(1-piperidino)-1-piperidino]carbonyloxy-camptothecin, a novel water-soluble derivative of camptothecin, against murine tumors. *Cancer Res.*, **47**, 5944–5947 (1987).

31. LeMen, J., Hayat, M., Mathé, G., Guillon, J. C., Chenu, E., Humblot, M., and Masson, Y. Methoxy-9-ellipticine lactate I. Experimental study. *Eur. J. Clin. Biol. Res.*, **15**, 534–541 (1970).

32. Mathé, G., Hayat, M., DeVassal, F., Schwarzenberg, L., Schneider, M., Schlumberger, J. R., Jasmin, C., and Rosenfeld, C. Methoxy-9-ellipticine lactate. III. Clinical screening. Its action in acute myeloblastic leukemia. *Eur. J. Clin. Biol. Res.*, **15**, 541–545 (1970).

33. Matsuzaki, T., Yokokura, T., Mutai, M., and Tsuruo, T. Inhibition of spontaneous and experimental metastasis by a new derivative of camptothecin, CPT-11, in mice. *Cancer Chemother. Pharmacol.*, **21**, 308–312 (1988).

34. Moertel, C. G., Schutt, A. J., Reitemeler, R. J., and Hahn, R. G. Phase II study of camptothecin (NSC-100880) in the treatment of advanced gastrointestinal cancer. *Cancer Chemother. Rep.*, **56**, 95–101 (1972).

35. Muggia, F. M., Creaven, P. J., Hausen, H. H., Cohen, M. H., and Selawry, O. S. Phase I clinical trial of weekly and daily treatment with camptothecin (NSC-100880): correlation with preclinical studies. *Cancer Chemother. Rep.*, **56**, 515–521 (1972).

36. Nitta, K., Yokokura, T., Sawada, S., Takeuchi, M., Tanaka, T., Uehara, N., Baba, H., Kunimoto, T., Miyasaka, T., and Mutai, M. Antitumor activity of a new derivative of camptothecin. *In* "Recent Advances in Chemotherapy. Anticancer Section. 1," ed. J. Ishigami, p. 28 (1985). Univ. Tokyo Press, Tokyo.

37. Sakai, R., Higa, T., Jefford, C. W. *et al.* Manzamine A, a novel antitumor alkaloid from a sponge. *J. Am. Chem. Soc.*, **108**, 6404–6405 (1986).

38. Suzuki, T., Suzuki, M., and Furusaki, A. Teurilene and thyrsiferyl 23-acetate, meso and remarkably cytotoxic compounds from the marine red alga *Laurencia obtusa* (Hudson) Lamouroux. *Tetrahedron Lett.*, **26**, 1329–1332 (1985).

39. Takahashi, M., Toyoda, Y., Yamamoto, H., Ishii, K., Mori, N., Yadomae, T., Takeya, K., and Itokawa, H. Effect of antitumor substance RA-700 on cultured cells. *Proc. Jpn. Cancer Assoc.*, 280 (1984) (in Japanese).

40. Tsuruo, T., Matsuzaki, T., Matsushita, M., Saito, H., and Yokokura, T. Antitumor effect of CPT-11, a new derivative of camptothecin, against pleiotropic drug-resistant tumors *in vitro* and *in vivo*. *Cancer Chemother. Pharmacol.*, **21**, 71–74 (1988).

41. Wall, M. E., Wani, M. C., Cook, C. E., Palmer, K. H., McPhail, A. T., and Sim, G. A. Plant antitumor agents: 1. Novel alkaloidal leukemia and tumor inhibitor from *Camptotheca acuminata*. *J. Am. Chem. Soc.*, **83**, 3888 (1966).

II. ADVANCES IN ANTITUMOR ANTIBIOTICS

BLEOMYCINS: BASIC RESEARCH

Tomohisa TAKITA,[*1] Yasuhiko MURAOKA,[*1] and Katsutosi TAKAHASHI[*2]

*Institute of Microbial Chemistry[*1] and Research Laboratories,*
*Pharmaceuticals Group, Nippon Kayaku Co., Ltd.[*2]*

Bleomycin is a group of antitumor glycopeptide antibiotic including phleomycins, bleomycins, and bleomycin analogs such as peplomycin and liblomycin. Bleomycin and peplomycin were established their status in the treatment of human tumors. Liblomycin is under clinical trial.

In this paper, we review the early studies on biology and chemistry of bleomycin, including the mechanism of the therapeutic action of bleomycins, studies on the chemical structure of bleomycin, and on the methods of preparation of bleomycin analogs.

A new bleomycin analog liblomycin is discussed on its biological and biochemical properties comparing with peplomycin and bleomycin. Liblomycin shows distinct characteristics in toxicity, activity, and mode of action.

Recent advances in understanding of the mechanism of cytotoxicity and behavior *in vivo* of bleomycin are reviewed. Possibilities of new analogs of bleomycin based in recent advances in chemical synthesis and increased knowledge are pointed out.

Discovery of Bleomycin

In 1956, the late Professor Hamao Umezawa and his co-workers discovered phleomycin (*17*) during a study of water-soluble basic antibiotics. Phleomycin was later found to exhibit strong antitumor activity against Ehrlich carcinoma with a high therapeutic index (*1, 46*). Soon thereafter, it was found that this antibiotic inhibited DNA synthesis in HeLa cells and *Escherichia coli* (*42*), however, it caused irreversible renal toxicity in dogs (*11*). Bleomycin was discovered after search for an antibiotic similar to phleomycin (*49, 50*).

Bleomycin is a group of antibiotics produced by a strain classified as *Streptomyces verticillus*. They are blue copper-containing substances which can be separated into about 10 active components by CM-Sephadex chromatography (*5*). Structurally, bleomycin is different from phleomycin in only one amino acid unit. In place of 2-[2-(2-aminoethyl)-Δ^2-thiazolin-4-yl]-thiazole-4-carboxylic acid of phleomycin, bleomycin contains 2'-(2-aminoethyl)-2,4'-bithiazole-4-carboxylic acid moiety (*36*); phleomycin is thus a dihydro-bleomycin (Fig. 1). Biologically, bleomycin exhibited strong antitumor activity similar to phleomycin, but it did not cause renal toxicity.

Copper-ion contained in bleomycin is removed as the precipitate of cupric sulfide by bubbling hydrogen sulfide gas through a bleomycin solution. Either with or without copper, bleomycin showed almost the same activity, but the toxicity was slightly greater

[*1] Kamiosaki 3-14-23, Shinagawa-ku, Tokyo 141, Japan (滝田智久, 村岡靖彦).
[*2] Shimo 3-31-12, Kita-ku, Tokyo 115, Japan (高橋克俊).

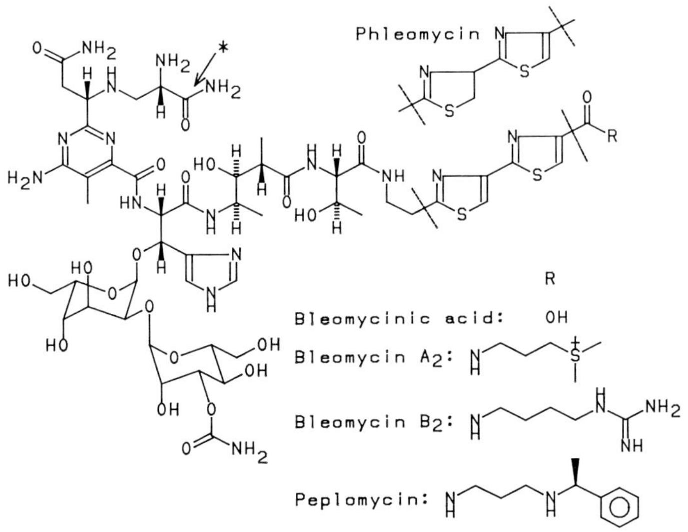

FIG. 1.   Structure of bleomycins and phleomycins
Bleomycin hydrolase cleaves bond marked (*).

in the form containing copper. Clinical studies were, therefore, begun on copper-free bleomycin in 1965, and the drugs therapeutic efficacy on squamous cell carcinoma was found by Professor T. Ichikawa *et al.* soon thereafter (*9*). Clinical use of bleomycin was permitted by the Ministry of Health and Welfare of Japan in 1968, and since then, bleomycin has been used in the treatment of lymphoma, testicular tumors and squamous cell carcinoma of skin, head, and neck, and cervix.

Early Studies on Biology and Chemistry of Bleomycin

Umezawa and his collaborators studied the mechanism of therapeutic action extensively. Distribution of ^{3}H-bleomycin in the organs of mice was studied by measuring the radioactivity and the antibacterial activity in organ extracts, and the antibiotic was found to be inactivated in organs and tissues in different degrees (*48*, *52*). This inactivation was slower in skin and lung than in other organs, especially in aged mice, and was found that this inactivation was due to the hydrolysis of a carboxamide bond in a bleomycin molecule by an enzyme called bleomycin hydrolase (Fig. 1). This enzyme also hydrolyzed L-lysine amide, L-arginine, and L-lysine β-naphthylamides, but it was different from known aminopeptidase B. It was also confirmed that the content of this enzyme in squamous cell carcinoma induced in mouse skin by methylcholanthrene was significantly lower than that in sarcoma of mouse skin induced by the same agent (*52*). Moreover, injected ^{3}H-bleomycin was distributed in the former at a higher concentration than in the latter. Thus, the selective effect on squamous cell carcinoma was shown to be due to the high distribution of the drug and the low content of the bleomycin-inactivating enzyme, resulting in a high concentration of the active antibiotic in this tumor.

This study has shown that the sensitivity of a human tumor to a drug can be predicted by the preferential distribution of the drug among various organs or tissues of an animal including tumors. This is a new approach to find a new antitumor compound useful in treating a certain kind of human tumor.

Umezawa and his collaborators determined the complicated chemical structures of all bleomycins (Fig. 1 shows the structure of bleomycins A_2 and B_2, major components of natural bleomycins) and elucidated that various bleomycins differ only in the terminal amine moiety (39). Clinically used bleomycin contains bleomycins A_2 and B_2 as major components. Addition of an amine to the culture medium caused production of bleomycin which contained the same added amine, thus, establishing a process of producing artificial bleomycins has been (4). Methods for preparing bleomycinic acid by an enzymatic hydrolysis of bleomycin B_2 (51) or by chemical cleavage of bleomycin demethyl-A_2 (35) have been developed, and semisynthetic bleomycins have been prepared starting from bleomycinic acid. Thus, more than 400 bleomycins have been obtained by fermentation or by chemical derivation of bleomycinic acid.

Peplomycin and Liblomycin

Bleomycin has already established its status as an important agent, especially in combination chemotherapy because of its lack of myelosuppressive properties. However, total dosage in cancer treatment is limited by the pulmonary toxicity. Therefore, the derivatives prepared by the above-described methods were closely evaluated to find a compound with has the same or stronger antitumor activity and lower pulmonary toxicity, and finally, peplomycin (Fig. 1) was selected as a candidate for clinical trials (18). Peplomycin showed strong activity against bleomycin-unresponsive tumors: chemically induced gastric and breast carcinomas in rats and two to four times weaker pulmonary toxicity than bleomycin in mice and dogs (3, 19). Thus, peplomycin has been used clinically since 1981. Its clinical efficacy has since been extended to prostatic (15) and breast cancer (14, 20, 23) in conformity with the broader antitumor spectrum observed in preclinical studies.

The pulmonary toxicity of peplomycin remained dose-limiting, however, so, a new screening program was started to find new, superior analogs. After examining over 200 analogs, liblomycin was selected as a candidate for clinical studies (53).

Liblomycin has a bulky lipophilic group at the end of the terminal amine which is introduced by reductive N-alkylation of a biosynthetic bleomycin (Fig. 2). Introduction of

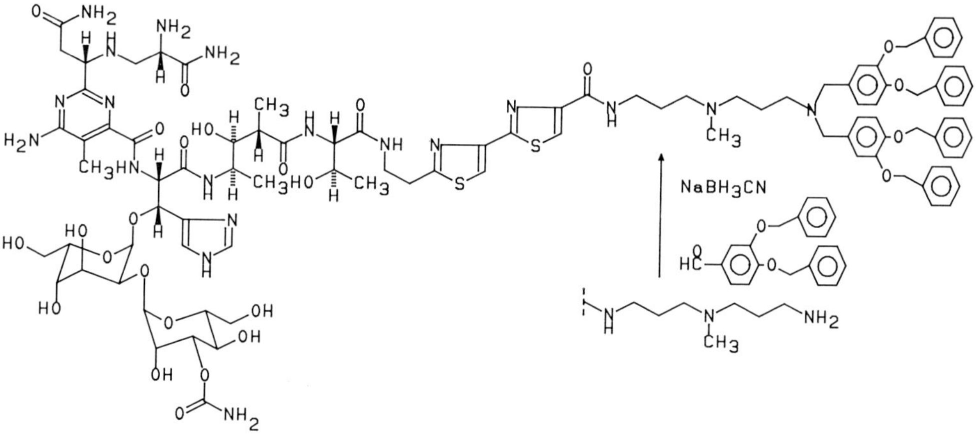

FIG. 2. Structure and preparation method of liblomycin

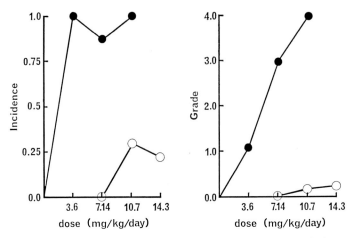

FIG. 3.   Pulmonary toxicities of liblomycin (○) and peplomycin (●) in mice
Drugs were administered i.v. to 9 week-old male ICR mice (5–10 mice in a group)
once daily for 7 days. Five weeks after the last injection, mice were sacrificed, lungs
were fixed with neutral formalin solution, and three histologic specimens (the left
lung, the superior and inferior lobes of the right lung) were prepared from each
mouse. The grade of pulmonary fibrosis was scored according to severity of toxicity,
as previously reported (18). Each point in the grade is a mean value of the scores of
all specimens observed in a group. Incidence is the percentage of mice with pulmonary fibrosis in a group.

TABLE I.   Subacute Toxicological Studies of Liblomycin and Peplomycin
in Dogs by Daily i.v. Injections for 91 Days

Drug	Sex	No. of animals	Dose (mg/kg/day)	Moribund sacrifice	Pulmonary fibrosis	Bone marrow toxicity
Liblomycin	Male	3	0.3	0/3	—	—
	Female	3	0.3	0/3	—	—
	Male	3	1.2	0/3	—	+
		3[a]	1.2	0/3	—[c]	↑[d]
	Female	3	1.2	1/3[b]	—	+
		3[a]	1.2	0/3	—[c]	↑[d]
Peplomycin	Male	3	0.6	1/3[b]	+	—
	Female	3	0.6	0/3	+	—

[a] Dogs were subjected to a recovery test for 35 days after the last injection.
[b] These two dogs became moribund after 88 daily injections.
[c] Results of histologic examination after a recovery test.
[d] Number of white blood cells and platelets showing recovery or return to normal levels after a recovery
     test.

this lipophilic group provides liblomycin with some distinct characteristics in toxicity,
activity, and mode of action (32): it showed much weaker pulmonary toxicity than peplomycin in mice (Fig. 3). At a lethal dose in a 91 day-subacute toxicity test in dogs, peplomycin caused pulmonary toxicity while liblomycin did not (Table I). However, liblomycin
showed moderate and reversible myelosuppression at this dose. Liblomycin is resistant
to inactivation by bleomycin hydrolase.
    Liblomycin showed antitumor activity against bleomycin and peplomycin-unres-

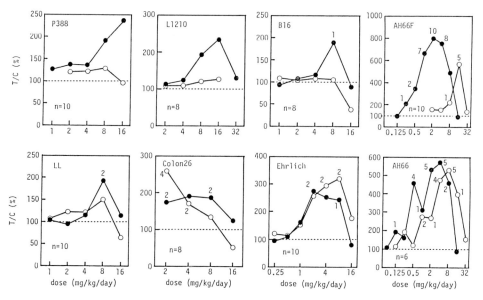

FIG. 4. Antitumor activities of liblomycin (●) and peplomycin (○) against murine transplantable tumors

The inoculum size and site, administration schedule, and observation period in each tumor system are as follows: P388 and L1210, 1×10^5 i.p., qld×9 (day 1) i.p., 60 days; B16, 5×10^4 i.v., qld×9 (day 1) i.p., 60 days; LL, 1×10^5 i.v., qld×9 (day 1) i.p., 60 days; Colon 26, 5×10^5 i.p., qld×9 (day 1) i.p., 60 days; Ehrlich, 1×10^6 i.p., qld×10 (2 hr) i.p., 75 days; AH66 and AH66F, 1×10^6 i.p., qld×10 (day 1) i.p., 60 days. T/C(%) values are calculated from median survival time in P388, B16, LL, and Colon 26 and from mean survival time in L1210, Ehrlich, AH66, and AH66F. Number (n) of animals used in a group and number of survivors are shown in the figure.

ponsive tumors such as L1210, P388 leukemias in mice, B16 melanoma in mice, and AH66F hepatoma in rats, as well as against responsive tumors (Fig. 4). Survival curves of rat hepatoma AH66 and AH66F cells treated with increasing doses of liblomycin for 1 hr were linear, while peplomycin showed curves with upward concavity similar to bleomycin (43) (Fig. 5). Over 100 times more liblomycin was taken up by these rat hepatoma cells than peplomycin, resulting in greater breakage of intracellular DNA (Fig. 6). In clinical Phase 1 studies, no pulmonary toxicity was observed, but myelosuppression was found to be dose-limiting (6).

Detailed Mechanism of Cytotoxicity of Bleomycin

The cytotoxicity of bleomycin appears to be due to its ability to bind and degrade DNA. In 1978, the structures of bleomycin (39) and its metal complex (37) were determined. On the basis of these structures, it became possible to elucidate the mechanism of bleomycin action on a molecular level. Bleomycin is a bifunctional compound that has DNA-binding and DNA-reaction sites (Fig. 7). In the binding of bleomycin to DNA, the bithiazole moiety seems to intercalate with double-stranded DNA (24, 25), and the terminal amine is also involved in the binding by electrostatic attraction (13). The reaction site forms the penta-dentate complex with ferrous ion. DNA degradation is caused

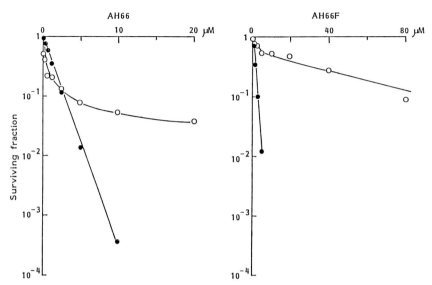

Fig. 5. Survival of AH66 and AH66F cells following 1 hr treatment with liblomycin (●) and peplomycin (○)
    AH66 and AH66F cells obtained from the peritoneal cavity of rats were cultured
with liblomycin or peplomycin in minimum essential medium (MEM) supplemented
with 10% foetal calf serum at 37°C or 1 hr in a 5% CO_2 incubator. After the incubation, the cells were washed twice with the medium by centrifugation and further
cultured in RPMI1640 medium containing 10% foetal calf serum, 50 μm 2-mer-
captoethanol and 0.1% noble agar at 37°C for 12 to 14 days. The number of colonies
formed was counted and the surviving fraction was obtained by dividing plating
efficiency of the drug-treated cells by that of the control cells. Each point is a mean
value of two replicate determinations.

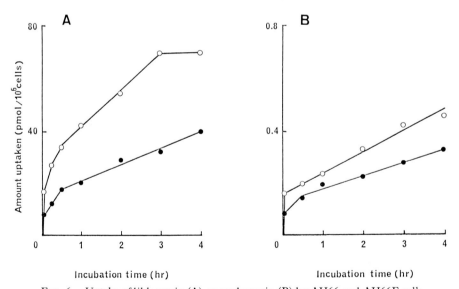

Fig. 6. Uptake of liblomycin (A) or peplomycin (B) by AH66 and AH66F cells
    AH66 (●) or AH66F (○) cells (1.2×106) were suspended in 0.5 ml of MEM
supplemented with 20 mM Hepes and 10% foetal calf serum, mixed with 0.1 ml of
the medium containing 24 μM copper complex of [³H]-liblomycin or [⁸H]-peplomy-
cin, and incubated at 37°C for various times. The cells were washed twice by centrifugation with 7 ml of phosphate buffered saline (PBS) (−) at 2,000 rpm for 30 sec,
and the cell pellets were solubilized in alkali for the determination of radioactivity.

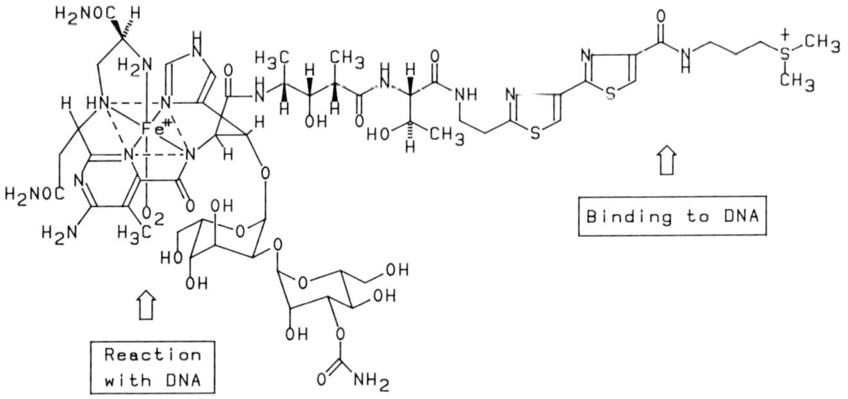

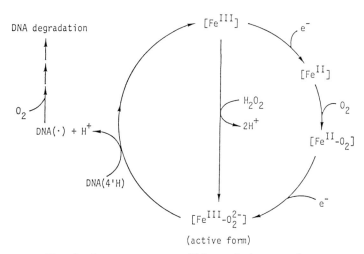

FIG. 7. The mechanism of bleomycin action on DNA

FIG. 8. Iron-oxygen states of bleomycin-iron complex

by activated oxygen formed on the bleomycin-iron complex. The reason the biological activity of bleomycin is lost by the inactivating enzyme is explained by metal-complex chemistry (30). The bleomycin-Fe^{2+}-O_2 complex binds to DNA and causes double-stranded scission (38). The active form of the complex involved in the DNA fragmentation has been suggested to be bleomycin-Fe^{3+}-O_2^{2-} ($2, 16$). It binds to DNA, and abstracts the hydrogen radical from the C-4 of the 2-deoxyribose moiety of DNA followed by the sequential reactions causing the DNA strand scission (8). Bleomycin-Fe(III) formed after the DNA strand scission is reduced to bleomycin-Fe(II) by intracellular reducing agents, and is again transformed to the active intermediate in the presence of oxygen. Thus, the bleomycin-iron complex acts as a kind of DNA nuclease in the presence of oxygen and reducing agents (Fig. 8). Reduction of bleomycin-Fe(III) to bleomycin-Fe(II) is suggested to be rate-determining in the intracellular enzyme-like action of bleomycin. The base sequence selective DNA cleavage by bleomycin has been intensively studied (29).

In 1979, Umezawa decided to prepare bleomycin by total chemical synthesis. Syn-

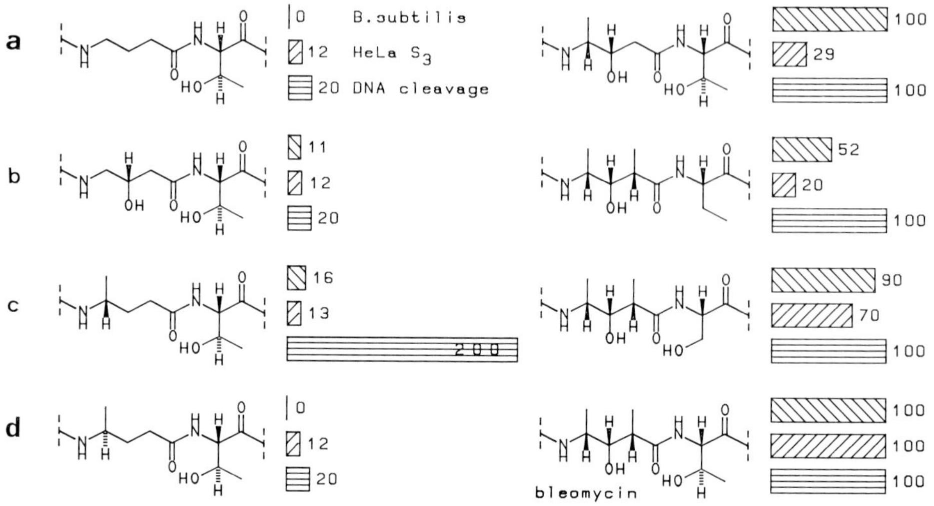

FIG. 9. Structure-activity relationship of synthetic bleomycins with different internal dipeptide moieties

Terminal amine of each compound is the same as that of bleomycin A_2. The antimicrobial activities (▧) were determined with *Bacillus subtilis* as a test organism. Growth inhibitory activities (▨) were determined with HeLa S3 cells. DNA cleaving activities (▤) were measured with pBR322 plasmid DNA. The activity of each compound is expressed as a value relative to the activity of bleomycin A_2 (100%).

theses of pyrimidoblamic acid, pyrimidine moiety of bleomycin (*54*), and deglycobleomycin A_2 (*40*) and the disaccharide moiety of bleomycin (*44*) had been achieved; finally, the total synthesis of bleomycin was accomplished in 1981 (*41*). Following this first successful total synthesis, an improved method was established (*26*), and several bleomycin analogues were synthesized using this method. Thus, the role of the functional groups in the bleomycin molecule responsible to the bioactivity can be elucidated more in detail by synthesis of new analogues. In this study, it was found that the (2S, 3S, 4R)-4-amino-3-hydroxy-2-methylpentanoic acid moiety of bleomycin is not only the connective chain between the DNA-reaction and DNA-binding sites in the bleomycin molecule, but also has an important role in antitumor activity. In particular, the methyl substituent, including its absolute configuration in this amino acid, is vital in the bioactivity (*53*) (Fig. 9).

Mechanism of In Vivo Activity of Bleomycin

Bleomycin forms an equimolar complex with cupric ion. The primary and secondary amino groups in the pyrimidoblamic acid, the nitrogen on the pyrimidine chromophore, the peptide nitrogen and imidazole nitrogen of the β-hydroxy histidine have been confirmed to be ligands of the bleomycin copper-complex (*10*, *37*). The DNA-cleaving activity of bleomycin *in vitro* (*31*) and the inactivation of bleomycin by bleomycin hydrolase (*47*) are inhibited by the Cu-complex formation.

The behavior of bleomycin *in vivo* has been identified as follows: the injected copper-free bleomycin forms a complex with cupric ion in blood (*12*), and after penetration into cells the copper of the complex is reductively removed by a sulfhydryl compound in cells; the cuprous ion thus liberated is transferred to a cellular protein which has the ability to bind with the cuprous ion (*34*); metallothionein, alcohol dehydrogenase, and other thiol compounds which have polythiol ligands, are suggested to act as the Cu(I)-trapping agents to yield metal-free bleomycin in cells (*33*). Copper-free bleomycin thus formed in cells is vulnerable to the action of bleomycin hydrolase. That which is not inactivated by the enzyme reaches the nucleus and binds and reacts with DNA molecules causing strand scission (*31*).

Bleomycin hydrolase is inhibited by bestatin, an inhibitor of aminopeptidase B and leucine-aminopeptidase, and by leupeptin, an inhibitor of endoprotease. Subcutaneous injection of a high dose (100 mg/kg) of bestain significantly increased the concentrations of active bleomycin in the skin and lungs of mice, and the addtion of this inhibitor to a culture medium increased the action of bleomycin in inhibiting growth of Yoshida rat sarcoma cells. The lack of myelosuppressive properties of bleomycin is suggested to be due to the high content of bleomycin hydrolase in the bone marrow. Leupeptin was found to increase cytotoxicity of bleomycin towards bone marrow cells (*55*). Recently, bleomycin hydrolase was highly purified and the inhibition of this enzyme by various agents was studied (*22, 27, 28*). The combination of bleomycin-hydrolase-inhibitor and bleomycin was thus again noted (*21*), and the involvement of bleomycin hydrolase in the inactivation of this antibiotic *in vivo* has been confirmed.

New Analogues Resistant to Bleomycin Hydrolase

Bleomycin analogues and derivatives resistant to bleomycin hydrolase are expected to show a stronger and broader anticancer spectrum than bleomycin. Liblomycin became resistant by modification of the terminal amine moiety. As described previously, bleomycin hydrolase hydrolyzes the α-aminocarboxamide bond of the pyrimidoblamyl moiety. So, chemical modification at the α-aminocarboxamide group was intensively studied.

By N-methylation of the α-amino group, the derivative became resistant to the enzyme, but, unfortunately, the therapeutic index of the derivative was lowered (*7*). When the amino group was acetylated, the bioactivity was completely lost. However, when this amino group was acylated with α-L-amino acids, the products showed some interesting properties (*53*). These derivatives could not degrade DNA *in vitro*, but they were cytotoxic and showed therapeutic effects. This is explained by ready removal of the aminoacyl group by aminopeptidase *in vivo*. In fact, aminoacyl bleomycin was converted to native bleomycin by incubation with various kinds of mouse tissue, revealing amino acyl bleomycin to be a kind of prodrug of bleomycin.

Modification of the carboxamide group gives the active derivatives, if the basicity of the α-amino groups is not significantly changed by the modification. As starting material of the modification, the free α-amino carboxylic acid, obtained by enzymatic hydrolysis by an aminopeptidase, was used. Amide-N-substituted derivatives of peplomycin were found to be resistant to bleomycin hydrolase and showed a low pulmonary toxicity (*45*). Their therapeutic indexes against Ehrlich carcinoma were as high as that of peplomycin.

Among these resistant bleomycin derivatives, a clinically useful bleomycin derivative might be expected.

REFERENCES

1. Bradner, W. T. and Pindell, M. H. Antitumour properties of phleomycin. *Nature*, **196**, 682–683 (1962).
2. Burger, R. M., Peisach, J., and Horwitz, S. B. Activated bleomycin: a transient complex of drug, iron, and oxygen that degrades DNA. *J. Biol. Chem.*, **256**, 11636–11644 (1981).
3. Ebihara, K., Nishikawa, K., Shibasaki, C., Takahashi, K., and Matsuda, A. Antitumor activity of peplomycin against 7,12-dimethylbenz(a)anthracene-induced rat mammary tumors. *Jpn. J. Antibiot.*, **40**, 1566–1570 (1987) (in Japanese).
4. Fujii, A., Takita, T., Shimada, N., and Umezawa, H. Biosyntheses of new bleomycins. *J. Antibiot.*, **27**, 73–77 (1974).
5. Fujii, A., Takita, T., Maeda, K., and Umezawa, H. New components of bleomycin. *J. Antibiot.*, **26**, 396–397 (1973).
6. Fukuoka, M., Ohta, K., Suzuki, A., Tamura, M., Hasegawa, K., Yoshida, K., Honma, T., Majima, H., Niitani, H., Ogawa, M., Ariyoshi, Y., Furuse, K., Kimura, I., Ohnoshi, T., and Ogura, T. Phase I clinical study of NK313, a new analogue of bleomycin. *Proc. Jpn. Cancer Assoc.*, 607 (1988) (in Japanese).
7. Fukuoka, T., Muraoka, Y., Fujii, A., Naganawa, H., Takita, T., and Umezawa, H. Chemistry of bleomycin. XXV. Reductive methylation of bleomycin, a chemical proof for the presence of the free secondary amine in bleomycin. *J. Antibiot.*, **33**, 114–117 (1980).
8. Giloni, L., Takeshita, M., Johnson, F., Iden, C., and Grollman, P. Bleomycin-induced strand-scission on DNA. Mechanism of deoxyribose cleavage. *J. Biol. Chem.*, **256**, 8608–8615 (1981).
9. Ichikawa, T., Matsuda, A., Yamamoto, K., Tsubosaki, M., Kaihara, T., Sakamoto, K., and Umezawa, H. Biological studies on bleomycin A. *J. Antibiot.*, **20**, 149–155 (1967).
10. Iitaka, Y., Nakamura, H., Nakatani, T., Muraoka, Y., Fujii, A., Takita, T., and Umezawa, H. Chemistry of bleomycin. XX. The X-ray structure determination of P-3A (Cu)-complex. A biosynthetic intermediate of bleomycin. *J. Antibiot.*, **31**, 1070–1072 (1978).
11. Ishizuka, M., Takayama, H., Takeuchi, T., and Umezawa, H. Studies on antitumor activity, antimicrobial activity and toxicity of phleomycin. *J. Antibiot.*, **19**, 260–271 (1966).
12. Kanao, M., Tomita, S., Ishihara, S., Murakami, A., and Okada, H. Chelation of bleomycin with copper *in vivo*. *Chemotherapy* (*Nippon Kagaku Ryoho Gakkai Kaishi*), **21**, 1305–1310 (1973) (in Japanese).
13. Kasai, H., Naganawa, H., Takita, T., and Umezawa, H. Chemistry of bleomycin. XXII. Interaction of bleomycin with nucleic acids, preferential binding to guanine base and electrostatic effect of the terminal amine. *J. Antibiot.*, **31**, 1316–1320 (1978).
14. Kimura, M., Koida, T., and Fukuda, T. Clinical effect of peplomycin on recurrent breast cancer. *Jpn. J. Cancer Chemother.*, **10**, 1665–1669 (1983) (in Japanese).
15. Koiso, K. and Niijima, T. Chemotherapy of advanced prostatic cancer with peplomycin. *Prostate* (Suppl.), **1**, 103–110 (1981).
16. Kuramochi, H., Takahashi, K., Takita, T., and Umezawa, H. An active intermediate formed in the reaction of bleomycin-Fe(II) complex with oxygen. *J. Antibiot.*, **34**, 576–582 (1981).
17. Maeda, K., Kosaka, H., Yagishita, K., and Umezawa, H. A new antibiotic, phleomycin. *J. Antibiot.*, *Ser. A*, **9**, 82–85 (1956).
18. Matsuda, A., Yoshioka, O., Ebihara, K., Ekimoto, H., Yamashita, T., and Umezawa, H. The search for new bleomycin. *In* "Bleomycin: Current Status and New Developments," ed. S. K. Carter, S. T. Crooke, and H. Umezawa, pp. 299–310 (1978). Academic Press, New York.
19. Matsuda, A., Yoshioka, O., Takahashi, K., Yamashita, T., Ebihara, K., Ekimoto, H., Abe, F., Hashimoto, Y., and Umezawa, H. Preclinical studies on bleomycin-PEP (NK-

631.) *In* "Bleomycin: Current Status and New Developments," ed. S. K. Carter, S. T. Crooke, and H. Umezawa, pp. 311–331 (1978). Academic Press, New York.

20. Nakanishi, Y., Hata, Y., Sato, N., Kawamura, A., Uenuma, T., Hasegawa, M., Miyakawa, K., Nakamura, T., Kawai, M., Kawamoto, K., Taneda, M., Nishimura, A., Kitayama, J., Oku, T., Kasai, Y., and Inoue, K. Anticancer effect of peplomycin on advanced recurrent breast cancer. *Jpn. J. Cancer Chemother.*, **11**, 1428–1433 (1984) (in Japanese).

21. Nishimura, C., Nishimura, T., Tanaka, N., and Suzuki, H. Potentiation of the cytotoxicity of peplomycin against Ehrlich ascites carcinoma by bleomycin hydrolase inhibitors. *J. Antibiot.*, **40**, 1794–1795 (1987).

22. Nishimura, C., Tanaka, N., Suzuki, H., and Tanaka, N. Purification of bleomycin hydrolase with a monoclonal antibody and its characterization. *Biochemistry*, **26**, 1574–1578 (1987).

23. Numata, M., Hosoe, S., and Hayashi, S. The use of peplomycin sulfate in recurrent or metastatic breast cancer. *Adv. Ther.*, **3**, 224–230 (1986).

24. Povirk, L. F., Hogan, M., and Dattagupta, N. Binding of bleomycin to DNA: Intercalation of the bithiazole ring. *Biochemistry*, **18**, 96–101 (1979).

25. Povirk, L. F., Hogan, M., Dattagupta, N., and Buechner, M. Copper (II) bleomycin and copper (II) phleomycin: comparative study of deoxyribonucleic acid binding. *Biochemistry*, **20**, 665–671 (1981).

26. Saito, S., Umezawa, Y., Yoshioka, T., Takita, T., Umezawa, H., and Muraoka, Y. An improved total synthesis of bleomycin. *J. Antibiot.*, **36**, 92–95 (1983).

27. Sebti, S. M., DeLeon, J. C., and Lazo, J. S. Purification, characterization and amino acid composition of rabbit pulmonary bleomycin hydrolase. *Biochemistry*, **26**, 4213–4219 (1987).

28. Sebti, S. M. and Lazo, J. S. Separation of the protective enzyme bleomycin hydrolase from rabbit pulmonary aminopeptidases. *Biochemistry*, **26**, 432–437 (1987).

29. Stubbe, J. and Kozarich, J. W. Mechanisms of bleomycin-induced DNA degradation. *Chem. Rev.*, **87**, 1107–1136 (1987).

30. Sugiura, Y., Muraoka, Y., Fujii, A., Takita, T., and Umezawa, H. Chemistry of bleomycin. XXIV. Deamido bleomycin from viewpoint of metal coordination and oxygen activation. *J. Antibiot.*, **32**, 756–758 (1979).

31. Suzuki, H., Nagai, K., Yamaki, H., Tanaka, N., and Umezawa, H. On the mechanism of action of bleomycin: Scission of DNA strands *in vitro* and *in vivo*. *J. Antibiot.*, **22**, 446–448 (1969).

32. Takahashi, K., Ekimoto, H., Minamide, S., Hishikawa, K., Kuramochi, H., Motegi, A., Nakatani, T., Takita, T., Takeuchi, T., and Umezawa, H. Liblomycin, a new analogue of bleomycin. *Cancer Treat. Rev.*, **14**, 169–177 (1987).

33. Takahashi, K., Takita, T., and Umezawa, H. The nature of thiol-compounds which trap cuprous ion reductively liberated from bleomycin-Cu(II) in cells. *J. Antibiot.*, **40**, 348–353 (1987).

34. Takahashi, K., Yoshioka, O., Matsuda, A., and Umezawa, H. Intracellular reduction of the cupric ion of bleomycin copper complex and transfer of the cuprous ion to a cellular protein. *J. Antibiot.*, **30**, 861–869 (1977).

35. Takita, T., Fujii, A., Fukuoka, T., and Umezawa, H. Chemical cleavage of bleomycin to bleomycinic acid and synthesis of new bleomycins. *J. Antibiot.*, **26**, 252–254 (1973).

36. Takita, T., Muraoka, Y., Fujii, A., Itoh, H., Maeda, K., and Umezawa, H. The structure of the sulfur-containing chromophore of phleomycin, and chemical transformation of phleomycin to bleomycin. *J. Antibiot.*, **25**, 197–199 (1972).

37. Takita, T., Muraoka, Y., Nakatani, T., Fujii, A., Iitaka, Y., and Umezawa, H. Chemistry of bleomycin. XXI. Metal-complex of bleomycin and its implication for the mechanism of bleomycin action. *J. Antibiot.*, **31**, 1073–1077 (1978).

38. Takita, T., Muraoka, Y., Nakatani, T., Fujii, A., Iitaka, Y., and Umezawa, H. Chemistry

of bleomycin. XXI. Metal-complex of bleomycin and its implication for the mechanism of bleomycin action. *J. Antibiot.*, **31**, 1073–1077 (1978).

39. Takita, T., Muraoka, Y., Nakatani, T., Fujii, A., Umezawa, Y., Naganawa, H., and Umezawa, H. Chemistry of bleomycin. XIX. Revised structures of bleomycin and phleomycin. *J. Antibiot.*, **31**, 801–804 (1978).

40. Takita, T., Umezawa, Y., Saito, S., Morishima, H., Umezawa, H., Muraoka, Y., Suzuki, M., Otsuka, M., Kobayashi, S., and Ohno, M. Total synthesis of deglyco-bleomycin A2. *Tetrahedron Lett.*, **22**, 671–674 (1981).

41. Takita, T., Umezawa, Y., Saito, S., Morishima, H., Umezawa, H., Muraoka, Y., Suzuki, M., Otsuka, M., Kobayashi, S., Ohno, M., Tsuchiya, T., Miyake, T., and Umezawa, S. Total synthesis of bleomycin. Peptides: Synthesis-Structure-Function (Proceedings of the 7th American Peptide Symposium), pp. 29–39 (1981).

42. Tanaka, N., Yamaguchi, H., and Umezawa, H. Mechanism of action of phleomycin: I. Selective inhibition of the DNA synthesis in *E. coli* and in HeLa cells. *J. Antibiot.*, *Ser A*, **16**, 86–91 (1963).

43. Terashima, T., Takabe, Y., Katsumata, T., Watanabe, M., and Umezawa, H. Effect of bleomycin on mammalian cell survival. *J. Natl. Cancer Inst.*, **49**, 1093–1100 (1972).

44. Tsuchiya, T., Miyake, T., Kageyama, S., Umezawa, S., Umezawa, H., and Takita, T. Total synthesis of the disaccharide of bleomycin. 2-O-(alpha-D-mannopyranosyl)-L-gulopyranose. *Tetrahedron Lett.*, **22**, 1413–1416 (1981).

45. Umezawa, H. Studies of microbial products in rising to the challenge of curing cancer. *Proc. R. Soc. Lond.* **B217** (The Leeuwenhoek Lecture, 1982), 357–376 (1983).

46. Umezawa, H., Hori, M., Ishizuka, M., and Takeuchi, T. Studies on antitumor effect of phleomycin. *J. Antibiot.*, **15**, 274–275 (1962).

47. Umezawa, H., Hori, S., Sawa, T., Yoshioka, T., and Takeuchi, T. A bleomycin-inactivating enzyme in mouse liver. *J. Antibiot.*, **27**, 419–424 (1974).

48. Umezawa, H., Ishizuka, M., Hori, S., Chimura, H., Takeuchi, T., and Komai, T. The distribution of ³H-bleomycin in mouse tissue. *J. Antibiot.*, **21**, 638–642 (1968).

49. Umezawa, H., Maeda, K., Takeuchi, T., and Okami, Y. New antibiotics, bleomycin A and B. *J. Antibiot.*, **19**, 200–209 (1966).

50. Umezawa, H., Suhara, Y., Takita, T., and Maeda, K. Purification of bleomycins. *J. Antibiot.*, **19**, 210–215 (1966).

51. Umezawa, H., Takahashi, Y., Fujii, A., Saino, T., Shirai, T., and Takita, T. Preparation of bleomycinic acid: Hydrolysis of bleomycin B₂ by a fusarium acylagmatine amidohydrolase. *J. Antibiot.*, **26**, 117–119 (1973).

52. Umezawa, H., Takeuchi, T., Hori, S., Sawa, T., Ishizuka, M., Ichikawa, T., and Komai, T. Studies on the mechanism of antitumor effect of bleomycin on squamous cell carcinoma. *J. Antibiot.*, **25**, 409–420 (1972).

53. Umezawa, H., Takita, T., Saito, S., Muraoka, Y., Takahashi, K., Ekimoto, H., Minamide, S., Nishikawa, K., Fukuoka, T., Nakatani, T., Fujii, A., and Matsuda, A. New analogs and derivatives of bleomycin. *In* "Bleomycin Chemotherapy," ed. B. I. Sikik, M. Rozencweig, and S. K. Carter, pp. 289–301 (1985). Academic Press, London.

54. Umezawa, Y., Morishima, H., Saito, S., Takita, T., Umezawa, H., Kobayashi, S., Otsuka, M., Narita, M., and Ohno, M. Synthesis of the pyrimidine moiety of bleomycin. *J. Am. Chem. Soc.*, **102**, 6630–6631 (1980).

55. Yoshioka, O., Amano, N., Takahashi, K., Matsuda, A., and Umezawa, H. Intercellular fate and activity of bleomycin. *In* "Bleomycin: Current Status and New Developments," ed. S. K. Carter, S. T. Crooke, and H. Umezawa, pp. 35–56 (1978). Academic Press, New York.

BLEOMYCINS: CLINICAL RESEARCH

Irwin H. KRAKOFF

*M. D. Anderson Cancer Center**

Bleomycin was developed by Umezawa and his colleagues in 1966 and found to have antitumor activity in cell culture, in transplanted tumors in mice and eventually in human beings with cancer. Its incorporation into combination regimens has produced a high rate of cures in advanced testicular cancer and Hodgkin's Disease, and complete and partial remissions in other tumors.

Bleomycin has been found to produce skin toxicity, severe, sometimes fatal pulmonary toxicity and, in some patients, fever. Pulmonary toxicity has limited its use; no effective preventive measure has been developed. Almost uniquely among anti-cancer drugs, bleomycin does not cause myelosuppression.

There have been continuing attempts to develop new, non-toxic bleomycins. Peplomycin and Tallysomycin S10b appear to have a spectrum of activity and toxicity very similar to those of the parent drug. However, liblomycin, the most recent analogue to be extensively studied, appears in animal systems to have a broader range of activity and to be free of pulmonary toxicity. Early clinical trials of liblomycin have been started.

The development of bleomycin as a therapeutic tool is a classic example of the orderly development of an anti-cancer drug from discovery through widespread clinical application. It was isolated from a strain of *Streptomyces verticillus* that was obtained from a soil sample collected from a Japanese coal mine. It was characterized by Umezawa *et al.* (*46*) who demonstrated that it was composed of a mixture of polypeptides (*47*). That mixture appeared to have better properties *in toto* than any of the fractions and it is the same mixture that is still used clinically.

The same group of investigators found that bleomycin inhibited DNA synthesis in HeLa cells, Ehrlich cells, and *Escherichia coli* (*43, 45*). It appears to cause both single and double strand breaks in DNA (*39*). The demonstrated activity against transplanted animal tumors led to its initial clinical trials which were done by Ichikawa (*21*). He and his colleagues demonstrated striking activity against squamous carcinomas of the penis and scrotum—logical targets since Ichikawa is a urologist—and subsequently in squamous tumors of the head and neck. In that initial clinical publication, the principal toxicities were also noted. Later studies in Europe (*4, 15*) and the United States (*50*) confirmed and amplified the therapeutic and toxicologic observations.

* Houston, Texas 77030, U.S.A.

Therapeutic Activity

1. Lymphoma

The most prominent antitumor activity of bleomycin has continued to be in the lymphomas, particularly Hodgkin's disease, in squamous carcinomas of the head and neck and in testicular cancer.

The demonstration of the activity of bleomycin as a single agent in Phase II studies was followed promptly by its incorporation into combination regimens. Wittes (*49*) has noted that the large number of uncontrolled trials has not permitted a rigorous assessment of the contributions of bleomycin to the efficacy of the various regimens. Nevertheless, bleomycin has become a component of *curative* combination chemotherapy in several types of cancer and there is compelling evidence that it is an important contributor to those cures. A logical step toward the use of bleomycin in combination chemotherapy was its addition to the highly active MOPP regimen of DeVita *et al.* (*13*) (Nitrogen mustard, vincristine, procarbazine, and prednisone). MOPP plus bleomycin was shown to be more active than MOPP alone (*10*) and the addition of doxorubicin further enhanced the activity of the five drug combination (*22, 24*). Carter (*9*) has diagrammed the historical flow of these combinations in a recent review (Fig. 1). As an approach to patients deemed to be resistant to MOPP, Bonadonna *et al.* (*6*) developed a new combination, ABVD (adriamycin, bleomycin, vincristine, and dacarbazine) which was shown to produce a high remission rate in patients resistant to MOPP. In later studies (*5, 38*) in which MOPP was alternated with ABVD, a significantly greater proportion of complete remissions was obtained than with MOPP alone. At this time, it appears that primary therapy with the alternating combination can produce a higher complete remission rate, a longer duration of relapse-free survival and probably a higher cure rate than can MOPP. Although further refinements of these regimens will undoubtedly occur, along with the incorporation of additional new drugs and irradiation into therapeutic regimens, it is clear that bleomycin has contributed substantially to improved outcomes in advanced Hodgkin's disease.

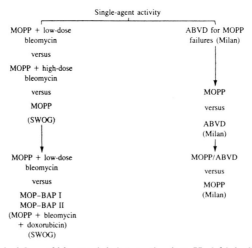

FIG. 1. Historical flow of bleomycin's integration into Hodgkin's disease combination chemotherapy for primary induction

Ref. *9* with permission of the author and publisher.

Patients with so-called poor-risk non-Hodgkin's lymphoma have also benefited from bleomycin. Addition of bleomycin to the well-established CHOP regimen (cyclophosphamide, doxorubicin, vincristine, and prednisone) has produced higher response rates and a significant proportion of cures (23, 41, 42).

2. Testicular cancer

This group of tumors was among the earliest in which combination chemotherapy was demonstrated to be more effective than treatment with single drugs (29). The response rates, however, were low and of relatively brief duration. The single agent activity of bleomycin (3) led logically to its incorporation into combination regimens (16, 35, 36) along with other agents of known activity, e.g., vinblastine (37) and cisplatin (20). Carter has also diagrammed the historical flow of testicular cancer treatment (Fig. 2). It is elucidating vis a vis the contributions of bleomycin to curative therapy in that group of tumors; however, it is also a paradigm of contemporary clinical investigation.

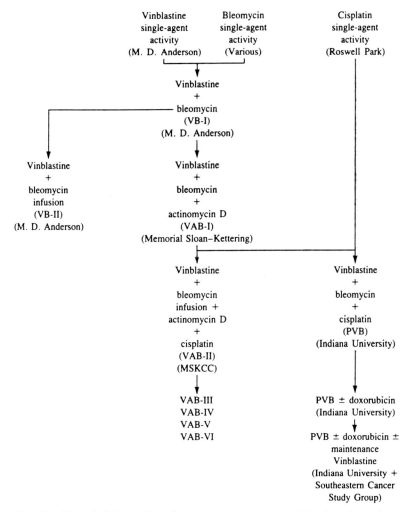

FIG. 2. Historical flow of modern testicular cancer combination chemotherapy Ref. 9 with permission of the author and publisher.

The diagram demonstrates the parallel, overlapping and intertwining activities of three institutions (M.D. Anderson Cancer Center, Memorial Sloan-Kettering Cancer Center and Indiana University) in the development of effective therapeutic programs. At this time, it is realistic to expect nearly 100% cures in patients with good risk, low bulk metastatic disease and more than 45% in the high bulk, poor risk group.

3. Squamous cancers

Tumors of the head and neck and of the uterine cervix were among those first reported to respond to bleomycin therapy and they continue to respond, particularly to regimens containing cisplatin, 5-fluorouracil, and methotrexate. Complete response rates, however, are generally low and of brief duration. There is, to date, no convincing evidence that combination chemotherapy with or without bleomycin prolongs survival significantly in these cancers.

A high rate of partial responses in squamous carcinoma of the skin has been reported (1, 18).

4. Other uses

Bleomycin has been demonstrated to be effective in the treatment of superficial bladder tumors when given by direct instillation into the bladder (7). It is also useful in preventing recurrence of pleural effusion when instilled into the pleural cavity (12, 34).

Toxicity

As noted above, skin toxicity, fever and pulmonary toxicity were observed in the course of the very first clinical study of bleomycin (21) and in the first reported European study (15). The first of the American studies (50) analyzed the toxicity in detail.

1. Skin toxicity

In the Phase I-II study reported by Yagoda et al. (50) all patients were treated with bleomycin daily until the occurrence of skin toxicity and thus, that was recorded as 100%. Characteristically, it occurred initially as erythema over pressure areas, progressing to shallow and then deeper ulcerations. Mucosal lesions followed the same course. Readministration of bleomycin after healing of the initial lesions produced recrudescence of the skin toxicity within 3–4 days. Anamnestic responses were produced in a few patients by the administration of methotrexate, mithramycin or BCNU as long as 6 weeks after a course of bleomycin and in a few patients bleomycin caused a skin reaction localized to the site of prior X-ray therapy. Many patients who received large cumulative doses of bleomycin displayed a loss of skin elasticity, probably due to the same phenomenon that resulted in pulmonary fibrosis.

Skin toxicity has not been a problem in clinical use since bleomycin is not used generally in intensive courses as was done in the early Phase I and II studies. In most protocol use, the agent is given for 3–5 days intermittently and those schedules have uncommonly produced skin reactions.

2. Pulmonary toxicity

A major limiting factor in the use of bleomycin is pulmonary toxicity. This occurs in 2–8% of patients treated. It is somewhat dose-dependent, appearing with increased incidence in patients who receive more than 300 mg/M^2 total cumulative dose. However, it may occur in patients with small cumulative doses and even during the first course. The pulmonary reaction occurs characteristically with cough and dyspnea. Radiographic changes were those of an interstitial, bilateral, basal infiltrate. In patients screened with pulmonary function studies, approximately one-third exhibit a decrease in total lung capacity and diffusion capacity. In patients with respiratory symptoms, these measurements of pulmonary function are consistently impaired—the abnormalities are progressive but, in some instances, may be reversed by the administration of adrenal cortical steroids. This pulmonary lesion may be fatal in approximately 1% of patients. Pathologically, there is interstitial fibrosis and alveolar squamous metaplasia and hyalinization. In animal models, the fibrosis is preceded by an acute inflammatory lesion.

The mechanism and pathogenesis of the pulmonary toxicity have been extensively studied (19, 25). Studies in rodents have demonstrated that the pulmonary lesion produced by bleomycin is accompanied by a marked increase in collagen synthesis; that measurable increase as well as the pulmonary function limitation and the pathologic picture can be prevented by prior or co-administration of the proline analogue, L-3,4-dehydroproline, without impairment of bleomycin's antitumor activity. Clinical trials of the ability of L-3,4-dehydroproline to prevent the pulmonary toxicity of bleomycin have not been carried out. It is of note that other manifestations of bleomycin toxicity (loss of skin elasticity, acute rheumatoid-like arthritis, Raynaud's phenomenon) are those which are or could be associated with abnormalities of collagen synthesis. A major impetus toward the development of new bleomycin analogues (see below) has been the limitations imposed on the parent agent by its pulmonary effects.

A distressing corollary of the pulmonary toxicity of bleomycin itself is its apparent propensity to exaggerate or be exaggerated by the administration of high concentrations of oxygen given during or following surgical anesthesia. Goldiner and Schweizer (17) reported a series of fatalities in patients undergoing surgical exploration following the apparently successful treatment of testicular cancer with a bleomycin-containing regimen. Those patients exhibited pulmonary changes identical to those who experienced toxicity during the administration of bleomycin. They have recommended restriction of oxygen concentrations to those approximating room air. Other investigators (30) have reported no apparent bleomycin/oxygen interactions in large series of patients given oxygen postoperatively.

3. Other toxicity

Fever is a common side effect of bleomycin administration. In a small proportion of patients, principally those with lymphomas, there is very high fever, hypertension and/or anaphylaxis. Pretreatment with antipyretics and antihistamines minimizes these side effects.

Other side effects occur with less frequency. Yagoda et al. (50) displayed the side effects and their frequency as shown in Fig. 3.

The nearly unique aspect of bleomycin toxicology is the very low rate and degree of myelosuppression. Although minor leukopenia and thrombocytopenia have been reported, this has rarely been dose-limiting. This property has facilitated the inclusion of bleomycin into combination regimens since it fulfills an important criterion for combination chemotherapy (26), i.e., a compound with a different target organ for toxicity. It can thus be incorporated into a regimen at full doses without the need for attenuation of

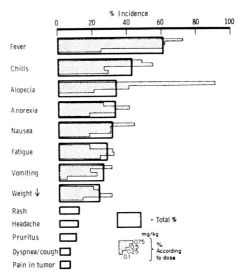

FIG. 3.   Incidence of clinical side effects in patients treated with bleomycin, showing the total incidence and that for each dose schedule for each side effect
Ref. *50* with permission of the authors and publisher.

dose of a companion, myelosuppressive drug. As noted above, these combinations have
resulted in a significant number of cures in a number of tumor types.

Pharmacokinetics

Bleomycin is water soluble, non-vesicant and stable in solution. It is eliminated from
the serum after bolus injection with a half-life of about 2 hr; after prolonged intravenous
infusion, its elimination half-life is 3–4 hr (*8*), 50–70% of the drug is excreted *via* the
kidneys and in patients with renal impairment, clearance is markedly decreased (*11*).
The dose therefore should be decreased in the face of renal functional impairment. The
short serum half-life and phase specificity led to a study (*27*) in which bleomycin was
given by continuous infusion. A subsequent study (*40*) demonstrated marked decrease
in pulmonary collagen content in mice when bleomycin was given by continuous infusion compared with the same dose given by repeated bolus injection. These two studies
have led to the conclusion that there is a more favorable therapeutic index when bleomycin is given by continuous infusion.

New Bleomycins

Its lack of myelosuppressive activity has made bleomycin an ideal drug for incorporation into combination regimens with other agents that are myelosuppressive. Unfortunately, its use has been limited by the pulmonary toxicity that becomes more frequent
with increasing cumulative doses. There has, therefore, been a great deal of effort devoted
to the development of new analogues which might have greater efficacy and/or a broader
spectrum of antitumor activity and which may be free of pulmonary toxicity.

1. Peplomycin

This compound was one of several synthesized in Umezawa's laboratories (16). It was selected as a second-generation bleomycin which might have greater efficacy, a broader antitumor spectrum and less pulmonary toxicity. Although it appeared to have some activity in prostate cancer, it proved to have the same general level of activity as bleomycin and, disappointingly, a similar level of pulmonary toxicity. It has essentially been abandoned in favor of other, more promising agents.

2. Tallysomycin S10b

This agent too was developed as a candidate second-generation bleomycin. Louie (31) has reviewed the relatively sparse Phase I clinical information available, concluding that its spectrum of toxicity was similar to that of bleomycin. Pulmonary toxicity in those limited studies was prominent. In later Phase II studies at the M.D. Anderson Cancer Center (unpublished data) similar toxicities were encountered. There were no responses in a heavily pre-treated group of patients with head and neck, colorectal, cervix, and non-small cell lung cancers. This compound is not presently under active clinical investigation.

3. Liblomycin

From several standpoints, this derivative, developed by Umezawa et al. (48) has characteristics that made it appear an outstanding candidate as a new bleomycin analogue.

In 1974, Umezawa et al. identified an enzyme in mammalian tissues that had the ability to inactivate bleomycin by hydrolysis at the free amino group; they termed this enzyme "bleomycin hydrolase" and demonstrated it to be a mechanism for resistance to bleomycin (2). Lazo et al. (44) demonstrated additional mechanisms in various bleomycin-resistant cell lines. Liblomycin is not a substrate for bleomycin hydrolase and appears to circumvent other mechanisms of resistance as well.

Liblomycin demonstrates activity against animal tumor lines *in vitro* and *in vivo* that is superior to that of bleomycin or peplomycin (48) and against a broader spectrum of human tumor cell lines in an *in vitro* stem cell assay (44).

In a detailed series of studies, Newman et al. (33) examined the pulmonary toxicity of intraperitoneally and intravenously administered liblomycin. They found no evidence of that effect as measured histopathologically, by lung collagen synthesis and by pulmonary function studies although pulmonary changes did occur when the drug was given intratracheally. Mice given liblomycin intraperitoneally exhibited hepatic capsular fibrosis; this did not occur when liblomycin was given intravenously. It was concluded that liblomycin has the ability to stimulate collagen synthesis locally but that the bulky lipophilic group at its terminal amine alters its distribution and biologic characteristics. In both Umezawa's (48) and Newman's (33) studies, myelosuppression was noted at the highest dose level.

Clinical Phase I studies of liblomycin have been initiated in Japan (H. Majima, personal communication) but a definite clinical assessment of this agent cannot yet be made.

CONCLUSION

After 20 years of clinical experience, it is apparent that bleomycin is a major antitumor agent and that it has contributed substantially to curative combination chemotherapy in several types of cancers. Pulmonary toxicity, long a limiting factor in its use remains a problem; however, the relatively recently advent of an analogue designed both to minimize that toxicity and to improve antitumor activity is a potentially very useful development.

REFERENCES

1. Agre, K. Overview of clinical evaluation in the United States. *In* "New Drug Seminar on Bleomycin," ed. W. T. Soper and A. B. Gott (1973). National Cancer Institute, Bethesda.
2. Akigama, S., Ikezaki, K., Kuramochi, H., Takahashi, K., and Kuwano, M. Bleomycin-resistant cells contain increased bleomycin-hydrolase activities. *Biochem. Biophys. Res. Commun.*, **101**, 55–60 (1981).
3. Blum, R. H., Carter, S. K., and Agre, K. A clinical review of bleomycin—A new antineoplastic agent. *Cancer*, **31**, 903–914 (1973).
4. Bonadonna, G., DeLena, M., Bartoli, C., Monfardini, S., and Guzzon, A., Molinari, R., Bajetta, E., Beretta, G., Fossati-Bellani, F., and Orefice, S. Studio Preliminare della Fase I della Bleomycino un Nuovo Famaco Antitumor. *Tumori*, **57**, 21–53 (1971).
5. Bonadonna, G., Santoro, A., Zucali, R., and Valagussa, R. Improved 5-year survival in advanced Hodgkin's disease by combined modality approach. *Cancer Clin. Trials*, **2**, 217–226 (1979).
6. Bonadonna, G., Zucali, R., Monfardini, S., *et al.* Combination chemotherapy of Hodgkin's disease with adriamycin, bleomycin, vinblastine and imidazole carboxamide *versus* MOPP. *Cancer*, **36**, 252–259 (1975).
7. Bracken, R. B., Johnscn, D. E., Rodrique, L., Samuels, M. L., and Ayala, A. Treatment of multiple superficial tumors of bladder with intravesical bleomycin. *Urology*, **9**, 161–163 (1977).
8. Broughton, A., Strong, J. E., Holoye, P. Y., and Bedrossian, C.W.M. Clinical pharmacology of bleomycin following intravenous infusion as determined by radioimmunoassay. *Cancer*, **40**, 2772–2778 (1977).
9. Carter, S. K. Bleomycin: more than a decade later. *In* "Bleomycin Chemotherapy," ed. B. I. Sikic, M. Rozencweig, and S. K. Carter, pp. 3–35 (1985). Academic Press, New York.
10. Coltman, C. A., Frei, E., III, and Delaney, F. Effectiveness of actinomycin D (CA), methotrexate (MTX) and vinblastine in prolonging the duration of combination chemotherapy (MOPP) induced remission in advanced Hodgkin's disease (HD). *Cancer Chemother. Rep.*, **57**, 109 (1973).
11. Crooke, S. T., Comis, R. L., Einhorn, L. H., Strong, J. E., Broughton, A., and Prestayko, A. W. Effects of variations in renal function on the clinical pharmacology of bleomycin administered as an IV bolus. *Cancer Treat. Rep.*, **61**, 1631–1636, (1977).
12. Cunningham, T. J., Horton, J., and Olson, K. B. Intra-cavitary bleomycin in the treatment of malignant effusions. *Proc. Am. Assoc. Cancer Res.*, **13**, 124 (1972).
13. DeVita, V. T., Jr., Serpick, H. A., and Carbone, P. P. Combination chemotherapy in the treatment of advanced Hodgkin's disease. *Ann. Intern. Med.*, **73**, 881–895 (1970).
14. Einhorn, L. and Donohue, J. P. Chemotherapy for disseminated testicular cancer. *Urol. Clin. N. Am.*, **4**, 407–426 (1977).
15. European Organization for Research on the Treatment of Cancer. Study of the clinical efficiency of bleomycin in human cancer. *Br. Med. J.*, **2**, 642–645 (1970).
16. Fujii, A., Takita, T., Shimada, N., and Umezawa, H. Biosyntheses of new bleomycins. *J. Antibiot.*, **27**, 73–77 (1974).

17. Goldiner, P. L. and Schweizer, O. The hazards of anesthesia and surgery in bleomycin-treated patients. *Semin. Oncol.*, **6**, 121–124 (1970).

18. Haas, C. D., Coltman, C. A., Gottlieb, J. A., Haut, A., Luce, J. K., Talley, R. W., Samal, B., Wilson, H. E., and Hoogstraten, B. Phase II evaluation of bleomycin. A Southwest Oncology Group Study. *Cancer*, **38**, 8–12 (1976).

19. Hacker, M. P. and Newman, R. A. The effect of L-3, 4-dehydroproline on the antitumor activity and toxicity of bleomycin. *Toxicol. Appl. Pharmacol.*, **69**, 102–109 (1983).

20. Higby, D. J., Wallace, H. J., Jr., Albert, D., and Holland, J. F. Diamminodichloroplatinum in the chemotherapy of testicular tumors. *J. Urol.*, **112**, 100–104 (1974).

21. Ichikawa, T., Nakano, I., and Hirokawa, I. Bleomycin treatment of the tumors of penis and scrotum. *J. Urol.*, **102**, 699–707 (1969).

22. Jones, S. E., Coltman, C. A., Grozea, P. N., Depersio, E. J., and Dixon, D. O. Conclusions from clinical trials of the Southwest Oncology Group. *Cancer Treat. Rep.*, **44**, 847–853 (1982).

23. Jones, S. E., Grozea, P. N., Metz, E. N., Hant, A., Stephens, R. L., Morrison, F. S., Butler, J. J., Byrne, G. E., Jr., Moon, T. E., Fisher, R., Haskins, C. L., and Coltman, C. A., Jr. Superiority of adriamycin-containing combination chemotherapy in the treatment of diffuse lymphoma. A Southwest Oncology Group Study. *Cancer*, **43**, 417–425 (1979).

24. Jones, S. E., Haut, A., Weick, J. K., Wilson, H. E., Grozea, P., and Fabian, C. J. Comparison of adriamycin-containing chemotherapy (MOP-BAP) with MOPP-bleomycin in the management of advanced Hodgkin's disease. *Cancer*, **51**, 1339–1347 (1983).

25. Kelley, J., Newman, R. A., and Evans, J. N. Bleomycin-induced pulmonary fibrosis in the rat: prevention with an inhibitor of collagen synthesis. *J. Lab. Clin. Med.*, **96**, 954–964 (1980).

26. Krakoff, I. H. Cancer chemotherapeutic agents. *CA-A Cancer J. Clin.*, **31**, 130–140 (1981).

27. Krakoff, I. H., Cvitkovic, E., Currie, V., Yeh, S., and LaMonte, C. Clinical pharmacologic and therapeutic studies of bleomycin given by continuous infusion. *Cancer*, **40**, 2027–2037 (1977).

28. Lazo, J. S., Braun, I. D., Labaree, D. C., Schisselbauer, J. C., Meandzija, B., Newman, R. A., and Kennedy, K. A. Characteristics of bleomycin-resistant phenotypes of human cell sublines and circumvention of bleomycin resistance by liblomycin. *Cancer Res.*, **49**, 185–190 (1989).

29. Li, M. C., Whitmore, W. F., Golbey, R., and Grabstaldt, H. Effects of combined drug therapy in metastatic cancer of the testis. *JAMA*, **174**, 1291–1299 (1960).

30. Logothetis, C. J. and Samuels, M. L. Surgery in the management of stage III germinal cell tumors. *Cancer Treat. Rev.*, **11**, 27–37 (1984).

31. Louie, A. C. Bleomycin: the search for other indications. *In* "Bleomycin Chemotherapy," ed. B. I. Sikic, M. Rozencweig, and S. K. Carter, pp. 277–287 (1985). Academic Press, New York.

32. Newman, R. A., Hacker, M. P., Kimberly, P. J., and Braddock, J. M. Assessment of bleomycin, tallysomycin and polyamine-mediated acute lung toxicity by pulmonary lavage angiotensin-converting enzyme activity. *Toxicol. Appl. Pharmacol.*, **41**, 469–474 (1981).

33. Newman, R. A., Siddik, Z. H., Travis, E. L. *et al.* Assessment of pulmonary and hematologic toxicities of liblomycin, a novel bleomycin analog. *Invest. New Drugs*, in press.

34. Ostrowski, M. J. and Halsall, G. M. Intracavitary bleomycin in the management of malignant effusions: A multicenter study. *Cancer Treat. Rep.*, **66**, 1903–1907 (1982).

35. Samuels, M. L., Holoye, P. Y., and Johnson, D. E. Bleomycin combination chemotherapy for metastatic testicular carcinoma. *Cancer Bull.*, **25**, 53–55 (1973).

36. Samuels, M. L., Holoye, P. Y., and Johnson, D. E. Bleomycin combination chemotherapy in the management of testicular neoplasia. *Cancer*, **36**, 318–326 (1975).

37. Samuels, M. L. and Howe, C. D. Vinblastine in the management of testicular cancer. *Cancer*, **25**, 1009–1017 (1970).

38. Santoro, A. and Bonadonna, G. Prolonged disease-free survival in MOPP-resistant Hodgkin's disease after treatment with adriamycin, bleomycin, vinblastine and dacarbazine (ABVD). *Cancer Chemother. Pharmacol.*, **2**, 101–105 (1979).

39. Sikic, B. I. Clinical pharmacology of bleomycin. *In* "Bleomycin Chemotherapy," ed. B. I. Sikic, M. Rozencweig, and S. K. Carter (1985). Academic Press, New York.

40. Sikic, B. I., Collins, J. M., Mimnaugh, E. G., and Gram, T. E. Improved therapeutic index of bleomycin when administered by continuous infusion in mice. *Cancer Treat. Rep.*, **62**, 2011–2017 (1978).

41. Skarin, A. T., Canellos, G. P., Rosenthal, D. S. *et al.* Improved prognosis of diffuse histiocytic and undifferentiated lymphomas by use of high dose methotrexate alternating with standard agents (M-BACOD). *J. Clin. Oncol.*, **1**, 91–98 (1983).

42. Skarin, A., Rosenthal, D. S., Moloney, W. C., and Frei, E., III. Combination chemotherapy of advanced non-Hodgkin lymphoma with bleomycin, adriamycin, cyclophosphamide, vincristine and prednisone (BACOP). *Blood*, **49**, 759–770 (1977).

43. Suzuki, H., Nagai, K., Yamaki, H., Tanaka, N., and Umezawa, H. Mechanism of action of bleomycin. Studies with growing culture of bacterial and tumor cells. *J. Antibiot.*, **21**, 379–386 (1968).

44. Tueni, E. A., Newman, R. A., Baker, F. L., Ajani, J. A., Fan, D., and Spitzer, G. *In vitro* activity of bleomycin, tallysomycin S10B and liblomycin against fresh human tumor cells. *Cancer Res.*, **49**, 1099–1102 (1989).

45. Umezawa, H., Ichizuka, M., Maeda, K., and Takeuchi, T. Studies on bleomycin. *Cancer*, **20**, 891–895 (1967).

46. Umezawa, H., Maeda, K., Takeuchi, T., and Okami, Y. New antibiotics, bleomycin A and B. *J. Antibiot.* (*A*) **19**, 200–209 (1966).

47. Umezawa, H., Suhara, Y., Takita, T., and Maeda, K. Purification of bleomycins. *J. Antibiot.* (*A*) **19**, 210–215 (1966).

48. Umezawa, H., Takita, T., Saito, S., Muraoka, Y., Takahashi, K., Ekimoto, H., Minamide, S., Nishikawa, K., Fukuoka, T., Nakatani, T., Fujii, A., and Matsuda, A. New analogs and derivatives of bleomycin. *In* "Bleomycin Chemotherapy," ed. B. I. Sikic, M. Rozencweig, and S. K. Carter, pp. 289–301 (1985). Academic Press, New York.

49. Wittes, R. Bleomycin: future prospects. *In* "Bleomycin Chemotherapy," ed. B. I. Sikic, M. Rozencweig, and S. K. Carter (1985). Academic Press, New York.

50. Yagoda, A., Mukherji, B., Young, C., Etcubanas, E., LaMonte, C., Smith, J. R., Tan, C.T.C., and Krakoff, I. H. Bleomycin an antitumor antibiotic. *Ann. Intern. Med.*, **77**, 861–870 (1972).

Gann Monograph on Cancer Research 36, 1989

RELATIONSHIP OF STRUCTURE TO ANTICANCER ACTIVITY AND TOXICITY IN ANTHRACYCLINES

Federico Arcamone[*1] and Sergio Penco[*2]

*Menarini Ricerche Sud[*1] and Farmitalia-Carlo Erba[*2]*

Although the anthracyclines show different types of interaction with cell constituents, nuclear and mitochondrial DNA seem to be the main targets of the drugs. This conclusion is deduced from physico-chemical and biochemical studies on different compounds either modified in the aglycone or in the sugar moiety. Both DNA sequence specificity and the geometry of the drug-DNA complex are proposed as determinants of optimal pharmacological properties. Redox reactions should not be of relevance in this context, as heart toxicity can also be explained by an interference with transcription processes. The importance of drug metabolism *in vivo* is shown on the basis of clinical pharmacology data concerning the new anticancer agents idarubicin and epirubicin.

Medical treatment of cancer is now possible because of the availability of a number of drugs that are generally used in combination or in combined modalities, such as is the case of adjuvant therapeutic approaches, and allow in many cases the control, and in some instances even the cure, of tumor diseases such as leukemias, lymphomas, sarcomas, cancer of the breast and of the bladder (*27*). A major class of anticancer chemotherapeutic agents is that of the anthracyclines and doxorubicin (adriamycin), introduced in clinical use worldwide in the early seventies, still the most frequently used, and clinically the most effective antitumor drug. Other related compounds in clinical use are daunorubicin, epirubicin, idarubicin, and aclacinomycin. Other compounds of clinical interest are esorubicin and 4'-deoxy-4'-iododoxorubicin (*1, 2, 7*). Chemical structures of the above mentioned compounds are presented in Fig. 1.

The different anthracyclines have different connotations as regards their use in clinical practice. Doxorubicin is considered the drug with the widest antitumor spectrum presently available and responsive tumors include the hematological malignancies, sarcomas, thyroid cancer, ovarian cancer, tumors of the breast, Wilm's tumor, and neuroblastomas. Daunorubicin is mainly used in drug combinations for the induction of remission in acute leukemias. Epirubicin has been developed and is currently employed as a doxorubicin analog endowed with a lower general toxicity and cardiotoxicity when used at dosage levels that are comparable, in efficacy, with standard dosages of doxorubicin (*13*). Idarubicin is a potent inducer of remission in relapsed or refractory adult and pediatric leukemias and is active in other tumor types also when given orally (*23*). However, the lack of activity against major diseases like non-small cell lung cancer, colorectal tumors, and malignant melanomas, to cite only a few, and the severity of side effects at the maximum tolerated dosages that are currently used, strongly indicate the need of improved

*1 00040 Pomezia (Rome), Italy.
*2 20146 Milan, Italy.

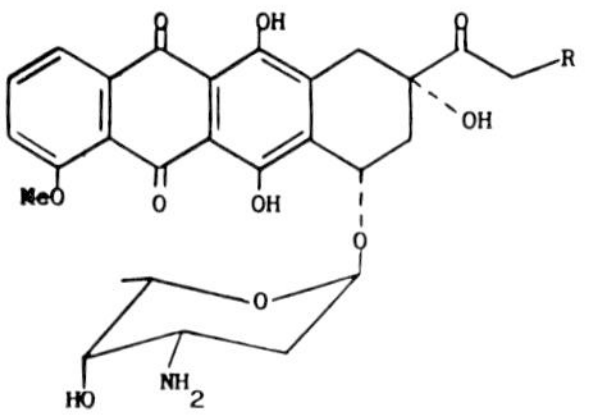

I : R = OH
II : R = H

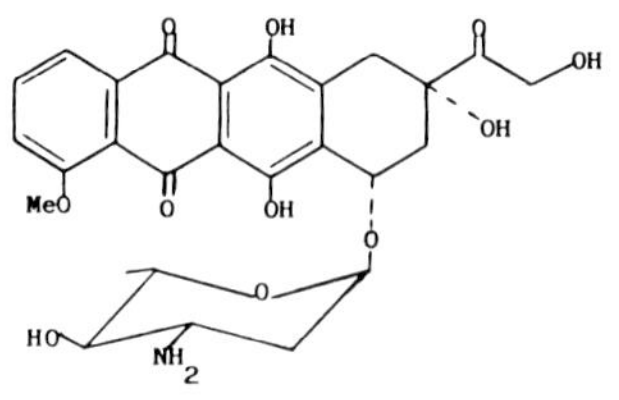

III

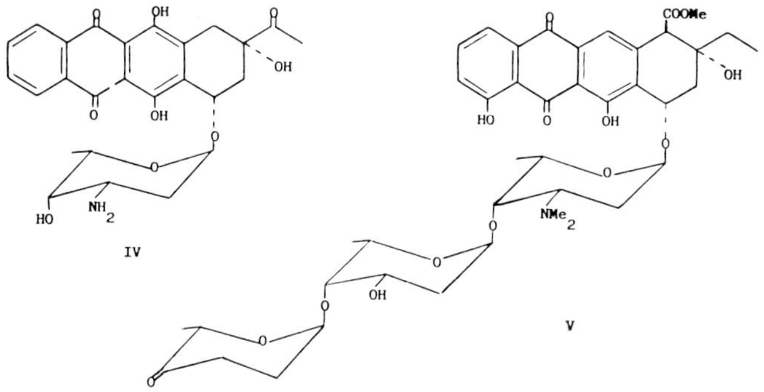

IV

V

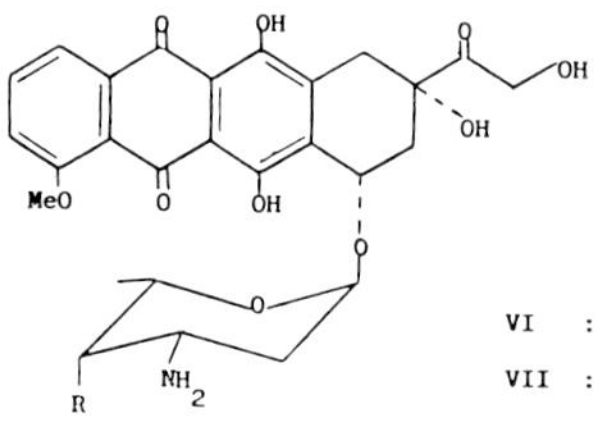

VI : R = H
VII : R = I

FIG. 1. Chemical structures of doxorubicin (I), daunorubicin (II), epirubicin (4'-epidoxorubicin, III), idarubicin (4-demethoxydaunorubicin, IV), aclacinomycin (V), esorubicin (4'-deoxydoxorubicin, VI), and 4'-deoxy-4'-iododoxorubicin (VII)

agents. The question that now arises is whether it will be possible to discover new anthracycline compounds possessing the required properties, namely a wider spectrum of activity (including efficacy in patients that were originally responsive and then became resistant to the drug) and/or a reduced toxicity allowing better tolerated treatment. This article aims at contributing elements for an answer to this question through a discussion covering aspects such as the mode of action, the molecular requirements for bioactivity, the mechanism of cardiotoxicity, and the effects of metabolism and pharmacokinetics on drug activity.

Mode of Action

The antitumor anthracyclines have been generally considered to act pharmacologically through a still imprecisely known molecular mechanism that, however, involves binding of the drug to cell nuclear DNA. Other hypothetical mechanisms have been proposed on the basis of (a) the chemical properties of the anthracyclines, or (b) biochemical findings still awaiting full explanation. To (a) belongs the property of the anthracyclines which are reduced at the quinone function and then react with molecular oxygen leading to toxic oxygen radical species (26). To (b) belong different observations concerning effects of these agents at the membrane level, the most important being the inhibition of plasma membrane redox enzyme systems linked to proton transport and to cell proliferation (43). However, work done in our laboratories confirms that DNA is the main pharmacological receptor of the antitumor anthracyclines.

Antitumor anthracyclines with high efficacy in experimental tumor systems such as I and VII (Fig. 1) exert their growth inhibitory effects on K562 human leukemia cells in culture through an identical mechanism that involves binding of the drugs to cell nuclei (24). In fact, intranuclear DNA bound drug concentrations at corresponding growth inhibitory concentrations in the medium, as measured by a sensitive, non-destructive microspectrofluorometric technique (25), were practically constant, that is, independent of cellular phenotype, whether sensitive or reistant, and, at least in the case of the two mentioned compounds, also of anthracycline structure. It appears, therefore, that intranuclear accumulation of DNA bound drugs represents a most relevant determinant of cytotoxicity for this class of drugs. The said studies also confirm that DNA bound drugs account for more than 99% of nuclear fluorescence (24, 43).

The hypothesis that double helical B DNA represents the main biological target of the antitumor anthracyclines and that this drug-receptor interaction is of relevance for clinical efficacy is in agreement with the observed relationship between affinity for calf thymus DNA and optimal therapeutic dosages in tumor bearing mice of different doxorubicin related compounds. It is also in agreement with the fact that those compounds that have reached the clinical stage after a careful pharmacological and toxicological selection belong to the group with the highest value of the DNA binding constant (45). On the other hand, aclacinomycin, a clinically useful anthracycline belonging to a structural type fundamentally different from doxorubicin, also displays a binding affinity towards calf thymus native DNA of the same order of magnitude as that of doxorubicin and daunorubicin (29).

If on general terms the above-mentioned relationship of anticancer activity with DNA binding affinity seems to be a true one, a comparison of cytotoxicity data in HeLa cell cultures with thermodynamic ones reveals no close correlation. In fact, although no cytotoxic anthracycline is known that exhibits bioactivity *in vitro* at concentrations below 100 nM and is devoid of DNA binding properties, it is possible that an anthracycline with strong DNA binding affinity be much less toxic to cultured HeLa cells than might be expected: see the case of 9-deoxydoxorubicin (Fig. 2) (6). This observation indicates that DNA binding alone does not result in a lethal effect on the cells. Therefore, either (1) a particular site and/or an optimal geometry of the anthracycline DNA complex is necessary for optimal biological activity, or (2) in addition to DNA binding a different interaction is required for cell death. In this context it should be kept in mind that multiple mechanisms are considered to be involved in anthracycline cytotoxicity on the basis of pharmacological observations (10) and conceivably not necessarily all of them are equally important for antitumor efficacy.

According to hypothesis (1), selective affinity towards one or more specific sites might be required for higher anticancer efficacy. Theoretical studies have convincingly

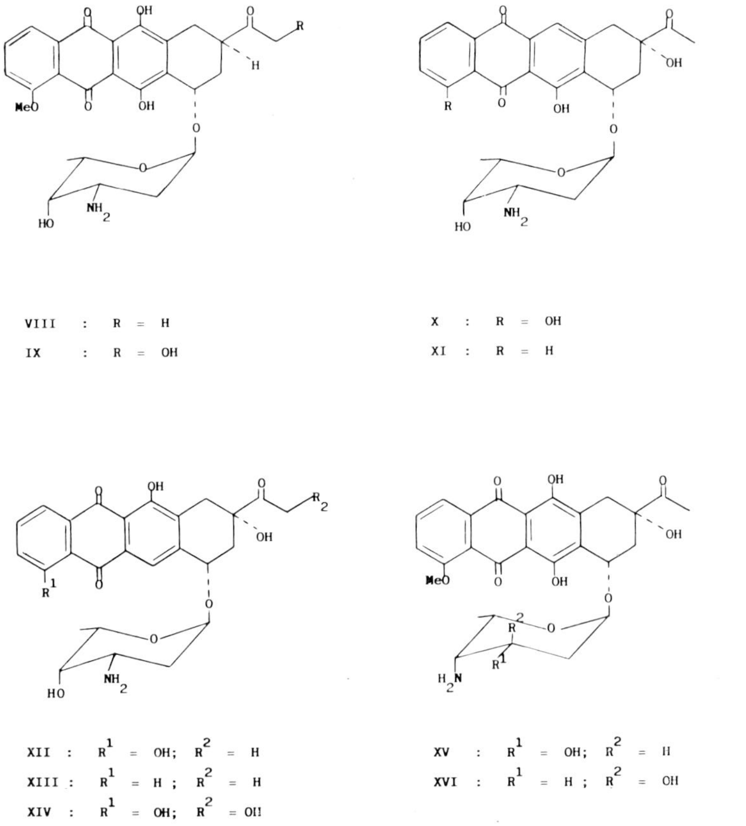

FIG. 2. Chemical structures of 9-deoxydaunorubicin (VIII), 9-deoxydoxorubicin (IX), 11-deoxycarminomycin (X), 11-deoxyidarubicin (XI), 6-deoxycarminomycin (XII), 6-deoxyidarubicin (XIII), 6-deoxy-14-hydroxycarminomycin (XIV), 4'-amino-3'-deamino-4'-deoxy-3'-hydroxydaunorubicin (XV), and its 3'-epi analog (XVI)

shown that the recognition site for doxorubicin is constituted by 3 base pairs, the one with the greatest affinity being the triplets CGA or CGT (17). This result has been confirmed by experimental studies, namely X-ray diffraction analysis of the complex of daunorubicin with the hexanucleotide d(CGTACG) (41) and foot-printing techniques (16). Oligonucleotide binding has been investigated in our laboratory using self-complementary hexanucleotides d(CGTACG) and d(CGCGCG), the former being identical to the one used for the X-ray study mentioned above. Both oligonucleotides showed the known preferential pattern in daunorubicin-DNA interaction, namely the purine-pyrimidine alternance. The different fluorescence yields of anthracycline intercalated at CpG or TpA sites (15) allowed the analysis of both equilibrium and kinetic properties of these systems. Doxorubicin and daunorubicin showed preferential intercalation at the 5'-CpG site of d(CpGpTpApCpG), the intercalation at the fluorescence preserving ApT site being more than ten times weaker. No preference was shown for an intercalation site within the three available ones in the d(CpGpCpGpCpG) duplex, the corresponding complexes showing a lower binding constant than the site in the d(CpGpTpApCpG) duplex. 9-Deoxydoxorubicin exhibited a considerably lower affinity towards both oligonucleotides, and showed evidence of intercalation at the TpA site. Also taking account of the energetics of sequence selectivity, it is concluded that the hydroxyl at C-9 is the main source of sequence selectivity, whereas the charged amino group on the sugar moiety is responsible for the extension of site specificity to 3 base pairs, in agreement with theoretical computations mentioned above. Another stabilization factor of DNA binding is represented by the 14-hydroxyl of doxorubicin, a compound that combines all three interacting groups and is the one showing the highest affinity. The conclusion is that DNA binding affinity coupled with CG affinity might correlate with antitumor activity (39).

Kinetics of the anthracycline-DNA interaction has received attention in our laboratory (40), also in relation to the work of others, according to which a correlation is demonstrated between the said kinetics and inhibition of the formation of the "open complex" by RNA polymerase and DNA during the transcription process (42). Moreover, the interpretation of the daunorubicin-DNA interaction in terms of a multi-step association mechanism (14) can be considered as evidence of binding site heterogeneity, clearly a necessary prerequisite to base-sequence specificity. Fluorescence stopped-flow experiments whose data were analysed by means of an appropriate computer program have been performed at low drug to nucleotide ratios (up to 100 base pairs per drug molecule). It was concluded that a five step mechanism is necessary for a complete interpretation of both association and dissociation kinetics (A=anthracycline; B1-B5=reaction products):

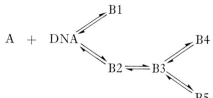

Interestingly, increased stabilization of B2 was found in the case of doxorubicin when compared with daunorubicin, and a destabilization in that of 9-deoxydoxorubicin. However, no direct correlation was found in general between the rate of complex dissociation and cytotoxicity of different anthracyclines, this suggesting that biological effects of different structurally related compounds result from the concomitant intervention of distinct mechanisms sharing DNA binding as a common step (40). The conclusion is in agreement with the biological findings (10), and is in line with the demonstrated importance of mechanisms other than direct inhibition of DNA replication and transcription, such as the effect ont opoisomerase II-DNA complexes, resulting in a stabilization of the "cleavable complex" that leads to an impairment of the breakage-reunion reaction and consequently to protein-linked DNA breaks (44). The association reactions of daunorubicin and doxorubicin with d(CpGpTpApCpG) were interpreted with only one exponential (40), the lack of slow exponential components indicating that slow kinetic steps observed with d(CpGpCpGpCpG), with the 9-deoxy or deaminated analogs and both oligonucleotides, as well as in the case of calf-thymus DNA represent redistribution of the bound drug in heterogeneous sites without intermediate dissociation.

Hypothesis (2) embraces different alternatives. The quinone system is a typical functionality of the anthracyclines. These compounds are therefore reduced enzymically to form semiquinones and/or hydroquinones. Microsomal NADPH-cytochrome P-450 reductase, mitochondrial NADH dehydrogenase and cytosolic xanthine oxidase can all function as catalysts of the reaction. The fate of the reduced forms should depend on the microenvironment in which they are produced and on the substitution pattern of the anthraquinone moiety. In fact, in the presence of oxygen the said forms can be reoxidized to the quinone generating oxygen centered radicals (26). In anaerobic conditions the reduced intermediate, semiquinone or hydroquinone, rearranges to give the free sugar, daunosamine, and the 7-deoxyaglycone *via* a C-7 carbon centered radical or a quinone methide. According to careful studies the true intermediate is the quinone methide, a species that, in principle, might also function as an alkylating agent *in vivo* and be responsible for the antitumor activity (22, 30).

Studies performed in our laboratory did not confirm the relevance of the redox reactions to pharmacological activity. Compound VIII (Fig. 2), possessing the same chromophore of II, gave, on enzymic reduction in anaerobic conditions the corresponding 7-deoxyaglycone, whereas X (Fig. 2) gave bis (7-deoxyaglycone-7-yl), in agreement with what has already been reported for 11-deoxyanthracyclines. On the other hand, XII (Fig. 2) did not exhibit fission of the glycoside bond under similar conditions and only 2% of the substrate was detectable as a stable semiquinone radical (6). However, XII (6-deoxycarminomycin) was markedly cytotoxic in cell culture. This observation would rule out the relevance of reductive bioactivation for this class of drugs. The conclusion is in agreement with the absence of bioactivity of VIII that has the same chromophoric system as II and is a good substrate for the so-called reductive bioactivation. The same applies to the result of the comparison between "isodaunorubicin" (XV, Fig. 2) and the corresponding L-xylo analog XVI, both showing the same chromophore and therefore redox properties. The former binds to DNA and is as active as the parent II, whereas the latter exhibits low affinity for DNA and is practically devoid of cytotoxicity (6). In

TABLE I.   Concentrations of Daunorubicin and Related Compounds Inhibiting by 50% the Viability of HeLa Cells in Culture after 24 hr Exposure to the Drug

Compound	IC_{50} (ng/ml)
Daunorubicin (II)	15
Idarubicin (IV)	4.2
9-Deoxydaunorubicin (VIII)	1,200
11-Deoxycarminomycin (X)	14
11-Deoxyidarubicin (XI)	25
6-Deoxycarminomycin (XII)	3.7
6-Deoxyidarubicin (XIII)	17
Isodaunorubicin (XV)	7
Isodaunorubicin, 3'-epi (XVI)	1,600

TABLE II.   Antitumor Activity of 6-Deoxy Derivatives against Gross Leukemia in Mice[a]

Compound	O.D. (mg/kg)	T/C %
Daunorubicin (II)	15	167, 183
6-Deoxycarminomycin (II)	2.5	175
Doxorubicin (I)	13	208
6-Deoxy-14-hydroxycarminomycin (XIV)	5	217

[a] CH3 female mice received 2×10^6 leukemia cells i.v. on day 0, and the drugs were injected i.v. on day 1. O.D.=optimal ($<LD_{10}$) dose. T/C %=survival time of treated animals expressed as % of untreated tumor controls.

Table I bioactivity of different daunorubicin analogs is compared with that of the parent compound, while Table II shows the *in vivo* activity of the 6-deoxyderivatives (*35*).

Molecular Requirements for Bioactivity

1. The aglycone moiety

The substitution of either the hydroxyl group at C-6 or that at C-11 on the daunorubicin B ring to give XVII and XVIII (Fig. 3) dramatically reduced affinity for DNA with little, if any, evidence of intercalation. Prevention of intercalation was explained on the basis of the steric effect of the bulky methoxy group (*37*). This structural modification was accompanied by the loss of antitumor activity (*50*). On the contrary, compound XIX (Fig. 3) was still able to give a DNA intercalation complex, the binding isotherm being typical of the intercalating anthracyclines. The compound exhibited a reduced affinity for calf thymus DNA and probably a different geometry of intercalation, together with noticeable bioactivity. However, the results of tests in murine experimental tumors did not encourage further development (*49*). Theoretical computations using the SIBFA

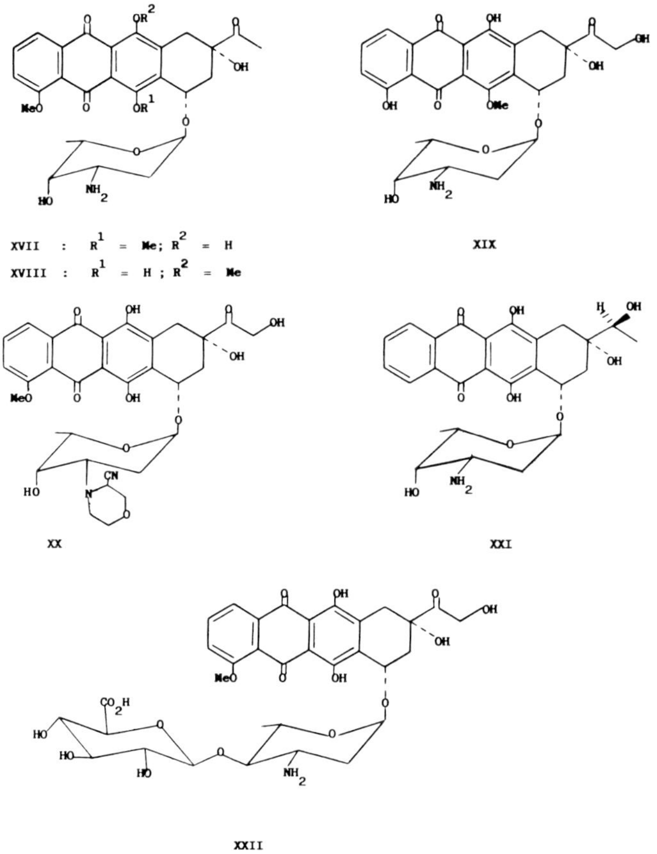

Fig. 3. Chemical structures of 6-O-methyldaunorubicin (XVII), 11-O-methyl-daunorubicin (XVIII), 4'-O-demethyl-6-O-methyldoxorubicin (XIX), 3'-deamino-3' (3-cyanomorpholin-4-yl) doxorubicin (XX), idarubicinol (XXI), and 4'-O-β-D-glucuronylepirubicin (XXII)

TABLE III.   Apparent Binding Constants for the Complex with Calf Thymus DNA and
Cytotoxicity against Cultured HeLa Cells of Anthracycline Glycosides

Compound	Kapp. $(10^6 \text{ M}^{-1})^a$	IC_{50} $(ng/ml)^b$
Daunorubicin (II)	55	12
Doxorubicin (I)	240	15
9-Deoxydaunorubicin (VIII)	54.5	1,200
9-Deoxydoxorubicin (IX)	50	230

[a] Determined according to ref. 45.
[b] After 2 hr exposure.

(sum of interactions between fragments computed *ab initio*) procedure have been performed in parallel with the determination of thermodynamic apparent binding constants
for the complexes of different anthracyclines with receptor models d(CpGpCpGpCpG)$_2$,
d(TpApTpApTpA)$_2$, and d(CpGpTpApCpGp)$_2$ (5). The results indicate that, when
compared with the three-dimensional model deduced from the X-ray diffraction analysis
(47), the introduction of the methyl group at O-6 as in XIX determines a preferred binding mode according to which the planar chromophore is significantly unstacked from the
base pairs of the intercalation site and shows a different orientation than that found for
daunorubicin. The change of complex geometry is assisted by the presence of the free
hydroxyl at C-4.

In the study of Wang *et al.* (47) evidence was provided of a stabilization of the intercalation complex derived, *inter alia*, from the formation of a hydrogen bond between
the hydroxyl at C-9 of daunorubicin and both the amino group and N-3 of guanine. In
the free anthracycline the 9-hydroxyl is involved in a hydrogen bond with the glycosidic
oxygen atom at C-7 (18, 32). Recent nuclear magnetic resonance (NMR) studies (38),
have shown that the preferred conformation of the N-trifluoroacetyl derivative of VIII
in CDCl$_3$ (and, according to preliminary data also in D$_2$O) is the same as that of N-
acetyl-daunorubicin, allowing the deduction that the 9-OH is, however, not important
for the orientation of the glycosidic bond (the latter is instead determined by steric interactions of the sugar and the aglycone moieties). Nor is the 9-OH important for the
formation of a stable DNA complex (Table III). However, the reduced cytotoxic activity of VIII and IX shown in the table and the absence of antitumor activity of IX when
given up to 22 mg/kg to mice bearing Gross leukemia point to the importance of the said
grouping for bioactivity. In fact, although cell uptake and retention of I and IX were
similar, IX induced very few DNA breaks that reached a maximum after 45 min incubation of the drug with the HeLa cells. On the contrary, DNA breaks induced by I continued to increase with time of exposure and persisted after drug removal, indicating a
key role of topoisomerase mediated reactions in the differential behavior of the two compounds and of the 9-OH in determining the different outcomes of the reaction. The
importance of the 14-OH for the stabilization of the DNA complex has already been
mentioned. Interestingly, this hydroxyl is involved in a linkage with DNA phosphate
groups (36).

2.   The sugar moiety

Modification at 4' as in III, VI, and VII has provided compounds of clinical interest.
On the other hand, consistent with a lower affinity for double stranded DNA, the analogs with a 3'-axial amino group, like the L-ribo and L-xylo analogs, were clearly less

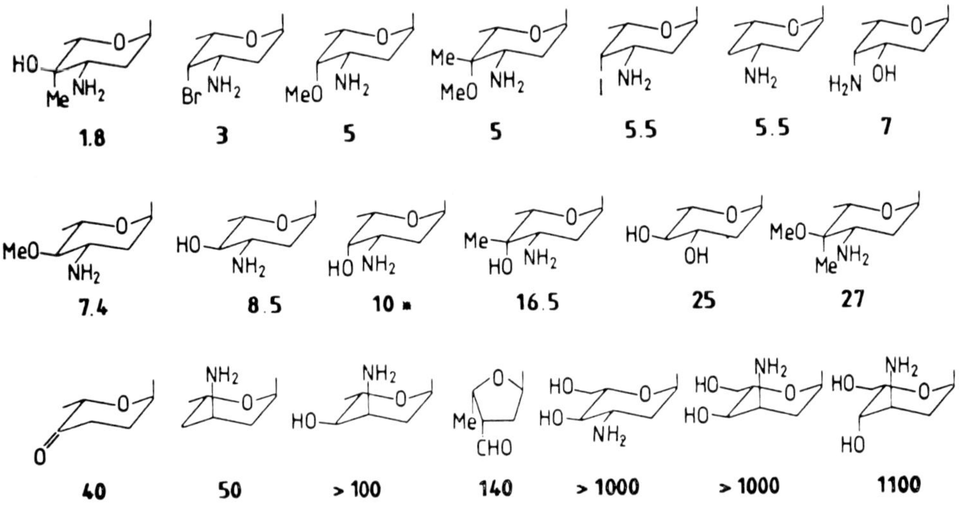

FIG. 4. Effect of sugar variations on the cytotoxicity of adriamycinone glycosides ID$_{50}$ values (ng/ml) in HeLa cell cultures after 24 hr exposure (* doxorubicin).

potent when compared with the parent in mice screening tests (3). In a study concerning the 4' C-methyl and O-methyl derivatives in the L-lyxo and L-arabino configuration, it was found that the said variations affected the potency but not the antitumor efficacy of the anthracyclines (8). The same conclusion was reached in an investigation of different deaminated analogs (11), both studies showing the superiority of adriamycinone over daunomycinone glycosides. The variation of potency against HeLa cells in culture in a series of doxorubicin analogs modified in the carbohydrate structure is presented in Fig. 4. The biological data are derived from references cited in this article. The conclusion drawn from the examination of this table is that orientation of the group at 3', namely the aminogroup or the hydroxyl group, is a main determinant for cytotoxic activity, suggesting that the said groups, oriented towards the outside of the DNA helix in the drug-receptor complex, are responsible for an interaction with a third component in the cell nucleus. Such component might be a protein that binds to selected regions of the DNA molecule, and whose function would be perturbed by the interaction with the 3' substituent when this is present in favorable orientation.

The considerations about the variations in potency are of relevance also for the problem of resistance. In fact, 4'-deoxy-4'-iododoxorubicin VII, although showing the same antitumor efficacy as doxorubicin in a number of murine tumors, showed higher activity against doxorubicin resistant tumors when compared with the parent drug (7). Particularly high potency, up to 500 times that of I, is exhibited by 3'-deamino-3'-(3-cyano-4-morpholinyl) doxorubicin (XX, Fig. 3), a compound possessing a potentially alkylating group with the equatorial orientation at 3' (48).

Cardiotoxicity

The hypothesis that radical formation is a major factor of chronic subcellular effects induced by repeated anthracycline dosages to the heart (41) is not supported, as we have seen above, by the structure-activity relationship data. On the other hand, an ultrastructural investigation of myocardial changes in the mouse induced by doxorubicin treatment showed nucleolar segregation and increased reactivity of the sarcoplasmic reticulum with the zinc iodide-osmium tetroxide (ZIO) technique within 6 hr after treatment. However, 24 hr after treatment nucleolar segregation appeared reversible, whereas the ZIO reactive material was the most prominent and persisting finding and appeared to be accompanied by a number of functional and morphologic changes clearly related with the observed cardiotoxic effects (9). The authors of the study point out that the ZIO method detects mainly disulfide bonds in polypeptides, cystine or oxidized glutathione. Other reactive substances are compounds containing free SH groups, unsaturated lipids, lipid peroxides (implicated in doxorubicin induced cardiotoxicity), and catecholamines, although "labile" S-S bonds have been found to react more promptly and, according to the cited authors, "seem to be suitable candidates as substrates of ZIO reactivity in the sarcoplasmic reticulum of doxorubicin-treated cardiocytes." Such observation would reveal the presence of an oxidative stress as already demonstrated by others (28, 33), a consequence of a higher than normal oxygen tension in the tissue. This condition would be in agreement with the higher inhibition of RNA synthesis in the heart with respect to the skeletal muscle induced by I, an effect that explains the decrease of myocardial RNA content in rats after I administration. The lower protein turnover correlated with the decreased transcription rate could lead to the observed cell damage by both (a) lowering the formation of contractile proteins and (b) interrupting aerobic metabolism (46). The latter effect would lead to a remarkable enhancement of the partial pressure of oxygen with consequent oxidative stress. Recently, Ellis et al. (20) have demonstrated the inhibition by doxorubicin of the transcription of mitochondrial DNA with related interference in the production of essential components of the oxidative phosphorlylation pathway leading to diminished ATP production, thus explaining the particular toxicity of doxorubicin for tissues characterized by a high energy demand.

Metabolism

Mammalian aldo-keto reductases, constitutive enzymes widely distributed in tissues, catalyze the reduction of the side chain carbonyl group typical of daunorubicin, doxorubicin, and related compounds such as epirubicin and idarubicin. The corresponding 13-dihydro derivatives, that are isolated from human urine, can also be obtained by microbial reduction of the parent drugs and show the (S) configuration at C-13 (34). The enzyme is known to be much more effective on daunorubicin than on doxorubicin analogs (21). The resulting 13-dihydro metabolites retain significant biologic activity and, in the case of idarubicin (IV), the plasma levels of idarubicinol (XXI, Fig. 3) in cancer patients are higher than those of the administered drug, contributing substantially to the pharmacological effects of IV (23).

The main human urinary metabolites of epirubicin (III) were identified as 4'-O-(β-D-glucuronyl)epirubicin (XXII), epirubicinol, and 4'-O-(β-D-glucuronyl)epirubicinol (12). The formation of the conjugated species, originally found in the plasma of patients treated with III (19), represent a unique characteristic of this drug. In fact, no other glucuronide conjugate of an anthracycline glycoside has been described. It is noteworthy that this metabolic reaction is found in man, but is clearly less important or absent in laboratory animals (4, 31). This property of III which differentiates this drug pharmacologically from I is related to the different orientation of the C-4' hydroxyl group that is equatorial instead of axial as in I.

CONCLUSION

It appears from the above that, although more than 20 years have elapsed since the discovery of the antitumor anthracyclines, more work must be done on these drugs. Clearly, there is room for (a) further exploration of the structure-activity relationships and (b) hopefully the development of pharmacologically improved analogs. As for (a), important information should be obtained from a careful analysis of the dependence of biological properties on the DNA sequence specificity of different anthracyclines and from the determination of the effect of structural variations on the reactions catalyzed by topoisomerase II, whose relevance for antitumor activity of different intercalating agents is unquestioned. As for (b), the rationalization resulting from the said studies should be of great help to the medicinal chemist in the design of better analogs. In addition, the awareness of the special effects of the anthracyclines on cardiac metabolism should encourage the use of remedies such as the enzyme superoxide dismutase in order to reduce toxicity. Also, investigations on the metabolism of different anthracycline derivatives and on the behavior of appropriate prodrugs might result in substantial improvements in the use of anthracyclines for the treatment of cancer diseases.

REFERENCES

1. Arcamone, F. "Doxorubicin, Anticancer Antibiotics," Medicinal Chemistry Series, ed. G. Stevens, Vol. 17 (1981). Academic Press, New York.
2. Arcamone, F. Antitumor anthracyclines: recent developments. *Med. Res. Rev.*, **4**, 153–188 (1984).
3. Arcamone, F. Structure-activity relationships in antitumor anthracyclines. *In* "X-Ray Crystallography and Drug Action," ed. A. S. Horn and C. De Ranter, pp. 367–388 (1984). Oxford University Press, Oxford, New York.
4. Arcamone, F., Lazzati, M., Vicario, G. P., and Zini, G. Disposition of ^{14}C-labelled 4'-epidoxorubicin and doxorubicin in the rat. A comparative study. *Cancer Chemother. Pharmacol.*, **12**, 157–166 (1984).
5. Arcamone, F., Menozzi, M., Tonani, R., and Pullman, B. A joint experimental and theoretical investigation of the comparative DNA binding affinities of intercalating anthracycline derivatives. *Mol. Pharmacol.*, in press.
6. Arcamone, F. and Penco, S. Chemical derivatives of anticancer antibiotics with different DNA binding properties. *In* "Molecular Mechanisms of Carcinogenic and Antitumor Activity," ed. C. Chagas and B. Pullman, pp. 225–241 (1987). Pontificia Academia Scientiarum.
7. Barbieri, B., Giuliani, F. C., Bordoni, T., Casazza, A. M., Geroni, C., Bellini, O., Suarato, A., Gioia, B., Penco, S., and Arcamone, F. Chemical and biological characterization of 4'-iodo-4'-deoxydoxorubicin. *Cancer Res.*, **47**, 4001–4006 (1987).
8. Bargiotti, A., Casazza, A. M., Cassinelli, G., Di Marco, A., Penco, S., Pratesi, G., Supino, R., Zaccara, A., Zunino, F., and Arcamone, F. Synthesis, biological and biochemical properties of new anthracyclines modified in the aminosugar moiety. *Cancer Chem. Pharmacol.*, **10**, 84–98 (1983).
9. Bellini, O. and Solcia, E. Early and late sarcoplasmic reticulum changes in doxorubicin cardiomyopathy. *Virchows Arch.* (*Cell Pathol.*), **49**, 137–152 (1985).
10. Capranico, G., Soranzo, C., and Zunino, F. Single strand DNA breaks induced by chromophore-modified anthracyclines in P388 leukemia cells. *Cancer Res.*, **46**, 5499–5503 (1986).

11. Cassinelli, G., Ballabio, M., Arcamone, F., Casazza, A. M., and Podesta', A. New anthracycline glycosides obtained by the nitrous acid deamination of daunorubicin, doxorubicin and their configurational analogues. *J. Antibiot.*, **38**, 856–867 (1985).

12. Cassinelli, G., Configliacchi, C., Penco, S., Rivola, G., Arcamone, F., Pacciarini, A., and Ferrari, L. Separation, characterization and analysis of epirubicin (4'-epidoxorubicin) and its metabolites from human urine. *Drug Metab. Disp.*, **12**, 506–510 (1984).

13. Cersosimo, R. J. and Hong, W. K. Epirubicin: a review of the pharmacology, clinical activity, and adverse effects of an adriamycin analogue. *J. Clin. Oncol.*, **4**, 425–439 (1986).

14. Chaires, J. B., Dattagupta, N., and Crothers, D. M. Kinetics of the daunomycin-DNA interaction. *Biochemistry*, **24**, 260–267 (1985).

15. Chaires, J. B. Equilibrium studies on the interaction of daunomycin with deoxypolynucleotides. *Biochemistry*, **22**, 4204–4211 (1983).

16. Chaires, J. B., Fox, K. R., Herrera, J. E., Britt, M., and Waring, M. J. Site and sequence specificity of the daunomycin-DNA interaction. *Biochemistry*, **26**, 8227–8236 (1987).

17. Chen, K.-X., Gresh, N., and Pullman, B. A theoretical investigation on the sequence selective binding of daunomycin to double-stranded polynucleotides. *J. Biomol. Struct. Dyn.*, **3**, 445–466 (1985).

18. Courseille, C., Busetta, B., Geoffre, S., and Hospital, M. Complex daunomycin-butanol. *Acta Cryst.*, **B35**, 764–767 (1979).

19. Deesen, P. G. and Jones, B. L. Sensitive and specific determination of the new anthracycline analog 4'-epidoxorubicin and its metabolites by high pressure liquid chromatography. *Drug Metab. Disp.*, **12**, 9–13 (1984).

20. Ellis, C. N., Ellis, M. B., and Blakemore, W. S. Effect of adriamycin on heart mitochondrial DNA. *Biochem. J.*, **245**, 309–312 (1987).

21. Felsted, R. C., Pichter, D. R., and Bachur, N. R. Rat liver aldehyde reductase. *Biochem. Pharmacol.*, **26**, 1117–1120 (1977).

22. Fisher, J., Abdella, B.R.J., and Melane, K. E. Anthracycline antibiotic reduction of spinach ferredoxin NADP reductase and ferredoxin. *Biochemistry*, **24**, 3562–3571 (1985).

23. Ganzina, F., Pacciarini, M. A., and Di Pietro, N. Idarubicin (4-demethoxydaunorubicin). A preliminary overview of preclinical and clinical studies. *Invest. New Drugs*, **4**, 85–105 (1986).

24. Gigli, M., Doglia, S. M., Millot, J.-M., Valentini, L., and Manfait, M. Quantitative study of doxorubicin in living cell nuclei by microspectrofluorometry. *Biochim. Biophys. Acta*, **950**, 13–20 (1988).

25. Gigli, M., Rasonaivo, T.W.D., Millot, J.-C., Jeannesson, P., Rizzo, V., Jardiller, J.-C., Arcamone, F., and Manfait, M. Correlation between growth inhibition and intranuclear doxorubicin and 4'-deoxy-4'-iododoxorubicin in living K562 cells by microspectrofluorometry. *Cancer Res.*, in press.

26. Gutierrez, P. L., Gee, M. V., and Bachur, N. R. Kinetics of anthracycline antibiotics, free radical formation and reductive glycosidase activity. *Arch. Biochem. Biophys.*, **223**, 68–75 (1983).

27. Hansen, H. H., Hoth, H. D., Lira Puerto, W., Olweny, C. L., and Tattersall, M. Essential drugs for cancer chemotherapy. Memorandum from WHO meeting. *Bull. WHO*, **63**, 999–1004 (1985).

28. Ishikawa, T. and Sies, H. Cardiac transport of glutathione disulfide and S-conjugates. Studies with isolated perfused rat heart during hydroperoxide metabolism. *J. Biol. Chem.*, **259**, 3838–3843 (1984).

29. Katenkamp, V., Stutter, E., Petri, I., Gollmick, F. A., and Berg, H. Interaction of anthracycline antibiotics with biopolymers. VIII. Binding parameters of aclacinomycin A to DNA. *J. Antibiot.*, **35**, 1222–1227 (1983).

30. Kleyer, D. L. and Koch, T. H. Mechanistic investigation of reduction of daunomycin

and 7-deoxydaunomycinone with bi-(3, 5, 5-trimethyl-2-oxamorpholin-3-yl). *J. Am. Chem. Soc.*, **106**, 2380–2387 (1984).

31. Maessen, P. A., Mrass, K. B., Pinedo, H. M., and Van der Vijgh, W.J.F. Metabolism of epirubicin in animals: absence of glucuronidation. *Cancer Chemother. Pharmacol.*, **20**, 85–87 (1987).

32. Mondelli, R., Ragg, E., Fronza, G., and Arnone, A. Nuclear magnetic resonance conformational study of daunomycin and related antitumor antibiotics in solution. The conformation of ring. A. *J. Chem. Soc. Perkin*, **II**, 15–26 (1987).

33. Olson, R. D., Mac Donald, J. S., Von Boxtel, C. J., Boerth, R. C., Harbison, R. D., Slonim, A. E., Freman, R. W., and Oates, J. A. Regulatory role of glutathione and soluble sulfhydryl groups in the toxicity of adriamycin. *J. Pharmacol. Exp. Ther.*, **215**, 450–454 (1980).

34. Penco, S., Cassinelli, G., Vigevani, A., Zini, P. A., Rivola, G., and Arcamone, F. Daunorubicin aldo-keto reductase: enantioface differential reduction of the side-chain carbonyl group of antitumor anthracyclines. Correction of stereochemistry at C-13 of 4-demethoxy-13-dihydrodaunorubicin. *Gazz. Chim. Ital.*, **115**, 195–197 (1985).

35. Penco, S., Malatesta, V., Barchielli, G., Sacchi, N., Bordoni, T., Bellini, O., and Arcamone, F. Enzymic reductive activation of anthracyclines: are the anthracycline redox properties determinant for the biological activity? *Biochem. Pharmacol.*, submitted for publication.

36. Pohle, W. and Flemming, J. Interaction of the C^{14}-OH group of adriamycin with DNA phosphate as spectroscopically evidenced. *J. Biomol. Struct. Dyn.*, **4**, 243–250 (1986).

37. Quadrifoglio, F., Cione, A., Manzini, G., Zaccara, A., and Zunino, F. Influence of some chromophore substituents on the intercalation of antibiotics into DNA. *Int. J. Biol. Macromol.*, **4**, 413–418 (1982).

38. Raggi, E., Mondelli, R., and Penco, S. Conformational analysis of 9-deoxydaunorubicin in solution. The application of quantitative transient 1H nuclear overhauser effect. *J. Chem. Soc. Perkin*, **II**, 1673–1678 (1988).

39. Rizzo, V., Battistini, C., Vigevani, A., Sacchi, N., Razzano, G., Arcamone, F., Garbesi, A., Colonna, F., Capobianco, M., and Tondelli, L. Anthracycline interaction with synthetic hexanucleotides: structural factors responsible for sequence specificity. Submitted to *Biochemistry* (1989).

40. Rizzo, V., Sacchi, N., and Menozzi, M. Kinetic studies of anthracycline-DNA interaction by fluorescence stopped flow confirm a complex mechanism. *Biochemistry*, in press.

41. Singal, P. K., Deally, M. R., and Weinberg, C. E. Subcellular effects of adriamycin in the heart, a concise review. *J. Mol. Cell Cardiol.*, **19**, 817–828 (1987).

42. Straney, D. C. and Crothers, D. M. Effect of drug-DNA interactions upon transcription initiation of the lac promoter. *Biochemistry*, **26**, 1987–1995 (1987).

43. Sun, I. L., Crane, F. L., Loew, H., and Grebing, C. Inhibition of plasma membrane NADH dehydrogenase by adriamycin and related anthracycline antibiotics. *J. Bioenerg. Biomembr.*, **16**, 209–221 (1984).

44. Tewey, K. M., Rowe, T. C., Yang, L., Halligan, B. D., and Liu, L. F. Adriamycin-induced DNA damage mediated by mammalian DNA topoisomerase. II. *Science*, **226**, 466–468 (1984).

45. Valentini, L., Nicolella, V., Vannini, E., Menozzi, M., Penco, S., and Arcamone, F. Association to anthracycline derivatives with DNA: a fluorescence study. *Il Farmaco Ed. Sci.*, **46**, 377–390 (1985).

46. Van Helden, P. D. and Wiid, J.J.F. Effects of adriamycin on heart and skeletal muscle chromatin. *Biochem. Pharmacol.*, **31**, 973–977 (1982).

47. Wang, A. H.-J., Ughetto, G., Quigley, G. T., and Rich, A. Interactions between an

anthracycline antibiotic and DNA: Molecular structure of daunomycin complexed to d (CpGpTpApCpG) at 1.2 Å resolution. *Biochemistry*, **26**, 1152–1163 (1987).

48. Wassermann, K., Zwelling, L. A., Mullins, T. D., Silberman, L. E., Andersson, B. S., Bakic, M., Acton, E. M., and Newmann, R. A. Effects of 3'-deamino-3'(3-cyano-4-morpholinyl)doxorubicin on the survival, DNA integrity, and nucleolar morphology of human leukemia cells *in vitro*. *Cancer Res.*, **46**, 4041–4046 (1986).

49. Zunino, F., Barbieri, B., Bellini, O., Casazza, A. M., Geroni, C., Giuliani, F., Cione, A., Manzini, G., and Quadrifoglio, F. Biochemical and biological activity of the anthracycline analog 4-demethyl-6-O-methyldoxorubicin. *Invest. New Drugs*, **4**, 17–23 (1986).

50. Zunino, F., Casazza, A. M., Pratesi, G., Formelli, F., and Di Marco, A. Effect of methylation of aglycone hydroxyl groups on the biological and biochemical properties of daunorubicin. *Biochem. Pharmacol.*, **30**, 1856–1858 (1981).

ACLARUBICIN AND PIRARUBICIN:
BASIC RESEARCH

Hiroshi Tone[*1] and Tomio Takeuchi[*2]

*Central Research Laboratories, Sanraku Incorporated[*1] and Institute
of Microbial Chemistry[*2]*

Aclarubicin (ACM) and pirarubicin (THP) are anthracycline antitumor
antibiotics discovered by Umezawa, Takeuchi, and their colleagues and
developed in Japan. They have high antitumor activity on various experimental tumors and lower cardiac toxicity than adriamycin. Aclarubicin
showed growth inhibitory effect on human stomach cancer in nude mice.
It binds to DNA, inhibits RNA synthesis at a lower concentration than
DNA synthesis, and blocks the late S phase of cell cycle. The level of
drug is much higher in the blood cell than the plasma, and it distributes
to the lung and spleen at a high concentration. THP suppressed metastasis
of Lewis lung carcinoma. This drug is incorporated into cells more rapidly
than adriamycin and blocks the G_2 phase of cell cycle. It is rapidly transferred from the plasma to tissues and has a shorter plasma level half-life
than does adriamycin. A higher drug level than the plasma is shown in
tissues, particularly in the lymph node.

Aclarubicin (ACM) is an antitumor agent included in a category of anthracycline
antibiotics. This drug was discovered by H. Umezawa *et al.* in 1975 (*29*) and is presently
used in Japan, France, Germany, and other countries with good efficacy against various
cancers, especially acute leukemia. Pirarubicin (THP) is a new anticancer drug, a derivative of adriamycin, on which the first paper was also published by Umezawa *et al.* in
1979 (*45*). The drug has demonstrated excellent efficacy against head and neck, breast,
urinary tract, and ovarian cancers, and also against acute leukemia, malignant lymphoma,
and some others. THP has been available in Japan since 1988 and is expected to be
used soon in Europe and the United States. In the present paper we review the basic
studies, including some unpublished data, on these two anthracycline anticancer drugs
discovered by Umezawa, Takeuchi, and their colleagues and developed in Japan.

Aclarubicin (Aclacinomycin A, ACM)

ACM was isolated from a culture broth of *Streptomyces galilaeus* MA144-M1 (*28*).
This antibiotic consists of aklavinone and three sugar moieties, L-rhodosamine, 2-deoxy-
fucose, and L-cinerulose (Fig. 1) (*27*).

1. Antitumor activity

ACM inhibits growth of various kinds of tumor cells *in vivo* and *in vitro*. Remarkable
increases in life span of tumor-bearing animals and growth inhibition of solid tumor was

---

[*1] Jonan 4-9-1, Fujisawa, Kanagawa 251, Japan (刀根　弘).
[*2] Kamiosaki 3-14-23, Shinagawa-ku, Tokyo 141, Japan (竹内富雄).

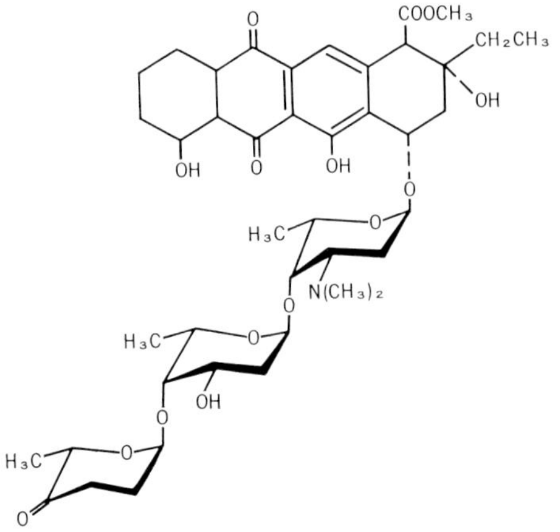

FIG. 1. Structure of ACM (*27*)

TABLE I. Antitumor Activity of ACM (*8, 26*)

Tumor	Treatment		Opt. dose (mg/kg/day)	ILS (%)	Inhibition (%)
	Route	Day			
Ascites type					
L1210 leukemia	i.p.	1–9	4	113	
	p.o.	1–9	10	69	
P388 leukemia	i.p.	1–9	5	108	
Ehrlich carcinoma	i.p.	1, 5, 9	4	133	
B16 melanoma	i.p.	1, 5, 9	3	43	
Lewis lung carcinoma	i.p.	1, 5, 9	1.6	50	
Rat hepatoma AH13	i.p.	3–12	2	168	
AH41C	i.v.	3–12	2	200	
Solid type					
Sarcoma 180	i.p.	1–10	6		94
CD mammary carcinoma	i.p.	1–9	6		100
Colon 38	i.p.	5, 12, 19	12		84
6C3Hed/OG lymphoma	i.p.	0–10	1		56

i.p., intraperitoneal; p.o., oral; i.v., intravenous.

demonstrated in the *in vivo* system with mouse leukemia L1210, P388, Ehrlich carcinoma, sarcoma 180, both in ascites- and solid-type, solid-type CD mammary carcinoma, Garder 6C3HED/OG lymphoma, Lewis lung carcinoma, and rat hepatomas (Table I) (*8, 26*). In addition to the effect on these experimental animal tumors, ACM showed significant inhibitory activity on growth of human xenografts, stomach cancer cells transplanted to nude mice (*19*).

Combination of ACM with other antitumor agents gives additive or synergistic activity. Marked synergistic effect on mouse leukemia L1210 was shown by administration of ACM in combination with cytosine arabinoside. Highly synergistic activity was also shown by combined administration with cyclophosphamide on mouse leukemia P388 (Table II) (*4, 41*). On solid-type sarcoma 180, the high combined effect of AMC was demonstrated with cysplatin (Table III).

TABLE II.   Effect of ACM in Combination with Other Antitumor Agents (4, 41)

Tumor	Drug	Dose (mg/kg/day)	Treatment Route	Treatment Day	ILS (%)	Survivor (/treated)
L1210	ACM	3	i.p.	1–10	80	0/6
	Cytosine arabinoside	10	i.p.	1–10	83	0/6
	ACM + Cytosine arabinoside	1.5 5	i.p.	1–10	459	4/6 (60 days)
P388	ACM	4	i.p.	q2d 1–19	66	0/6
	Cyclophosphamide	200	i.p.	Single 1	359	1/6
	ACM + Cyclophosphamide	4 200	i.p. i.p.	q2d 1–19 Single	460	5/6 (80 days)

TABLE III.   Combined Effect of ACM and Cysplatinum on Solid-type Sarcoma 180

Drug	Dose (mg/kg/day)	Inhibition of tumor growth (%)
ACM	2	19
Cysplatinum	1	47
	1.5	34
ACM + Cysplatinum	2 1	57
ACM + Cysplatinum	2 1.5	80

Intravenous injection from days 3–12.

2. Other actions

ACM has other effects on biological systems in addition to its cytocidal action. The drug stimulated antibody formation and potentiated immune responses (13, 32). Sartorelli and Moris (33) reported induction of human leukemia cell differentiation by ACM. Its effect on adriamycin-resistant Friend leukemia cells has been studied by Tapiero et al. (38). Pretreatment with ACM enhanced adriamycin accumulation in the cells and also the cytotoxicity of adriamycin. ACM enhanced cell killing by X-ray irradiation (24), which suggests another application of this drug in clinical use.

3. Mode of cytocidal action

ACM inhibits growth of tumor cells in vitro. L-cells (B929-L2J), grown for 4–5 hr, were treated with ACM, adriamycin or daunomycin for 1 hr and then the survival rate was measured. ACM exhibited a characteristic sigmoidal dose-response curve, while adriamycin and daunomycin gave a simple exponential one, which indicated the action mechanism of ACM is different from that of the others. The sigmoidal profile given by ACM was changed to a simple exponential curve by prolonged treatment for 24 hr. ACM blocks the cell cycle at the G_1-S border and the late S phase, while adriamycin reportedly blocks the G_2 phase (37). This supports that the ACM mode of cytocidal action differs from that of adriamycin.

ACM inhibits nucleic acid synthesis, which is believed to be the main mechanism of its cytocidal action. The drug reduced the amount of [^{14}C]uridine incorporated into mouse leukemia L1210 cells. Incorporation of [^{14}C]thymidine was also inhbited but the effective concentration of ACM for inhibition was much lower in case of uridine intake than thymidine intake (9). In other words, ACM inhibits RNA synthesis at a lower concentration than DNA synthesis. A similar inhibition pattern of nucleic acid synthesis was demonstrated in Novikoff hepatoma cells (1).

Crook et al. (1) and Egorin et al. (3) extensively studied anthracyclines from the view point of their nucleic acid synthesis inhibition pattern, subcellular distribution and cardiac toxicity in relation to their chemical structures. They grouped the anthracyclines into two classes: ACM was placed in Class II as a compound which inhibits RNA synthesis more highly than DNA synthesis. These compounds are distributed at a higher concentration to the cytoplasm than the nuclei, and have lower cardiac toxicity. Meanwhile, the compounds assigned to Class I including adriamycin inhibit DNA and RNA synthesis at a similar drug level; they are present in the nuclei, and show higher cardiac toxicity. The inhibition of RNA synthesis by ACM was also demonstrated by a molecular biological method. Treatment of tumor cells with ACM gave a characteristic sedimentation pattern of nuclear RNA fractions in ultracentrifugation, demonstrating that 45S preribosomal RNA synthesis was affected and that the synthesized RNA was significantly smaller than that synthesized in untreated cells (1).

ACM inhibited RNA polymerase II from mouse Ehrlich carcinoma cells with calf thymus double stranded DNA or synthetic poly (dAdT) as a template. Kinetic study revealed that the inhibition was competitive with the template DNA. This drug binds DNA molecules in vitro. Double stranded DNA possessed one binding site for ACM per 4 base pairs, according to an equilibrium experiment, while one binding site per 3 base pairs for adriamycin (17, 49).

From these results, the following action mechanism is suggested: ACM binds DNA and RNA synthesis is inhibited by the binding because the template activity of DNA is decreased. Thereby, DNA synthesis is also inhibited but RNA synthesis is more highly affected at the same drug concentration. Cell growth is blocked at the G_1-S border and late S phase of the cell cycle and then the cell is killed. This is one possible main mechanism for the cytocidal action of ACM.

4. Cardiac and other toxicities

ACM has a lower cardiac toxicity than adriamycin. The effect of ACM on the heart was thoroughly studied in hamsters, rats, and rabbits (2, 6, 48). High dosing of ACM showed the T wave flat in electrocardiogram (ECG), and a lethal dose gave ST segment depression and lengthening of the QT interval in addition to the abnormal T wave. These abnormalities caused by ACM were less severe than those by adriamycin, that is, similar ECG changes were caused by the latter drug even at a lower drug level. With cessation of ACM dosing the abnormal ECG recovered to normal (Table IV). Milder ultrastructural changes in the myocardium were demonstrated by treatment with ACM than with adriamycin. One of the reasons why the cardiac toxicity of ACM is lower than that of adriamycin may be the difference in elimination of the drug from the myocardium. ACM level in the heart muscle was higher than adriamycin level 5 min after intravenous

TABLE IV. Subacute Cardiac Toxicity of ACM and Adriamycin Abnormal ECG in Hamsters (6)

ECG parameters	ACM (mg/kg)			
	1.5		2.0	
	Dosing period	Observation period	Dosing period	Observation period
Heart rate	—	—	—	—
PR, PRc interval	—	—	—	—
QRS duration	↗	—	—	—
R wave	—	—	—	—
S wave	—	—	—	—
T wave	↓	—	↓	—
QT, QTc interval	—	—	—	—
Others	—	—	—	—

ECG parameters	Adriamycin (mg/kg)			
	0.17		0.5	
	Dosing period	Observation period	Dosing period	Observation period
Heart rate	—	—	—	—
PR, PRc interval	—	↗	—	↗
QRS duration	—	—	—	—
R wave	—	↗	↑	↑
S wave	—	—	—	↘
T wave	—	—	—	—
QT, QTc interval	—	—	—	—
Others	—	—	—	Arrhythmia

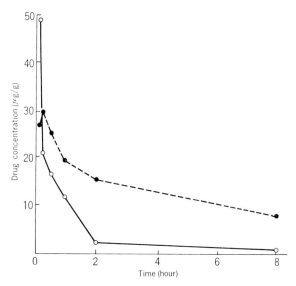

FIG. 2.   Heart muscle level of ACM (○) and adriamycin (●) in hamsters
    ACM or adriamycin was injected intravenously at a respective dose of 5 mg/ kg and drug level in the heart muscle was measured periodically from 5 min after injection.

injection to hamsters at 5 mg/kg. But these levels were reversed after only 15 min. ACM was reduced to an almost negligible concentration 2 hr after administration while adriamycin still remained at 8 μg/g even 8 hr later (Fig. 2).

LD_{50} value of ACM was 32–33 mg/kg in mice and 25–28 mg/kg in rats both by intravenous injection. Roughly twice higher LD_{50} value was obtained by oral administration than intravenous injection. The maximum tolerated dose by single intravenous injection was about 12 mg/kg for rats and 3 mg/kg for dogs, respectively. Subacute and chronic toxicity studies demonstrated that maximum tolerated dose by daily injection was 54 mg/kg for rats and 180 mg/kg for dogs, respectively (18, 34, 35, 41). Therefore, ACM can be administered at 4.5–60 times higher total dose by daily injection than single administration.

No mutagenicity of ACM was shown by Ames' test at a concentration of 5–100 nmol/plate, while adriamycin was mutagenic even at a 100-fold lower concentration (47).

In teratological studies in rats and rabbits (14–16), no malformation was caused by ACM administration during the gestation, prenatal or postnatal periods.

5. Pharmacodynamics

The blood level profile of ACM has two specific characteristics. The first is that the plasma level is lower than the blood cell level and the second is the very rapid elimination from the plasma. When ACM was injected intravenously to mice or dogs, the blood cell level was 2–3 times higher than the plasma level. The observed plasma levels were analyzed according to a three-compartment open model. The half lives of alpha, beta, and

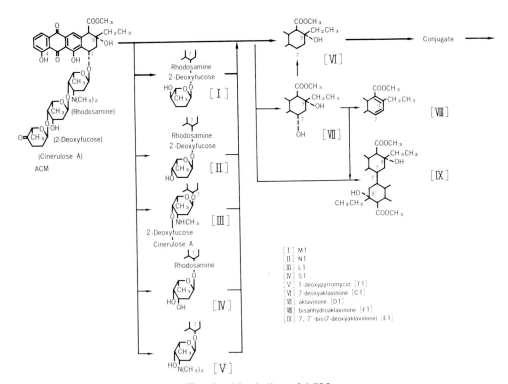

FIG. 3.   Metabolism of ACM

gamma phases were 0.0078 hr (28.1 sec), 0.113 hr (6.78 min), and 4.81 hr, respectively, in dogs. This very short half life of alpha phase is interpreted as being due to the immediate transfer of ACM from the blood to tissues of various organs, because the tissue level is much higher than the plasma level when the drug is injected intravenously (9).

The metabolism of ACM *in vivo* and *in vitro* has been studied (10, 30). Microsomal and cytosol reductases and other enzymes act on the drug under both anaerobic and aerobic conditions (31). Many metabolites were isolated and identified: M1, N1, L1, S1, T1, aklavinone, C1, E1, and F1. The glycoside compounds (M1, N1, L1, S1, and T1) showed antitumor activity but aglycones (aklavinone, C1, E1, and F1) were inactive. A possible pathway is presented (Fig. 3).

ACM and its metabolites were distributed at much higher concentration to various tissues than plasma (9). The plasma level in dogs was about 0.02μg/ml 2 hr after injection, while the average tissue level was roughly 2 μg/g or more. The tissue level was about 100 times higher than the plasma concentration; the lungs, spleen, and lymph nodes had high drug levels. In the liver, the metabolite level was higher than the ACM level, which indicates that a large part of ACM was decomposed in this organ.

Only about 2% of a dose of ACM was recovered in the urine as ACM and metabolites by 72 hr after injection. But in an experiment with [^{14}C]ACM 66% of the radioactivity was recovered in the urine and 20% in the feces (9, 10).

Pirarubicin ((2″R)-4′-O-tetrahydropyranyladriamycin, THP)

THP is a new anthracycline antitumor antibiotic which was derived chemically from adriamycin by introducing a tetrahydropyranyl group to the 4′-position through an ether linkage (Fig. 4) (46).

1. Activity on experimental tumors

THP has antitumor activity *in vivo* and *in vitro* equal to or greater than adriamycin. Notable increase in life span (ILS) and tumor growth inhibition activity *in vivo* were demonstrated on experimental mouse tumors such as L1210, P388, colon 26 in ascites type, and sarcoma 180, Ehrlich carcinoma, Lewis lung carcinoma, B16 melanoma, and colon 38 in solid type. Rat tumor Yoshida sarcoma was also susceptible to this drug (Table V). On L1210 leukemia is particular, a great ILS was achieved and many 60 day-survivors were observed (7, 23, 44, 45).

Administration of THP in combination with some other anticancer drugs gives synergistic activity. The effect of combination therapy of THP and other antitumor agents was examined on L1210 mice leukemia according to three dose schedules: in schedule A, THP and another drug were given intraperitoneally on days 1 to 10. In schedule B, THP was given on days 1 to 10 and the combined drug on days 1, 3, 5, 7, and 9, both intraperitoneally. In schedule C, THP and the combined drug were given intravenously on days 1, 3, 5, 7, and 9. The combination index (CI) is the ratio of combination ILS to the sum of THP and combined drug ILS values in their individual use. Combination of THP with cytosine arabinoside, 6-mercaptopurine or cyclophosphamide was particularly effective (Table VI) (23).

THP inhibited metastasis of Lewis lung carcinoma in mice much more effectively than adriamycin (44). Tumor cells were inoculated subcutaneously to mice and tumor nodules formed in the lungs by metastasis were counted microscopically. Metastasis in

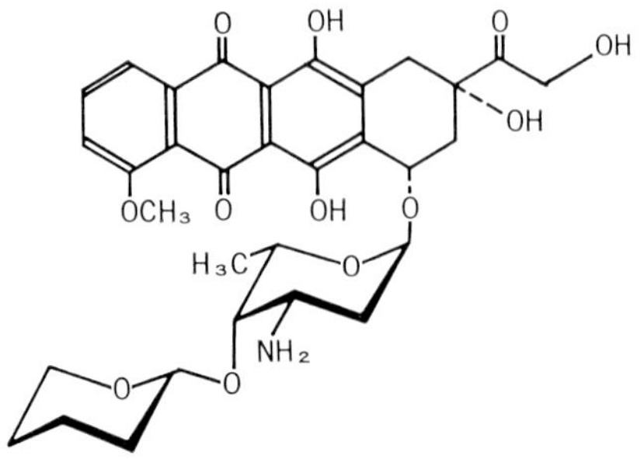

FIG. 4.   Structure of THP (46)

TABLE V.   Antitumor Activity of THP (7, 23, 44, 45)

Tumor	Drug administration		THP			Adriamycin		
	Route	Schedule	Opt. dose (ng/kg/ day)	ILS (%)	No. of survivor	Opt. dose (mg/kg/ day)	ILS (%)	No. of survivor
L1210 leukemia	i.p.	i.p. day 1–9	2.5	>147	1/12	2.5	118	0/12
	i.p.	i.p. day 1, 5, 9	8	>270	6/6	2	>190	2/6
	i.p.	i.v. day 1, 2	6.25	>183	4/6	6.25	113	0/6
P388	i.p.	i.p. day 1–9	2.5	>157	1/12	2.5	147	0/12
Colon 26	i.p.	i.p. q2d×5 (day 1–)	5	>95	2/10	1.25	>105	5/10
Ehrlich carc.	s.c.	i.p. day 1–7	3	61[a]	8/8	2	78[a]	8/8
Sarcoma 180	s.c.	i.p. day 1–7	4	77[a]	8/8	2	58[a]	8/8
Lewis lung carc.	s.c.	i.p. q2d×5 (day 1–)	5	58	0/10	1.25	27	0/10
B16 melanoma	s.c.	i.p. q2d×5 (day 1–)	5	39	0/10	2.5	−3	0/10
Colon 38	s.c.	i.p. q2d×5 (day 1–)	5	42	0/10	1.25	−6	0/10
Yoshida sarcoma	i.p.	i.p. day 1	10	>298	3/5	5	>277	2/5
Walker C.S. 256	s.c.	i.p. day 1	10	5[a]	4/5	5	−15[a]	5/5

[a] Inhibition ratio (%).

TABLE VI.   Antitumor Effect of THP on L1210 in Combination
with Various Antitumor Agents (23)

Combined drug	Schedule A THP, comb. drug days 1–10		Schedule B THP, day 1–10 comb. drug days 1, 3, 5, 7, 9 i.p.		Schedule C THP, comb. drug days 1, 3, 5, 7, 9	
	ILS	CI	ILS	CI	ILS	CI
Cytosine arabinoside	498	3.5	492	2.6	475	4.4
6-Mercaptopurine	444	3.4	—	—	—	—
Methotrexate	233	1.4	246	1.2	—	—
5-Fluorouracil	188	1.4	209	—	69	0.6
Cyclophosphamide	490	2.4	624	2.2	302	1.6
Mitomycin C	164	1.3	398	1.9	—	—
Vincristine	310	2.1	174	—	47	0.8
ACNU	386	2.2	—	—	—	—

ILS, increase in life span (%); CI, combination index = (combination therapy: ILS)/THP: ILS+comb.
drug: ILS); Dose: 1/(2–3) of opt. dose for each drug.

the control, which was without drug treatment, was calculated at 100%. Treatment with THP at a dose of 5 mg/kg/day on days 1, 2, 5, 7, and 9, gave only 1.1% metastasis; that is, about 99% of the metastasis was inhibited. On the other hand, the best value with adriamycin was 33.4% metastasis, or 66.6% inhibition at 2.5 mg/kg/day with a toxic effect.

2. Mode of action

THP is rapidly incorporated into tumor cells. Mouse lymphoma L5178Y cells were incubated with THP or adriamycin *in vitro*. The uptake velocity of THP was about 170 times higher than that of adriamycin. About 74% of THP or adriamycin was distributed to the nuclei fraction after 10 min of incubation (20). According to Munck *et al.* (25) over 95% of the incorporated THP or adriamycin was localized in the nuclei fraction in a similar experiment with Friend leukemia cells.

THP inhibited the growth of animal and human tumor cells *in vitro*; specifically, it inhibited the incorporation of thymidine or uridine into the nucleic acid fraction (23). In a flow cytometry experiment (36), treatment of human leukemia cell RPMI8402 with THP showdd an accumulation of cells of the G_2 and M stage at the concentration where the cell growth was suppressed. Therefore THP was distributed to the nuclei after rapid incorporation into cells and they might be killed after G_2 block of cell cycle.

3. Toxicity

The toxicity of THP is lower than that of adriamycin. LD_{50} values in acute toxicity of THP were 14.5 and 14.1 mg/kg in male and female mice, respectively; the LD_{50} of adriamycin was 9 to 10. A long-term toxicity study confirmed that this new drug was less toxic than adriamycin (21, 22, 42, 43).

Cardiac toxicity, a well-known adverse effect of anthracycline antitumor agents, was examined in hamsters. Intravenous injection of THP at a dose of 25 mg/kg caused almost equal ECG changes to those caused by adriamycin at a dose of 3.13 mg/kg. The acute cardiac toxicity of THP was thus shown to be roughly 7 times lower than that of adriamycin. The toxic effect of THP on the cardiac function was also lower than adriamycin in a subacute experiment in which the drugs were injected to hamsters for 15 days (39).

4. Pharmacokinetics and metabolism

THP-plasma levels in mice and dogs were measured by high performance liquid chromatography beginning 20 min after intravenous injection. The data were then processed by computer according to a three compartment model and several kinetic parameters were obtained. The plasma level of THP decreased rapidly in both animals with half-lives in the alpha phase of 0.45 min in mice and 0.7 min in dogs. When adriamycin was injected, the times were 0.77 min and 2.7 min, respectively (Fig. 5). These data show that THP disappeared from the plasma in dogs about 4 times faster than adriamycin. In the beta and gamma phases, the *t*-halves of THP were about 3 to 4 times shorter than those of adriamycin (11, 12).

High THP concentration was detected in the lung, spleen, kidney, and lymph nodes 2 hr after intravenous injection. The tissue level of THP was much higher than the plasma level. For example, the lung level was about 15 μg/g 2 hr after injection, while the plasma level had decreased to less than 0.1 μg/ml 30 min after administration. Concentrations in tissue such as the lung and spleen thus reached about 300 times higher than those in the

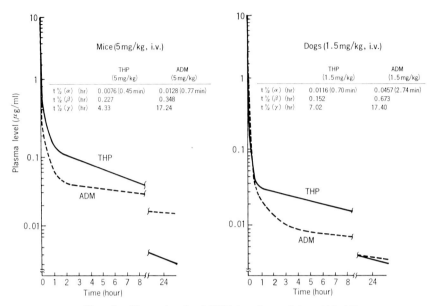

FIG. 5.   Plasma levels of THP in mice and dogs (*11, 12*)

THP or adriamycin (ADM) was respectively injected intravenously to mice or dogs at the indicated doses. The obtained plasma levels were analyzed with the NONLIN computer program according to a three-compartment model.

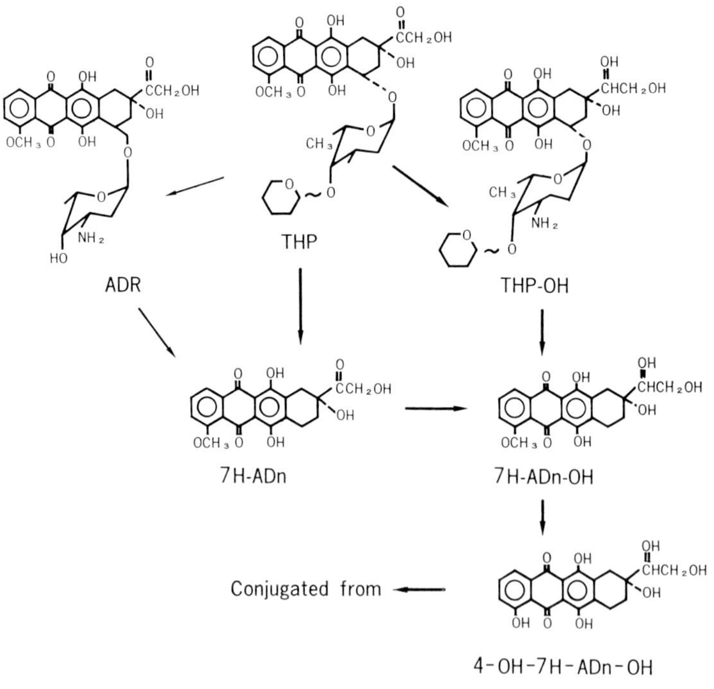

FIG. 6.   A possible metabolic pathway of THP

THP-OH, 13-dihydro-THP; 7H-ADn, 7-deoxyadriamycinone; 7H-ADn-OH, 7-deoxy-13-dihydroadriamycinone; 4-OH-7H-ADn-OH, 4-O-demethyl-7-deoxy-13-dihydroadriamycinone; ADR, adriamycin.

plasma. As shown by the short *t*-half, THP is transferred from the plasma to tissues very rapidly.

The distribution pattern was somewhat different from that of adriamycin. In addition, THP levels in these tissues decreased faster than those of adriamycin, as shown by the differences between the levels after 2 and 8 hr. Some drug accumulation occurred in the thymus, lymph nodes, and bone marrow, however (*12*).

Based on experimental results such as the metabolite analysis of tissues and urines (*11, 12*), radioisotope experiments (*40*), and enzymatic and *in vitro* degradation of THP (*5*), the possible metabolic pathway of THP was presumed (Fig. 6). THP is degraded to aglycones by the removal of the sugar moiety directly from THP or after reduction at the 13-position. The formation of aglycone is thought to be the main path for several reasons. Aglycone levels in most tissues were much higher when THP was given than when adriamycin was injected. High levels of aglycones were also detected during *in vitro* degradation, but almost no glycosides were found; therefore, a large part of the THP injected was metabolized according to this pathway. But a low level of adriamycin was detected in some tissues after THP injection; there may thus be a minor path of adriamycin formation in some tissues, such as the liver. Adriamycin was detectable because of its very slow tissue clearance.

These two anthracycline antitumor antibiotics, ACM and THP, are quite interesting basically and clinically. Particularly high efficacy is shown against adult myelocytic leukemia by ACM and against head and neck cancer and ovarian tumor by THP. Both have minimal side effects and little cardiac toxicity. Anthracycline resistance, immune response, and cell differentiation are also affected by ACM.

REFERENCES

1. Crooke, S. T., Duvernay, V. H., Galvan, L., and Prestayko, A. W. Structure-activity relationships of anthracyclines relative to effects on macromolecular syntheses. *Mol. Pharmacol.*, **14**, 290–298 (1978).

2. Dantchev, D., Slioussartchouk, V., Paintrand, M., Hayat, M., Bourut, C., and Mathé, G. Electron microscopic studies of the heart and light microscopic studies of the skin after treatment of golden hamsters with adriamycin, detorubicin, AD-32 and aclacinomycin. *Cancer Treat. Rep.*, **63**, 875–888 (1979).

3. Egorin, M. J., Clawson, R. E., Ross, L. A., Schlossberger, N. M., and Bachur, N. R. Cellular accumulation and disposition of aclacinomycin A. *Cancer Res.*, **39**, 4396–4400 (1979).

4. Fujimoto, S., Inagaki, J., Horikoshi, N., and Ogawa, M. Combination chemotherapy with a new anthracycline glycoside, aclacinomycin-A, and active drugs for malignant lymphomas in P388 mouse leukemia system. *Gann*, **70**, 411–420 (1979).

5. Fujita, H., Tone, H., Iguchi, H., and Shoumura, T. Pharmacodynamics of anticancer agents. Adriamycin, THP-adriamycin and aclacinomycin. *Oncologia*, **7**, 92–106 (1983) (in Japanese).

6. Hirano, S., Tone, H., and Sunaga, T. Cardiotoxic study of aclacinomycin A. Subacute cardiotoxicity of aclacinomycin A and its recovery in hamsters. *Jpn. J. Antibiot.*, **33**, 268–280 (1980) (in Japanese).

7. Hisamatsu, T., Suzuki, K., Sakakibara, S., Komuro, K., Nagasawa, M., Takeuchi, T., and Umezawa, H. Antitumor spectrum of a new anthracycline, (2″R)-4′-O-tetrahydropyranyladriamycin, and effect on the cellular immune response in mice. *Jpn. J. Cancer Res. (Gann)*, **74**, 1008–1020 (1985).

8. Hori, S., Shirai, M., Hirano, S., Oki, T., Inui, T., Tsukagoshi, S., Ishizuka, M., Takeuchi, T., and Umezawa, H. Antitumor activity of new anthracycline antibiotics, aclacinomycin A and its analogs, and their toxicity. *Gann*, **48**, 685–690 (1977).

9. Iguchi, H., Matsushita, Y., Ohmori, K., Hirano, S., Kiyosaki, T., Hori, S., Tone, H.,
   and Oki, T. Studies on the absorption, excretion and distribution of aclacinomycin A:
   absorption, excretion and distribution of aclacinomycin A in mice, rabbits and dogs by
   photometric assay. *Jpn. J. Antibiot.*, **33**, 179–191 (1980) (in Japanese).

10. Iguchi, H., Seryu, Y., Kiyosaki, T., Hori, S., Tone, H., and Oki, T. Studies on the ab-
    sorption, excretion and distribution of aclacinomycin A: absorption, excretion and distri-
    bution of ^{14}C- or ^{3}H-aclacinomycin A in mice, rats and rabbits. *Jpn. J. Antibiot.*, **33**, 169–
    178 (1980) (in Japanese).

11. Iguchi, H., Tone, H., Ishikura, T., Takeuchi, T., and Umezawa, H. Pharmacokinetics
    and disposition of 4′-O-tetrahydropyranyladriamycin in mice by HPLC analysis. *Cancer
    Chemother. Pharmacol.*, **15**, 132–140 (1985).

12. Iguchi, H., Tone, H., Kiyosaki, T., and Ishikura, T. Pharmacokinetics and disposition of
    (2″R)-4′-O-tetrahydropyranyladriamycin in dogs. *Jpn. J. Antibiot.*, **39**, 638–652 (1986)
    (in Japanese).

13. Ishizuka, M., Takeuchi, T., Masuda, T., Fukasawa, S., and Umezawa, H. Enhancement
    of immune responses and possible inhibition of suppressor cells by aclacinomycin A.
    J. Antibiot., **34**, 331–340 (1981).

14. Kamata, K., Tomizawa, S., Sato, R., and Kashima, M. Teratological studies on aclacino-
    mycin A: Effect of aclacinomycin A on rat fetus. *Pharmacometrics*, **19**, 783–790 (1980)
    (in Japanese).

15. Kamata, K., Tomizawa, S., Sato, R., and Kashima, M. Teratological studies on aclacino-
    mycin A: effect of aclacinomycin A on reproductive performance and teratogenicity in
    rats. *Pharmacometrics*, **19**, 875–885 (1980) (in Japanese).

16. Kamata, K., Tomizawa, S., Sato, R., and Kashima, M. Teratological studies on aclacino-
    mycin A: effect of aclacinomycin A on rabbit fetus. *Pharmacometrics*, **19**, 887–894 (1980)
    (in Japanese).

17. Katenkamp, U., Stretter, E., Petri, I., Gollmick, F. A., and Berg, H. Interaction of an-
    thracycline antibiotics with biopolymers. VII. Binding parameters of aclacinomycin A
    to DNA. *J. Antibiot.*, **36**, 1222–1227 (1983).

18. Kawamura, K., Tomizawa, S., Sato, H., Sato, M., and Kashima, M. Chronic toxicity of
    aclacinomycin A in dogs. *Pharmacometrics*, **19**, 756–781 (1980) (in Japanese).

19. Kubota, T., Shimosato, Y., Moon, Y., H., Matsumoto, S., Ishibiki, K., and Abe, O.
    Experimental cancer chemotherapy of human stomach and colon carcinomas serially
    transplanted in nude mice. IV. Anthracyclines. *Jpn. J. Cancer Chemother.*, **5**, 535–543
    (1978) (in Japanese).

20. Kunimoto, S., Miura, K., Takahashi, Y., Takeuchi, T., and Umezawa, H. Rapid uptake
    by cultured tumor cells and intracellular behavior of 4′-O-tetrahydropyranyladriamycin.
    J. Antibiot., **34**, 312–317 (1983).

21. Kurebe, M., Sasaki, H., Niizato, T., Miki, M., and Kajita, T. Toxicological studies on
    (2″R)-4′-O-tetrahydropyranyladriamycin, a new antitumor antibiotic. Its acute toxicity
    in rats. *Jpn. J. Antibiot.*, **39**, 259–263 (1986) (in Japanese).

22. Kurebe, M., Yokota, M., Chesterman, H., Massay, J. E., and Gopinath, C. Studies on
    (2″R)-4′-O-tetrahydropyranyladriamycin, a new antitumor antibiotic. Its subacute toxi-
    city in dogs. *Jpn. J. Antibiot.*, **39**, 351–386 (1986) (in Japanese).

23. Matsushita, Y., Kumagai, H., Yoshimoto, A., Tone, H., Ishikura, T., Takeuchi, T., and
    Umezawa, H. Antitumor activities of (2″R)-4′-O-tetrahydropyranyladriamycin (THP)
    and its combination with other antitumor agents on murine tumors. *J. Antibiot.*, **38**, 1408–
    1419 (1985).

24. Miyamoto, T., Wakabayashi, M., and Terashima, T. Aclarubicin (aclacinomycin A) and irradiation: Evaluation using HeLa cells. *Radiology*, **149**, 835–839 (1983).

25. Munck, J. N., Fourcade, A., Bennoun, M., and Tapiero, H. Relationship between the intracellular level and growth inhibition of a new anthracycline 4'-O-tetrahydropyranyl-adriamycin in Friend leukemia cell variants. *Leuk. Res.*, **9**, 289–296 (1985).

26. Oki, T. New anthracycline antibiotics. *Jpn. J. Antibiot.*, **30** (Suppl.), s70–s84 (1977) (in Japanese).

27. Oki, T., Kitamura, I., Matsuzawa, Y., Shibamoto, N., Ogasawara, T., Yoshimoto, A., Inui, T., Naganawa, H., Takeuchi, T., and Umezawa, H. Antitumor anthracycline antibiotics, aclacinomycin A and analogues. II. Structure determination. *J. Antibiot.*, **32**, 801–819 (1979).

28. Oki, T., Kitamura, I., Yoshimoto, A., Matsuzawa, Y., Shibamoto, N., Ogasawara, T., Inui, T., Takamatsu, A., Takeuchi, T., Masuda, T., Hamada, M., Suda, H., Ishizuka, M., Sawa, T., and Umezawa, H. Antitumor anthracycline antibiotics, aclacinomycin A and analogues. I. Taxonomy, production, isolation and physico-chemical properties. *J. Antibiot.*, **32**, 791–800 (1979).

29. Oki, T., Matsuzawa, Y., Yoshimoto, H., Numata, K., Kitamura, I., Hori, S., Takamatsu, A., Umezawa, H., Ishizuka, M., Naganawa, H., Suda, H., Hamada, M., and Takeuchi, T. New antitumor antibiotics, aclacinomycin A and B. *J. Antibiot.*, **28**, 830–834 (1975).

30. Oki, T., Shibamoto, N., Iguchi, H., and Shirai, M. Metabolism of aclacinomycin A. *Jpn. J. Antibiot.*, **33**, 163–168 (1980) (in Japanese).

31. Oki, T., Komiyama, T., Tone, H., Inui, T., Takeuchi, T., and Umezawa, H. Reductive cleavage of anthracycline glycosides by microsomal NADPH-cytochrome *C* reductase. *J. Antibiot.*, **30**, 613–615 (1977).

32. Orbach-Arbouys, S., Andrade-Mena, C. E., Berardet, M., and Mathé, G. Potentiated immune responses after administration of aclacinomycin. *Int. Arch Allergy Appl. Immunol.*, **68**, 117–121 (1982).

33. Sartorelli, A. C. and Morin, M. J. Inhibition of glycoprotein biosynthesis by the inducers of HL-60 cell differentiation, aclacinomycin A and marcellomycin. *Cancer Res.*, **44**, 2807–2812 (1984).

34. Shirai, M., Ohmori, K., Hirano, S., Iguchi, H., and Hori, S. Chronic toxicity of aclacinomycin A in rats. *Jpn. J. Antibiot.*, **33**, 294–319 (1980) (in Japanese).

35. Shirai, M., Ohmori, K., Hirano, S., Iguchi, H., Hori, S., and Sato, H. Acute toxicity of aclacinomycin A in mice, rats and dogs. *Jpn. J. Antibiot.*, **33**, 138–149 (1980) (in Japanese).

36. Takamoto, S. and Ota, K. Flow cytometric analysis of the effect of THP-adriamycin on the cell cycle traverse of PRMI-8402 cells. *Jpn. J. Cancer Chemother.*, **13**, 1868–1875 (1986) (in Japanese).

37. Tanabe, M., Miyamoto, T., Nakajima, Y., and Terashima, T. Lethal effect of aclacinomycin A on cultured mouse L cells. *Gann*, **71**, 699–703 (1980).

38. Tapiero, H., Boule, D., Trincal, G., Fourcade, A., and Lampidis, T. J. Potentiation of adriamycin accumulation and effectiveness in adriamycin-resistant cells by aclacinomycin A. *Leuk. Res.*, **12**, 411–418 (1988).

39. Tone, H., Hirano, S., Shirai, M., Kumagai, H., Okajima, Y., and Wakabayashi, T. Effect of (2''R)-4'-O-tetrahydropyranyladriamycin, a new antitumor antibiotic, on the cardiac function of hamsters. *Jpn. J. Antibiot.*, **39**, 547–568 (1986) (in Japanese).

40. Tone, H., Iguchi, H., Fujigaki, M., Nishio, M., Esumi, Y., Takeichi, M., Tsutsumi, S., and Yokoshima, T. Pharmacokinetics and disposition of a new anticancer antibiotic (2''R)-4'-O-tetrahydropyranyladriamycin in rats. Distribution and excretion after a single administration. *Jpn. J. Antibiot.*, **39**. 612–628 (1986) (in Japanese).

41. Tone, H., Nishida, H., Takeuchi, T., and Umezawa, H. Experimental studies on aclacinomycin. *Drugs Res. Exp. Clin.*, **11**, 9–15 (1985).

42. Tone, H., Shirai, M., Danks, A. P., Lee, P., Finn, J. P., and Ashby, R. Toxicological studies on (2″R)-4′-O-tetrahydropyranyladriamycin, a new antitumor antibiotic. Subacute toxicity study in rats. *Jpn. J. Antibiot.*, **39**(2), 327–350 (1986) (in Japanese).

43. Tone, H., Shirai, M., Onoue, F., and Kumagai, H. Toxicological studies on (2″R)-4′-O-tetrahydropyranyladriamycin, a new antitumor antibiotic. Acute toxicity study in mice. *Jpn. J. Antibiot.*, **39**, 250–258 (1986) (in Japanese).

44. Tsuruo, T., Iida, H., Tsukagoshi, S., and Sakurai, Y. 4′-O-Tetrahydropyranyladriamycin as a potential new antitumor agent. *Cancer Res.*, **42**, 1462–1467 (1982).

45. Umezawa, H., Takahashi, Y., Kinoshita, M., Naganawa, H., Masuda, T., Ishizuka, M., Tatsuta, K., and Takeuchi, T. Tetrahydropyranyl derivatives of daunomycin and adriamycin. *J. Antibiot.*, **32**, 1082–1084 (1979).

46. Umezawa, H., Takahashi, Y., Takeuchi, T., Nakamura, H., Iitaka, Y., and Tatsuta, K. The absolute structures of THP-adriamycins. *J. Antibiot.*, **37**, 1094–1097 (1984).

47. Umezawa, K., Sawamura, M., Matsushima, T., and Sugimura, T. Mutagenicity of aclacinomycin A and daunomycin derivatives. *Cancer Res.*, **38**, 1782–1784 (1978).

48. Wakabayashi, T., Oki, T., Tone, H., Hirano, S., and Ohmori, K. A comparative electron microscopic study of aclacinomycin and adriamycin cardiotoxicities in rabbits and hamsters. *J. Electron Microsc.*, **29**, 106–118 (1980).

49. Yamaki, H., Suzuki, H., Nishimura, T., and Tanaka, N. Mechanism of action of aclacinomycin A1. The effect on macromolecular synthesis. *J. Antibiot.*, **31**, 1149–1154 (1978).

COMPARATIVE EXPERIMENTAL STUDY AND EVALUATION OF CARDIOTOXICITY AND SKIN TOXICITY OF TWELVE ANTHRACYCLINE ANALOGS AND ONE ANTHRACENEDIONE

D. Dantchev, A. Anjo, C. Bourut, M. Reynes, and G. Mathé

*Institut de Cancérologie et d'Immunogénétique (Univ. Paris-Sud, CNRS UA 04-1163, Ass. Cl. Bernard and ARC), Hôpital Paul-Brousse**

Golden hamsters were submitted three times a week for 4 weeks to intraperitoneal (i.p.) administration of one anthracenedione, the mitoxantrone (MTN), and 12 different anthracyclines: adriamycin (ADM), daunorubicin (DNR), detorubicin (DTR), 4'-epi-adriamycin (e-ADM), rubidazon (RBZ), aclacinomycin (ACM), N-trifluoroacetyladriamycin-14-valerate (AD-32), tetrahydropyranyladriamycin (THP-ADM), N-L-leucyldaunorubicin (1-DNR), carminomycin (CAM), rubicyclamin (RBC), and N-trifluoroacetyladriamycin-14-9-hemiadipate (AD-143), at doses equivalent to 3/4 of those which are optimally oncostatic on murine L1210 leukemia. The electron microscopic study of the myocardium showed that all studied drugs are cardiotoxic, but the degree of this cardiotoxicity is different. A histopathological study of the skin detected degenerative lesions with different degree of alopecia.

According to the degree of their cardiotoxicity, skin toxicity, and general toxicity or mortality, all studied drugs were classified into three groups: 1st group, ADM, DNR, 1-DNR, and RBZ, causing very severe cardiac alterations and alopecia (grade 2–3), and very high mortality; 2nd group, e-ADM, DTR, CAM, RBC, and MTN, causing less severe cardiac alterations and alopecia (grade 1–2), and always high mortality, and 3rd group, ACM, THP-ADM, AD-32, and AD-143, causing less severe myocardial alterations (grade 1), without alopecia (grade 0), and extremely low mortality and general toxicity.

Cardiotoxicity and alopecia are the two main limiting factors for the use of anthracyclines in antitumor chemotherapy. At the suggestion of Professor G. Mathé, we set up with him as early as 1976 an experimental hamster model to study by electron microscopy (EM), the cardiotoxicity and, by photon microscopy, the toxicity of the skin, of anthracyclines and some other drugs.

In this paper, we summarize the methods used and the results of 12 studied anthracyclines and one anthracenedione, the mitoxantrone, as published in previous reports (2–6). We describe also the application of this method for the classification of studied drugs taking into account cardiotoxicity, dermal toxicity and mortality or general toxicity.

---

* 94804-Villejuif, France.

Experiments were conducted as follows: twenty-four adult female golden hamsters were used for testing each drug, 12 of which were used for evaluation of mortality. They received an intrapertitoneal (i.p.) administration 3 times a week for 4 weeks, a dose equivalent to 3/4 of the optimal oncostatic dose on murine L1210 leukemia, injected at days 1, 5, and 9 after tumor cell inoculation (7). Each week, 3 hamsters for each drug and 3 controls were sacrificed, and the tissues of interest were quickly removed, the ventricular cross (apices) being immediately fixed for transmission EM study; other tissues, particularly skin were collected for light microscopic (LM) examination. Table I shows the studied drugs and doses used. Using equivalent doses and always under the same experimental conditions, our method permitted us to make comparative evaluations on the *mortality* due to general toxicity, the *cardiotoxicity*, and the *skin-toxicity* of each drug.

TABLE I. Drug Studied and Dose Used in Hamster

Drug	Dose used in hamster (mg/kg)
Adriamycin (ADM)	3
Daunorubicin (DNR)	3
Detorubicin (DTR)	3
4′epi-adriamycin (e-ADM)	3
Rubidazone (RBZ)	9
Aclacinomycin (ACM)	6
N-trifluoroacetyladriamycin-14-valerate (AD-32)	30
Tetrahydropyranyladriamycin (THP-ADM)	3
L-1-Leucil-daunorubicin (1-DNR)	6
Carminomycin (CAM)	0.15
Mitoxantrone (MTN)	1
Rubicyclamine (RBC)	7.5
N-trifluoroacetyladriamycin-14-O-hemiadipate (AD-143)	30

TABLE II. Mortality Due to Toxicity of Drug-treated Animals (12 animals per group) with the Number of Surviving Animals at the End of Each Week

	No. of animals surviving at the end of:			
	1st week	2nd week	3rd week	4th week
ADM	12	7	0	0
DNR	12	7	0	0
DTR	12	7	4	0
e-ADM	12	12	7	0
RBZ	12	6	0	0
ACM	12	12	11	11
AD-32	12	12	12	11
THP-ADM	12	12	12	12
1-DNR	12	8	0	0
CAM	12	11	4	0
MTN	12	11	5	0
RBC	11	11	9	7
AD-143	12	12	12	12

Mortality Due to General Toxicity

Table II shows the mortality of drug-treated animals due to toxicity with the number of surviving animals at the end of each week. The mortality was very high for the animals treated with 9 of the 13 drugs: adriamycin (ADM), detorubicin (DTR), daunorubicin (DNR), 4'-epi-adriamycin (e-ADM), rubidazon (RBZ), N-L-leucyldaunorubicine (1-DNR), carminomycin (CAM), rubicyclamin (RBC), mitoxantrone (MTN); almost all animals were dead before the end of the 4th week, with more or less loss of hair, of body weight and with severe digestive troubles. On the contrary, mortality was very low or null for the animals receiving acracinomycin (ACM), tetrahydropyranyladriamycin (THP-ADM), N-trifluoroacetyladriamycin-14-valerate (AD-32), and N-trifluoroacetyl-adriamycin-14-9-hemiadipate (AD-143); all these animals preserved their good general status, without loss of body weight, without digestive troubles, and without loss of hair.

Electron Microscopic Alterations of the Myocardium

In order to establish a comparative appreciation of the degree change in myocardium as shown by EM ,we used a grading system derived from that of Billingham *et al.* (*1*). Grade 0 was used for a normal cardiac morphology; grade 1 was cases with moderate alterations; grade 2 was used when more than 50% of myocardial cells showed severe alterations, and grade 3 when the myocardium was diffusely affected by very severe cell alterations. We also used the intermediate grades 0–1, 1–2, and 2–3 to indicate that about half of the myocardial cells showed the morphologic structure or changes of each of the two grades. Table III summarizes the degree of myocardial EM alterations according to our semiquantitative grading system.

Photo 1 shows an example of normal EM structure of the myocardium classified as grade 0 and observed at the end of the 1st week of treatment with ACM: sarcomeres, myofilaments, mitochondria, and intercalated disks are in as good condition as those of controls.

Photo 2 illustrates an example of moderate myocardial alterations classified as grade 1 and observed at the end of the 1st week of treatment with DTR, with a swelling of mitochondria, clearing of their matrices and lysis of their crests, separation and lysis of myofilaments, and disruption of Z-band registry.

Photo 3 shows an example of severe myocardial alterations classified as grade 2 and observed at the end of the 1st week of treatment with DNR, with swelling of mitochondria, clearing of their matrices and lysis of the crests, clumping of the chromatine into electron-dense masses adjacent to the nuclear membrane and to the nucleoli, separation of the fascia adherence of the intercalated disks and formation of myelinic figures.

TABLE III.   Degree of Myocardial Electron Microscopic Alterations at the End of
Each Week According to a Semi-quantitative Grading System

Grade 0:	no pathologic alterations
Grade 1:	moderate cell alterations
Grade 2:	severe cell alterations
Grade 3:	very severe cell alterations

Intermediate grades of 0–1, 1–2, and 2–3 indicate that about half of myocardial cells showed the morphologic structure or alterations of each of the two grades.

112   D. DANTCHEV ET AL.

TABLE IV. Degree of Cardiotoxicity for Each Drug at the End of Each Week

| | Degree of toxicity at the end of: | | | |
	1st week	2nd week	3rd week	4th week
ADM	1–2	2–3	—	—
DNR	1–2	2–3	—	—
DTR	0–1	1–2	1–2	—
e-ADM	0–1	1–2	2	—
RBZ	1–2	2–3	—	—
ACM	0–1	1	1	1
AD-32	0–1	1	1	1
THP-ADM	0–1	0–1	1	1
1-DNR	1	1–2	2–3	—
CAM	0–1	1–2	2–3	—
MTN	0–1	1	1–2	—
RBC	0–1	1	1–2	1–2
AD-143	0–1	1	1	1
Controls	0	0	0	0

TABLE V. Classification in Three Groups of Studied Drugs According to the Degree of Their Cardiotoxicity and General Toxicity or Mortality

| | | Degree of myocardial alterations at the end of: | | | |
		1st week	2nd week	3rd week	4th week
First group:					
Very severe myocardial alterations	ADM	1–2	2–3	—	—
(Gr 2–3) and very high mortality	DNR	1–2	2–3	—	—
	1-DNR	1	1–2	2–3	—
	RBZ	1–2	2–3	—	—
Second group:					
Less severe myocardial alterations	e-ADM	0–1	1–2	2	—
(Gr 1–2) and high mortality	DTR	0–1	1–2	1–2	—
	CAM	0–1	1–2	2	—
	MTN	0–1	1	1–2	1–2
	RBC	0–1	1	1–2	—
Third group:					
Less severe myocardial alterations	ACM	0–1	1	1	1
(Gr 1) and very low mortality	THP-ADM	0–1	0–1	1	1
	AD-32	0–1	0–1	1	1
	AD-143	0–1	0–1	0–1	1

Photo 4 shows an example of very severe myocardial alterations classified as grade 3 and observed at the end of the 2nd week of treatment with DNR, with dilatation of sarcoplasmic reticulum, separation and lysis of myofilaments, condensation of the chromatine into electron-dense masses, separation of intercalated disks, formation of empty spaces, myelinic figures and vacuolisation.

Table IV shows the degree of cardiotoxicity for each studied drug at the end of each week. It is evident that, under our experimental conditions, all studied anthracycline analogs and the mitoxantrone were cardiotoxic, but the degree of this cardiotoxicity differed.

According to the degree of their cardiotoxic effect and their mortality or general toxicity, it is possible to classify all studied drugs into three groups.

The *first group* causes very severe myocardial alteration (grade 2–3) and very high mortality, and includes ADM, DNR, 1-DNR, and RBZ.

The *second group* causes less severe myocardial alterations (grade 1–2), but always very high mortality or general toxicity, and includes e-ADM, DTR, CAM, RBC, and MTN.

The *third group* causes moderate myocalrdial alterations (grade 1), and very low mortality and general toxicity, and includes ACM, THP-ADM, AD-32, and AD-143. Almost all animals treated with the last four drugs survived after the 4 weeks of treatment (Table II) with well-preserved general status, and two months after cessation of the treatment the EM study of their myocardium revealed a recovery of myocardial alterations.

Table V summarizes this classification with the degree of cardiotoxicity at the end of each week and for each drug.

Histopathologic Lesions of the Skin

The study of the skin histology permits us to detect degenerative lesions associated with alopecia. Using the same grading system and classification of the drugs, a comparative study indicated a close correlation between the cardiac and skin toxic effects in the three drug groups. All the very cardiotoxic drugs classified in the first group (ADM, DNR, 1-DNR, and RBZ) were also very toxic for the skin and caused atrophy of all epidermal layers and a marked loss of hair. Photo 5 A shows an example of this histopathological structure of the skin at the end of the 2nd and 3rd week of treatment with ADM, with severe atrophy of epidermal layers and disappearance of the hair.

The five drugs included in the second group (e-ADM, DTR, CAM, RBC, and MTN), which are less cardiotoxic, also showed less skin toxicity and only moderate alopecia. Photo 5 B shows an example of moderate degenerative alterations of epidermal

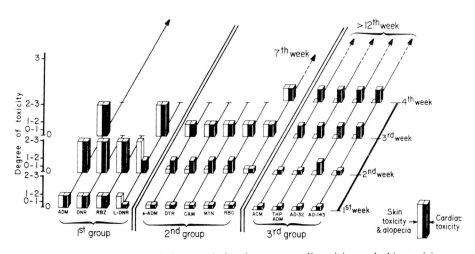

FIG. 1. Histograms of the correlation between cardiotoxicity and skin toxicity (alopecia) in the three drug groups of our classification

cells and the morphologic structure of the hair which still looked like those of controls at the end of the 2nd week of treatment with MTN.

The four anthracyclines included in the third group (ACM, THP-ADM, AD-32, and AD-143), which are also less cardiotoxic and with a very low general toxicity and mortality, do not cause skin toxicity. Photo 5C shows an example of normal histologic structure of the skin, without alopecia, at the end of the 4th week of treatment with ACM.

Figure 1 shows the histograms of these correlations between cardiac and skin toxic effects in the three drug groups of our classification.

CONCLUSION

In conclusion, in golden hamsters, after i.p. administration of 12 anthracyclines and one anthracenedione, MTN, an EM study of the myocardium showed that all these drugs were cardiotoxic, however, the degree of this cardiotoxicity varied. The comparative study of the degree of the cardiotoxicity, skin toxicity, and general toxicity or mortality, was the basis for classification of the drugs into three groups. ACM, THP-ADM, AD-32, and AD-143 were classified as the least cardiotoxic and almost without skin toxicity. If with this lower toxicity the clinical observations of those drugs confirm a good antitumor activity, they will be an important contribution to the chemotherapy of neoplasias.

Acknowledgments

The authors express their gratitude to Mrs. G. Martin for the iconographic reproduction and to Nicole Vriz for the preparation of the manuscript.

REFERENCES

1. Billingham, M. A., Mason, J. W., Briston, M. R., and Daniel, J. R. Anthracycline cardiomyopathy monitored by morphologic changes. *Cancer Treat. Rep.*, **62**, 865–872 (1978).
2. Dantchev, D., Slioussartchouk, V., Paintrand, M., Hayat, M., Bourut, C., and Mathé, G. Electron microscopic studies of the heart and light microscopic studies of the skin after treatment of golden hamsters with adriamycin, detorubicin, AD-32 and aclacinomycin. *Cancer Treat. Rep.*, **63**, 875–878 (1979).
3. Dantchev, D., Slioussartchouk, V., Paintrand, M., Bourut, C., Hayat, M., and Mathé, G. Ultrastructural study of the cardiotoxicity and light-microscopic findings of the skin after treatment of golden hamsters with seven different anthracyclines. *In* "Cancer Chemo- and Immunopharmacology. 1. Chemopharmacology," ed. G. Mathé and F. M. Muggia, pp. 223–249 (1980). Springer-Verlag, Heidelberg and New York.
4. Dantchev, D., Paintrand, M., Bourut, C., Pignot, I., Maral, R., and Mathé, G. Comparative experimental study and evaluation of the degree of cardiotoxicity and alopecia of twelve different anthracyclines using the golden hamster model. *In* "Anthracyclines: Current Status and Future Developments," ed. G. Mathé, R. de Jager, and R. Maral, pp. 25–36 (1983). Masson Publ., New York.
5. Dantchev, D., Paintrand, M., Bourut, C., Pignot, I., Maral, R., and Mathé, G. Cardiac and skin toxicity of mitoxantrone in comparison with anthracyclines. *In* "Current Drugs and Methods of Cancer Treatment," ed. G. Mathé, E. Mihich, and P. Reizenstein, pp. 27–39 (1983). Masson Publ., New York.
6. Dantchev, D., Balercia, G., Bourut, C., Anjo, A., Maral, R., and Mathé, G. Comparative

microscopic study of cardiotoxicity and skin toxicity of anthracycline analogs. *Biomed. Pharmacother.*, **38**, 322–328 (1984).

7. Freireich, E. J., Gehan, E. A., Rall, D. P., Schmidt, L. M., and Skipper, H. E. Quantitative comparison of toxicity of anticancer agents in mouse, rat, hamster, dog, monkey and man. *Cancer Chemother. Rep.*, **50**, 219–245 (1966).

EXPLANATION OF PHOTOS

PHOTO 1. Myocardium of a golden hamster 7 days after treatment with ACM (6 mg/kg/injection i.p. three times a week) classified as grade 0. Sarcomeres, mitrochondria, myofilaments, and intercalated disks are in good condition, as are those of the controls.

PHOTO 2. Myocardial alterations of a golden hamster 7 days after treatment with DTR 3 mg/kg/injection i.p. three times a week) classified as grade 1, with swelling of mitochondria, clearing of their matrices and lysis of their crests, separation, loss of parallel orientation and lysis of myofilaments with disruption of Z-band registry.

PHOTO 3. Myocardial alterations of a golden hamster 7 days after treatment with DNR (3 mg/kg/injection i.p. three times a week) classified as grade 2, with swelling and clearing of mitrochondria and lysis of their crests, clumping of the chromatin into electron-dense masses, separation of the fascial adhesions of the intercalated disks, and formation of myelinic figures.

PHOTO 4. Myocardial alterations from a golden hamster 14 days after treatment with DNR (2 mg/kg/injection i.p. three times a week) classified as grade 3, with dilatation of the sarcoplasmic reticulum, separation and lysis of myofilaments, condensation of the chromatin into electron-dense masses, separation of intercalated disks, formation of empty space and myelinic figures.

PHOTO 5.   A: histopathological structure of the skin at the end of the 2nd week of treatment with ADM, with very severe atrophy of epidermal layers and disappearance of the hair (alopecia).

B: histopathological structure of the skin at the end of the 2nd week of treatment with MTN, with moderate degenerative alterations of epidermal cells and of the hair.

C: normal histopathological structure of the skin at the end of a 4 weeks' treatment with ACM.

116

D. DANTCHEV ET AL.

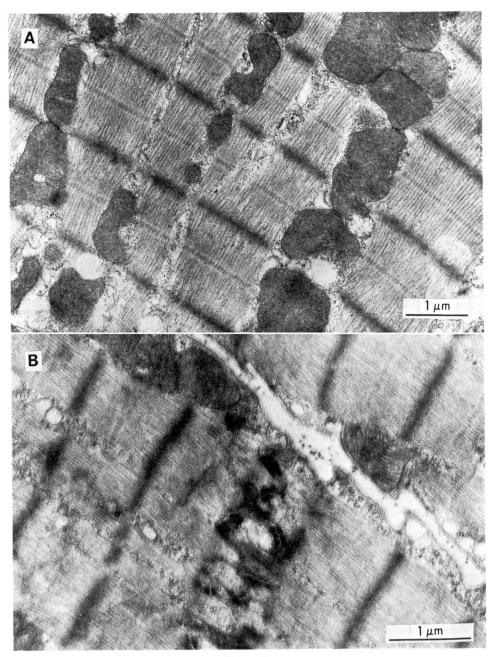

Photo 1

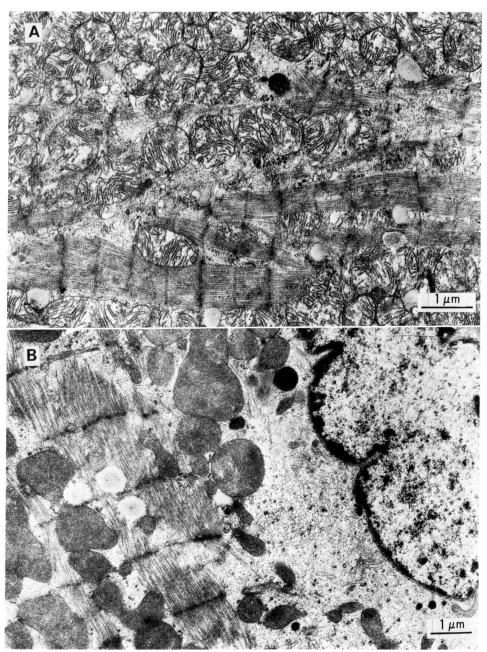

Photo 2

118   D. DANTCHEV ET AL.

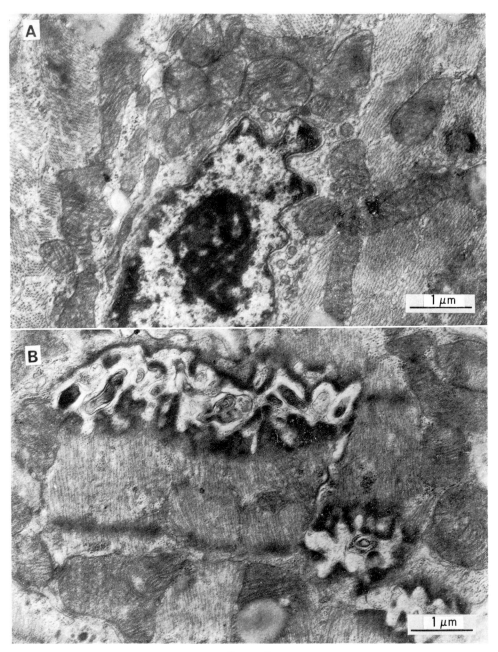

PHOTO 3

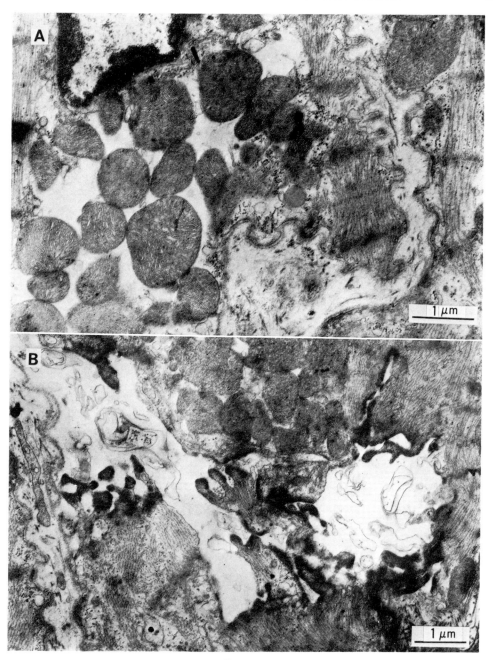

PHOTO 4

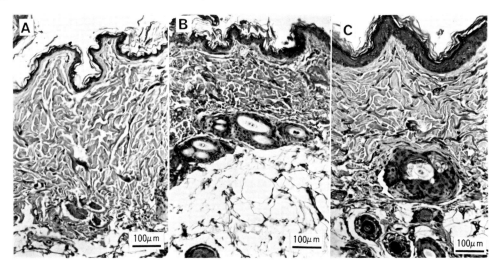

PHOTO 5

ACLARUBICIN IN ACUTE LEUKEMIA IN ADULTS

Kazumasa YAMADA

*Department of Medicine, Branch Hospital, Nagoya University
School of Medicine**

Aclacinomycin A (ACM) is a new anthracycline isolated from *Streptomyces galilaeus*. Sixty-two adults with acute leukemias entered a Phase II trial with ACM (15 mg/m² by continuous infusion for 14 days). Of the 21 previously untreated patients, 38% responded with complete remission (CR). Of the 41 patients who had had prior treatment with chemotherapy, 17% responded with CR. Thus, CR responses were at an overall rate of 24.4%.

Hemotologic toxicity was essentially leukopenia. Other side effects observed were nausea and vomiting (38%), anorexia (32%), and diarrhoea (12%). Only one patient of the 62 had alopecia, and electrocardiogram (ECG) changes were recorded in 11% of the 62. It is to be emphasized that ACM is not necessarily cross-resistant with either daunorubicin (DNR) or doxorubicin (DXR).

Based on the results obtained in the Phase II trial, a Phase III trial of a four-drug combination (ACM, N⁴-behenoyl-1-β-D-arabinofuranosylcytosine, 6-mercaptopurine, and prednisolone (BH-AC·AMP) for adults with acute non-lymphocytic leukemia was initiated. BH-AC·AMP produced a 66.7% CR in 60 previously untreated patients and a 63% CR in 55 previously treated patients. The established therapeutic effectiveness, comparable to that of DNR and DXR, and very low cardiac and alopecic toxicity indicate that ACM is a promising agent in the treatment of hemotological malignancies.

Aclacinomycin A (ACM) is a new anthracycline isolated from *Streptomyces galilaeus* by Oki *et al.* (*9, 10*). It consists of a tetracyclic quinoid aglycone, aklavinone, linked to an aminosugar, L-rhodosamine, and to two other deoxysugars, 2-deoxy-L-fucose, and L-cinerulose A (Fig. 1).

The compound has shown wide antitumor activity against ascitic and solid forms of various experimental tumors (*5, 11*): L1210 and P388 leukemias, B16 melanoma, and others. The antitumor activity of ACM in L1210 and P388 leukemias was comparable to that of daunorubicin (DNR), but at twice the dose level of adriamycin (ADM). The animal toxicology (*5, 10*) showed that LD_{50} of ACM was 2 to 3 times as high as those of DNR and ADM, and both acute and subacute cardiotoxicity of ACM measured in terms of electrocardiogram (ECG) patterns, histological and electron microscopical changes of the myocardium proved far less than that of ADM (*3, 15*). ACM also showed a greater inhibition effect on RNA synthesis than did DNR and ADM (*2, 11*), and no mutagenic activity, while DNR and ADM are highly mutagenic (*14*).

Hence, after Phase I trials in man (*4, 8, 9, 12, 13, 17*), a Phase II-III study of ACM

---

* Daiko-minami 1-1-20, Higashi-ku, Nagoya 461, Japan (山田一正).

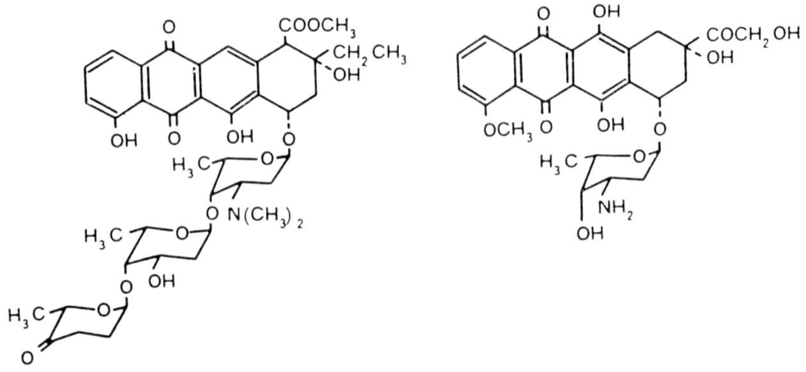

Aclacinomycin A   Adriamycin

FIG. 1.   Structures of ACM-A and ADM

in adult patients with acute leukemia was conducted by the Cooperative Study Group on the Treatment of Leukemia through a grant-in aid for Cancer Research from the Ministry of Health and Welfare of Japan.

Phase II Study on ACM in Patients with Acute Leukemias

Any adults with acute leukemia was eligible for inclusion in the study regardless of morphologic type, clinical status, or other considerations.

ACM was supplied by the Sanraku-Ocean Co. Ltd. (Tokyo) in 20 mg vials. It was dissolved in 500 ml of physiological saline and administered intravenously for 1 hr. The protocol chosen for leukemia was the continuous daily administration at a dose of 15 mg/m^2/day. The aim throughout was to continue the drug administration during the induction phase until the maximum tolerable amount was reached, and thus the administration of ACM resulted in a hypoplastic marrow or complete remission (CR). Throughout the study, supportive therapy, including leukocyte and platelet transfusion was used when needed. Evaluation during study included the monitoring of hematologic values, hepatic and renal functions and ECG. CR was defined as a state of less than 5% blasts in the bone marrow nuclear cells, normal hematopoietic components and no signs attributable to leukemia. In the results to be discussed, only CR is considered significant.

1. Clinical response

Of the total of 62 adult patients with acute leukemia, 41 had had prior treatment with chemotherapy and 21 were previously untreated. There were 37 males and 25 females with a mean age of 39 years and a range of from 15 to 81 years.

Of the 21 previously untreated patients, 38% responded with CR (Table I). There were 5 CRs in 12 patients with acute myelogenous leukemia (AML), and 1 CR in each of 6 patients with acute myelomonocytic leukemia, 2 patients with erythroleukemia, and 1 patient with acute lymphoblastic leukemia.

Of the 41 patients who had had prior treatment with chemotherapy 17% responded with CR (Table II). Thus, responses with CR were noted at an overall rate of 24.2%.

A median total of 200 mg/m^2 with a range of 93 to 275 mg/m^2 and a median total

TABLE I.   Phase II Study of ACM-A in Acute Leukemia in Previously Untreated Patients

Type	No. of patients	CR	PR	Failure	CR rate (%)
AML	12	5	0	7	41.7
AMoL	6	1	2	3	16.7
EL	2	1	0	1	50.0
ALL	1	1	0	0	100.0
Total	21	8	2	11	38.0

PR, practical remission.

TABLE II.   Phase II Study of ACM-A in Acute Leukemia in Previously Treated Patients

Type	No. of patients	CR	PR	F	CR rate (%)
AML	24	4	5	15	16.7
AMoL	7	0	1	6	0
APL	2	2	0	0	100.0
ALL	8	1	0	7	12.5
Total	41	7	6	28	17.0

TABLE III.   Side Effects in ACM-A Treatment of Acute Leukemia (62 cases)

Side effect	Rate (%)	Side effect	Rate (%)
Nausea and vomiting	38	Hepatic dysfunction	6
Anorexia	32	Tarry stool	5
Stomatitis	32	Renal dysfunction	3
Hematuria	13	Precordial oppression	3
Diarrhea	12	Alopecia	1
Phlebitis	10	Changes of ECG	16.6

of 16 days with a range of 7 to 21 days were necessary for induction of CR. In one group who received a total dose of not more than 200 mg, the CR rate was only 9.1%, yet it increased to a level of 26 to 28% respectively in those who received 201 to 300 mg or in those with more than 301 mg in total.

2.   Toxicity

The incidence and degree of drug toxicity (Table III) were measured during and after the study, the predominant effects being those related to marrow depression. The nadir of the peripheral leukocyte ranged from 200 to 6,700/cmm with a median of 1,200/cmm, which was reached on the median day of 20. The nadir of the platelet ranged from 2,000 to 46,000/cmm with a median of 9,000/cmm, reached on the median day of 18. Hematuria (13%) and tarry stool (5%) were noted. Gastrointestinal effects were seen in nausea and vomiting (38%), anorexia (32%), and diarrhoea (12%), and other side effects of stomatitis (15%), phlebitis (10%), etc. were noted. Liver impairment with elevation of alkaline phosphatase, glutamic-oxaloacetic transaminase and glutamic-pyruvic transaminase were found in 6% of the patients. In most of these, hepatic enzymes returned to normal level after cessation of treatment. It is to be emphasized that only one patient of the 62 had alopecia. ECG changes were recorded in 7 patients (11%) of the 62; the abnormalities noted were sinus tachycardia and the flattening or inversion of T-waves. In 5 cases, the changes were transient and drug administration was continued. In 2 cases, in whom administration of the drug was discontinued, the observed alterations were completely reversed and normalcy was restored.

Phase III Study

A Phase III study of ACM-A, in combination with N^4-behenoy-1-β-D-arabinofuranosylcytosine (BH-AC), 6-mercaptopurine (6-MP), and prednisolone was initiated (BH-AC·AMP regimen). The dosage schedule of each drug was as follows: ACM-A, 14 mg/m² per day intravenous infusion; BH-AC, 170 mg/m² per day intravenously; 6-MP, 80 mg/m² per day orally, and prednisolone, 20 mg/m² per day orally. Doses were increased or reduced according to the patient's response and to achieve hypoplastic marrow during the 15-day treatment period.

Of the total of 125 adult patients with acute non-lymphocytic leukemia (ANLL), 60 had had no prior treatment with chemotherapy and 65 had been previously treated. There were 76 males and 49 females with a median age of 46 years and a range of from 15 to 72 years.

Of the 60 previously untreated patients, 66.7% responded with CR. There were 27 CRs in 37 patients with AML, 10 CRs in 14 patients with AMoL, 2 CRs in 3 patients with acute promyelocytic leukemia (APL), and 1 CR in 6 patients with erythroleukemia (EL).

Of the 65 patients who had had prior chemotherapy treatment, 66.7% responded with CR. There were 25 CRs in 41 patients with AML, 5 CRs in 10 patients with acute monocytic leukemia (AMoL), and 11 CRs in 13 patients with APL.

DISCUSSION AND CONCLUSION

In a Phase II study, ACM was tested for antitumor activity and clinical toxicity in 62 adult patients with acute leukemia. The observed CR rate of 38% in the previously untreated patients is comparable to that reported for ADM and DNR with the various dose regimens (*16, 17*).

The CR rate of 17% in the previously treated patients appears encouraging, because most of the responders were considered to be resistant to either DNR or ADM. In fact, there are some patients who had CR to ACM after completely failing to respond to an adequate trial of DNR or ADM. This evidence supports the claim that ACM is not necessarily cross resistant with either DNR or ADM, although animal experiments using DNR-resistant L1210 and ADM-resistant P388 leukemias indicated that ACM had cross-resistance to both agents (*5, 11*).

The major limiting factors for the use of either DNR or ADM are alopecia and cardiotoxicity. In our series of 62 patients, only one had alopecia. Mathé *et al.* (*6*) reported that none of the 12 patients in their Phase II study of ACM had hair loss. Danchev *et al.* (*2*) systematically submitted anthracycline analogues to electron microscope study of the myocardium of golden hamsters and reported that ACM was found to be the least in inducing cardiotoxicity. Hori *et al.* (*4*) and Wakabayashi *et al.* (*14*) reported that cardiotoxicity of ACM in rabbits and hamsters was less than one-fifteenth that of ADM. In our clinical studies, 11% of the 62 patients showed ECG changes such as tachycardia or

ST-T changes, in all of whom the alterations were completely restored during continuation of the treatment. No one had a clinical sign of congestive heart failure attributable to ACM treatment. Mathé also reported that only one patient of the 20 in whom the effect of ACM on the heart was evaluable presented a cardiac intolerance with negative T-waves after a total dose of 42 mg, and this was normalized after discontinuation of the drug.

Yamagata et al. (17) reported that palpitation and sinus tachycardia were seen in 3 patients who received a cumulative dose of 1,000 mg of ACM. Oki (8) reported ECG changes in 10 of 197 patients in a Phase I-II study of ACM. A recent survey of cardiotoxicity in the Cooperative Group Study on ACM showed that ECG changes were recorded in 18 (6%) of the 270 patients in whom ECG was monitored during the treatment (11). A variety of changes such as tachycardia, auricular fibrillation, low voltage, ST-T changes and unspecified arrhythmia during ACM treatment are considered non-specified and to occur at various dose levels irrespective of dosage schedule. There was no clinical sign of congestive heart failure or of cardiomyopathy, even in a group of 40 patients who received a cumulative does of 500 mg/m² of ACM. Thus, it was estimated that clinical cardiotoxicity of ACM appears much less than that reported for ADM and DNR (6).

In our clinical pharmacology study of ACM, the plasma levels declined rapidly after intravenous administration suggesting rapid uptake into tissues. In the meantime, rapid elevation and long persistence of the active metabolites indicate that enzymatic keto reduction to the pharmacologically active products, MA144M1 and MA144N1, is a major step in biotransformation of ACM.

Ogawa et al. (7) reported objective responses in patients with malignant lymphoma in their Phase I study of ACM.

The established therapeutic effectiveness, comparable to that of DNR and ADM, and the very low cardiac and alopecic toxicity indicate that ACM deserves the further clinical trials now under way for Phase III study in acute leukemia as well as for Phase II-III study in malignant lymphoma.

Acknowledgments

We gratefully acknowledge the support of Sanraku-Ocean Co., Ltd. in supplying the ACM-A used in this study, and of Drs. H. Umezawa and T. Oki in supplying the experimental data on which these studies were based as well as valuable advice.

REFERENCES

1. Crooke, S. P., Duvernary, V. H., Galvan, L., and Prestayko, A. W. Structural activity relationships of anthracyclines relative to effect on macromolecular synthesis. *Mol. Pharmacol.*, **14**, 290–298 (1978).

2. Dantchev, D., Slioussartchouk, V., Paintrand, M., Hayat, M., Bourat, C., and Mathé, G. Electron microscopic studies of the heart and light microscopic studies of the skin after treatment of golden hamsters with adriamycin, detorubicin, AD-32, and aclacinomycin. *Cancer Treat. Rep.*, **63**, 875–888 (1979).

3. Furue, H., Komita, T., Nakao, I., Furukawa, I., Kanko, T., and Yokoyama, T. Clinical experiences with aclacinomycin A. *Recent Results Cancer Res.*, **63**, 242–246 (1978).

4. Hori, S., Shirai, M., Hirano, S., Oki, T., Inui, T., Tukagoshi, S., Ishizuka, M., Takeuchi, T., and Umezawa, H. Antitumor activity of new anthracycline antibiotics, aclacinomycin-A and its analogs, and their toxicity. *Gann*, **68**, 685–690 (1977).

5. Lenaz, L. and Page, J. A. Cardiotoxicity of adriamycin and related anthracyclins. *Cancer Treat. Rev.*, **3**, 111–120 (1976).
6. Mathé, G., Bayssas, M., Gouveia, J., Danchev, D., Ribaud, P., Machover, D., Misset, J., Schwarzemberg, L., Jasmin, C., and Hayat, M. Preliminary results of a phase II trial of aclacinomycin in acute leukemia and lymphosarcoma. *Cancer Chemother. Pharmacol.*, **1**, 259–262 (1978).
7. Ogawa, M., Inagaki, J., Horikoshi, N., Inoue, K., Chinen, T., Ueoka, H., and Nagura, E. Clinical study of aclacinomycin A. *Cancer Treat. Rep.*, **63**, 931–934 (1979).
8. Oka, S. A review of clinical studies on aclacinomycin A. Phase I and preliminary phase II evaluation of ACM-A. *Sci. Rep. Res. Inst. Tohoku Univ. Ser. C*, **25**, 37–49 (1978).
9. Oki, T., Matsuzawa, Y., Yoshimoto, A., Numata, K., Kitamura, I., Hori, S., Takamatsu, A., Umezawa, H., Ishizuka, M., Naganawa, H., Suda, H., Hamada, M., and Takeuchi, T. New antitumor antibiotics, aclacinomycin A and B. *J. Antibiot.*, **28**, 830–834 (1975).
10. Oki, T. A new anthracycline antibiotic. *Jpn. J. Antibiot.*, **30** (Suppl.), 70–84 (1977) (in Japanese).
11. Sakano, T., Okazaki, N., Ise, T., Kitaoka, K., and Kimura, K. Phase I study of aclacinomycin A. *Jpn. J. Clin. Oncol.*, **8**, 49–53 (1978).
12. Suzuki, H., Kawashima, K., and Yamada, K. Aclacinomycin A, a new antileukemic agent. *Lancet*, **i**, 870–871 (1979).
13. Umezawa, K., Sawamura, M., Matsushima, T., and Sugimura, T. Mutagenicity of aclacinomycin A and daunomycin derivatives. *Cancer Res.*, **38**, 1782–1784 (1978).
14. Wakabayashi, T., Oki, T., Tone, H., Hirano, S., and Omori, K. A comparative electron microscopic study of aclacinomycin and adriamycin cardiotoxicities in rabbits and hamsters. *J. Electron Microsc.*, **29**, 106–118 (1980).
15. Well, M., Glidewell, J., Jacquillat, C. *et al.* Daunorubicin in the therapy of acute granulocytic leukemia. *Cancer Res.*, **33**, 921–928 (1973).
16. Wiernik, P. H. Use of adriamycin (NSC-123127) in hematologic malignancies. *Cancer Chemother. Rep.*, **3**, 369–373 (1975).
17. Yamagata, S., Niimoto, M., Hamai, Y., and Hattori, T. Clinical study of aclacinomycin A (Abstr.). *Proc. 26th Annu. Meet Chemother.*, 137 (1978) (in Japanese).

COMBINATION CHEMOTHERAPY WITH ACLARUBICIN FOR ACUTE MYELOID LEUKEMIA IN ADULTS

Paris S. Mitrou

Department of Internal Medicine, Division of Haematology,
*J. W. Goethe-Universität**

Aclarubicin (ACM) was effective in single agent therapy of relapsing or refractory acute myelocytic leukemia (AML). In recent work ACM was combined with cytosine arabinoside (Ara-C) or VP 16-213 (etoposide) in the treatment of previously untreated or refractory AML. In patients older than 50 years of age with *de novo* previously untreated AML the remission rate was 41% with ACM and Ara-C. Encouraging results have been achieved with combinations of ACM with etoposide or Ara-C in relapsing or refractory leukemias. Preliminary results of a randomized study suggest that ACM combined with Ara-C is superior to daunorubicin (DNR) and Ara-C in remission induction. The results of these studies are difficult to compare and extrapolate owing to different doses and schedules of ACM and patient characteristics. Despite the growing experience with ACM in the treatment of AML the optimal dose and schedule are controversial. Large cumulative doses per cycle seem to cause a higher level of non-hematologic toxicity, particularly mucositis and diarrhoea. The data of the randomized study cited above suggest that higher doses of ACM (225 mg/m² per cycle) are equally as cardiotoxic as DNR.

The results with ACM in combination with other antileukemic agents published so far are encouraging. Further studies are needed to evaluate the findings and to determine the optimal dose and schedule of ACM in the treatment of AML.

Anthracycline antibiotics and cytosine arabinoside (Ara-C) are the most commonly used cytotoxic agents in the treatment of acute myeloid leukemia (9). Since the long-term administration of anthracyclines is limited by their cumulative cardiotoxicity, an effort has been made to detect analogs, which do not have the cardiotoxic effect. Aclacinomycin A, or aclarubicin (ACM) differs from other antracycline antibiotics with respect to chemical structure and biological activities (13). ACM seems to be less cardiotoxic than daunorubicin (DNR) or doxorubicin (1, 3, 13) in animal experiments, although careful cardiac studies have not yet been performed in men to determine its cardiotoxicity. The cellular uptake of ACM occurs more rapidly than that of doxorubicin (4). ACM is an inhibitor of RNA synthesis and interferes with the late S/G_2-phase and the G_1-phase of the cell cycle (2, 13, 18, 19).

In Phase I and Phase II-studies ACM showed a significant anti-leukemic activity, particularly in acute nonlymphoblastic leukemia (ANLL) (10, 11, 14, 16, 17, 20, 21). The experimental and clinical results of single agent therapy with in ANLL were summarized in a recent report (12). The present report summarizes the experience with ACM in

---

* Theodor-Stern-Kai 7, D-6000 Frankfurt/M. 70, F.R.G.

TABLE I. Patient Characteristics

No. of patients	61
Female	39
Male	22
Age, median (range)	62 (52–78 yrs.)
AML classification	
M1, M2	36
M3	4
M4	12
M5	8
M6	1

TABLE II. Chemotherapy

Induction	
ACM 12 mg/m^2/day×7 i.v.	
Ara-C 100 mg/m^2/day×7 CIVI	1–2 courses
Early consolidation	
One cycle of ACM and Ara-C	
Late consolidation	
1. m-AMSA	50 mg/m^2/day×5 i.v.
VP 16-213	75 mg/m^2/day×5 i.v.
Ara-C	75 mg/m^2/day×5 i.v.
every 12 hr	
2. Ara-C 600 mg/m^2 2-hr-infusion	
every 12 hr, days 1–4	

combined chemotherapy of acute nonlymphoblastic leukemia. First, we describe the preliminary results of a multicenter Phase II-study with ACM and Ara-C in previously untreated patients with *de novo* acute myelocytic leukemia (AML) followed by the results of combination chemotherapy of other groups in previously treated or untreated AML patients.

Prospective Phase II-study of the Süddeutsche Hämoblastosegruppe

Between May 1987 and November 1987 patients with *de novo* ANLL were treated in a prospective cooperative study with an age adapted protocol. ACM and Ara-C were combined for the treatment of patients over 50 years of age with previously untreated *de novo* AML. Other patient characteristics are outlined in Table I. Ineligibility criteria were preceding myelodysplastic syndrome, a subacute course of AML or antineoplastic treatment for diseases other than AML.

Leukemias were classified according to the cytological and cytochemical criteria of the FAB* classification by a review comittee. All patients had adequate cardiac, renal, and hepatic function. The pretreatment evaluation included a haemogramm, bone marrow aspiration and biopsy, cytochemical examination, electrocardiogram (ECG), and X-ray examination of the chest and paranasal sinuses. Patients were monitored with blood cell cell counts daily and biochemical profile twice a week. Continuous ECG monitoring or radionuclide cardiac scanning were not performed.

---

* French-American-British Working Group for Leukemia Classification.

1.   Treatment

Induction chemotherapy included ACM 12 mg/m² daily for 7 days and Ara-C 100 mg/m² as continuous intravenous infusion (CIVI) for 7 days. The study design allowed a second cycle of ACM and Ara-C if the bone marrow showed unequivocal residual leukemia. Patients entering complete remission received a consolidation course with ACM and Ara-C and two courses of late consolidation (Table II) without further maintenance treatment.

Evaluation of antileukemic response was based on CALG-B criteria (5). Treatment toxicity was quantitated using the WHO grading system.

2.   Therapeutic effects

Fifty-eight out of 61 patients received 1–2 courses of induction chemotherapy. In 3 cases treatment was interrupted during the first course of treatment. Response is outlined in Table III. Twenty-nine of the patients responded, 25 with a complete response. The median overall survival was 7 months (Fig. 1) and the median relapse-free survival 7.5 months (Fig. 2). Patients receiving late consolidation had a median survival of 16.5 months (Fig. 3) and a median relapse free survival of 12.5 months (Fig. 4). The proportion of long-term survivor cannot yet be determined. Forty-six patients died; the time of death is shown in Table IV.

3.   Toxicity

The main non-hematologic side effects are summarized in Table V. In general, toxicity was rather mild. Cardiac complications were observed in old patients. The median

TABLE III.   Results of Induction Chemotherapy

	No.	%
Less than one cycle	3	5
Complete remission	25	41
Partial remission	4	6.5
Treatment failure	15	24.5
Early death	14	23

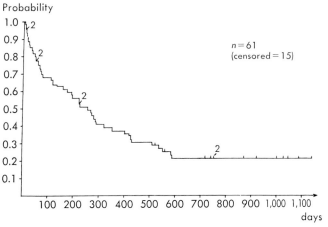

FIG. 1.   Survival patients
>50 years (5/85)

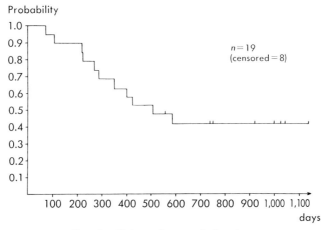

FIG. 2. Relapse-free survival patients
>50 years (5/85)

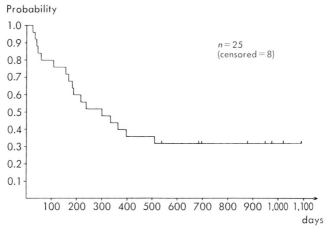

FIG. 3. Survival patients with late consolidation
>50 years (5/85)

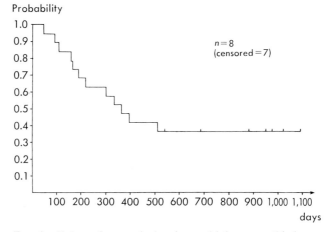

FIG. 4. Relapse-free survival patients with late consolidation
>50 years (5/85)

TABLE IV. Time of Death

During induction	14
Primary treatment failure	11
During early consolidation	1
During late consolidation	3
During complete remission	1
During partial remission	4
Relapse	11
Unknown	1
Total	46

TABLE V. Non-hematologic Toxicity of the First Course with ACM+Ara-C

Side effect	Grade (WHO)			
	0	1–2	3	4
Nausea/vomiting	19	36	6	0
Diarrhea	40	17	3	1
Stomatitis	37	19	5	0
Hepatic toxicity				
SGOT/SGPT	42	19	0	0
Bilirubin	53	7	0	1
Cardiac toxicity				
Rhythm	56	4	1	0
Function	58	1	1	1

duration of severe leucopenia with less than 250 granulocytes/μl was 16 days for all patients and that of severe thrombocytopenia ($<$25,000 platelets/μl) 13 days. Severe infections or septicemia were observed in 3 and 7 patients, respectively.

Other Prospective Studies

There is a limited number of studies with ACM in the combined chemotherapy of acute myeloid leukemia. Rowe *et al.* (*15*) used higher doses of ACM (60 mg/m² for 5 days) in combination with VP16-213 in the treatment of refractory AML. Twelve of the 35 patients entered complete remission. It is remarkable that 2 out of 4 patients with primary treatment failure due to DAT (DNR, Ara-C, 6-thioguanine (6-TG)) went into complete remission. However, severe gastrointestinal toxicity and mucositis were common side effects of this regimen.

In a prospective randomized study (*7*) two "3+7 protocols" with DNR or ACM were compared. The dosage of ACM was 75 mg/m² on three consecutive days in this protocol. From the preliminary results it seems that ACM induced more complete remissions than DNR (70 *vs.* 45%). Seventy-eight percent of the patients treated with ACM obtained a complete response with one course of treatment, whereas only 56% of those on DNR entered a complete remission after the first chemotherapy cycle. Severe cardiac dysfunction and arrhythmias were observed in both arms of the protocol (3% with ACM, 1.5% with DNR).

Holowiecki and Lutz (*8*) performed three consecutive studies with ACM combined with Ara-C$\pm$6-TG. In the first study 50 patients with relapsed or resistant AML were treated with ACM, 25 mg/m² for 7 days combined with Ara-C and 6-TG. A complete response rate of 42% was achieved. The same combination included a complete response rate of 31% in 13 patients over 50 years of age. This study was stopped because of the high mortality caused by infections and bleeding. In a third continued study ACM 20 mg/m²$\times$7 combined with Ara-C induced 59% complete remissions in patients younger than 60 years of age with previously untreated AML.

CONCLUSIONS

Acrarubicin was used as the sole agent in previously treated patients with relapsed or resistant acute myeloid leukemias with a complete response rate of 13 to 44% (10, 11, 13, 14, 16, 17, 21). The best results were obtained in patients treated at first relapse without prior reinduction with drugs other than ACM (11). From the results it appears that the introduction of ACM in combined chemotherapy is justified.

In our study ACM was combined with Ara-C in the treatment of previously untreated AML-patients over 50 years of age. Complete remission rate, overall survival and remission duration are similar to those achieved with other combinations (6). The dosage of ACM was rather low in comparison to the dosage of 300 mg/m² (15) or 215 mg/m² (7) in other studies. The combination of high-dose ACM with etoposide showed encouraging results in patients with refractory AML (15). Similar results were reported by a European group (8) with lower doses of ACM combined with Ara-C and 6-TG in the treatment of patients with refractory or relapsing AML. The randomized study of this Danish group provides some answers to questions on the activity and side effects of ACM in comparison to the most commonly used anthracycline, DNR in the treatment of AML. From the results published so far it would appear that ACM is superior to DNR in remission induction. However, there is no information about the overall survival and remission duration in the two treatment arms of this study.

The optimal dose and schedule of ACM are controversial. Low doses of ACM (12 to 25 mg/m² daily) for 7 days had a low non-hematologic toxicity provoking moderate remission induction as shown in our study and in the studies of Holowiecki and Lutz (8). High doses to 300 mg/m² showed more severe side effects with grade 3 mucositis in half and severe diarrhea in one third of the pretreated patients (15). The non-hematologic toxicity of 75 mg/m² for 3 days did not differ from that of DNR in the study of the Danish group (7). The data of the ACM studies in single agent and combined chemotherapy suggest that 175–225 mg/m² per cycle may be an effective dosage in combined chemotherapy with an acceptable toxicity.

The apparent lower cardiotoxicity of ACM (1, 13) was an important reason for the introduction of this drug in the treatment of AML. In studies with ACM in single agent or combined chemotherapy arrhythmias have been reported in 5–10% of the patients (10, 11, 14, 15, 20) who have previously received doxorubicin or DNR.

In our present study cardiotoxic effects were observed in elderly patients with preexisting cardiac disease. In the prospective and randomized study of the Danish group (7), cardiotoxicity was comparable in the two arms. There are not at present convincing data that ACM is substantially less cardiotoxic than DNR in a clinical situation.

Single agent therapy with ACM induced complete remissions in AML refractory to DNR and/or doxorubicin (10). Similar results have been reported with the combination of ACM and etoposide or Ara-C in a small group of patients with primary treatment failure to DAT (*8, 15*). These results suggest some degree of non-cross-resistance with DNR.

In conclusion, ACM is an active agent in the treatment of AML and can be successfully combined with other antileukemic agents. Further studies are required to determine the optimal dose and schedule of ACM in the treatment of AML.

Acknowledgments

The author wishes to acknowledge the cooperation of Drs. G. Ehninger, M. Freund, G. Heil, D. Hoelzer, E. Kurrle, H. Link, S. Öhl, W. Queißer G. Schlimok, and H. Wendt in the multicenter study, whose results are part of those presented in this paper.

REFERENCES

1. Bouhour, J. B., Fumoleau, P., and De Lajartre, A. Y. Comparative ultrastructural study on cardiotoxicity of adriamycin *versus* aclacinomycin A in the rat. Proc. 13th Int. Cancer Congr., Seattle (1982) (Abstr. No. 2326).

2. Crooke, S. T., Duvernay, V. H., Galvan, L., and Prestayko, A. W. Structure activity relationships of anthracyclines relative to effects on macromolecular syntheses. *Mol. Pharmacol.*, **14**, 290–298 (1978).

3. Dantchev, D., Slioussartchouk, V., Paintrand, M., Hayat, M., Bouret, C., and Mathé, G. Electron micrsocopic studies of the heart and light-microscopic studies of the skin after treatment of golden hamsters with Adriamycin, Detorubicin, AD-32, and Aclacinomycin. *Cancer Treat. Rep.*, **63**, 875–888 (1979).

4. Egorin, M. J., Clawson, R. E., and Ross, L. A. Cellular accumulation and disposition of aclacinomycin A. *Cancer Res.*, **39**, 4396–4400 (1979).

5. Ellison, R. R., Holland, J. F., and Weil, M. Arabinosyl cytosine: A useful agent in the treatment of acute leukaemia in adults. *Blood*, **32**, 507–523 (1968).

6. Gale, R. P. and Foon, K. A. Therapy of acute myelogenous leukemia. *Sem. Hematol.*, **24**, 40–54 (1987).

7. Hansen, O. P., Ellegaard, J., Madsen, P. B., Brincker, H., Christensen, B. E., Killmann, S. A., Laursen, M. L., Karle, H., Drivsholm, A., Jensen, M. K., Laursen, B., Jans, H., Hippe, E., Pedersen-Bjergaard, J., Nissen, N., Thorling, K., and Jensen, K. B. Combination chemotherapy with Aclarubicin (ACR) plus Cytosine Arabinoside (CA) *versus* Daunorubicin (DNR) plus Cytosine Arabinoside in *de novo* acute myelocytic leukemia (AML). A Danish national trial. *Proc. ASCO*, **7**, 175 (1988) (Abstr. No. 675).

8. Holowiecki, J. and Lutz, D. The current status of Aclarubicin in the combination chemotherapy of untreated and relapsed or resistant ANLL—a multicenter study. Biennial Conference on Chemotherapy of Infectious Diseases and Malignancies, Munich (1987) (Abstr. No. 223).

9. Lister, T. A. and Rohatiner, A.Z.S. The treatment of acute myelogenous leukaemia in adults. *Blood*, **19**, 172–192 (1982).

10. Machover, D., Gastiaburu, J., and Delgado, M. Phase I–II study of aclacinomycin for treatment of acute myeloid leukemia. Proc. 13th Int. Congr. Chemother., Vienna (1983) (Abstr. SY 84/6).

11. Mitrou, P. S., Kuse, R., Anger, H., Herrmann, R., Bonfert, B., Pralle, H., Thiel, E., Westerhausen, M., Mainzer, K., and Bartels, H. Aclarubicin (Aclacinomycin A) in the treatment of relapsing acute leukaemias. *Eur. J. Cancer Clin. Oncol.*, **21**, 919–924 (1985).

12. Oka, S., Mathé, G., and Mitrou, P. S. Aclacinomycin A. *Cancer Treat. Rev.*, **11**, 299–302 (1984).

13. Oki, T. Aclacinomycin A. *In* "Anthracyclines: Current Status and New Developments," ed. S. T. Crooke and S. D. Reich, pp. 323–342 (1980). Academic Press, New York.

14. Pedersen-Bjergaard, J., Brincker, H., Ellergaard, J., Drivsholm, A., and Freund, L. Phase II trial of aclacinomycin A in acute non-lymphocytic leukemia refractory to treatment with daunorubicin. *Proc. ASCO*, **3**, 208 (1984).

15. Rowe, J. M., Chang, A.Y.C., and Bennett, J. M. Aclacinomycin A and etoposide (VP-16-213): An effective regimen in previously treated patients with refractory acute myelogenous leukaemia. *Blood*, **71**, 992–996 (1988).

16. Sampi, K., Abe, R., Hayashi, Y., and Hattori, M. Preliminary phase II study of aclacinomycin A in patients with adult acute leukemia. *Jpn. J. Clin. Oncol.*, **11**, 75–80 (1981).

17. Suzuki, H., Kawashima, K., and Yamada, K. Phase I and preliminary phase II studies on aclacinomycin A in patients with acute leukemia. *Jpn. J. Clin. Oncol.*, **10**, 111–118 (1980).

18. Tone, H., Takeuchi, T., and Umezawa, H. Experimental studies on aclacinomycin. Proc. 13th Int. Congr. Chemother., Vienna (1982) (Abstr. SY 84/1).

19. Traganos, F., Staiano-Coico, L., Darzynkiewitz, Z., and Melamed, M. R. Effects of aclacinomycin on cell survival and cell cycle progression of cultured mammalian cells. *Cancer Res.*, **41**, 2728–2737 (1981).

20. Warrell, R. P., Arlin, Z. A., Kempin, S. J., and Young, C. W. Phase I–II evaluation of a new anthracycline antibiotic, Aclacinomycin A, in adults with refractory leukemia. *Cancer Treat. Rep.*, **66**, 1619–1623 (1982).

21. Yamada, K., Nakamura, T., Tsuruo, T. *et al.* A phase II study of aclacinomycin A in acute leukemia in adults. *Cancer Treat. Rev.*, **7**, 77–82 (1980).

PIRARUBICIN: CLINICAL RESEARCH

Tatuo SAITO

*Kyoundo Hospital, Sasaki Institute**

The results of a Phase II study on intravenous use of pirarubicin, which is the generic name of (2″R)-4′-O-tetrahydropyranyladriamycin (THP) for treatment of 756 solid tumor patients were presented. Pirarubicin dosages were 40 to 60 mg/b.w. or 30 to 40 mg/b.w. for 2 consecutive days every 3 to 4 weeks, 20 to 30 mg/body once a week, and 10 to 20 mg/body for 5 consecutive days every 3 weeks.

There were 10 complete responses (CRs) and 67 partial responses (RPs) in 499 evaluable cases and the total response rate (PR and CR) was 15.4%. Clsasified by tumor, the efficacy rates were 13.1% for stomach cancer, 18.8% for head and neck cancer, 21.4% for breast cancer, 26.8% for ovarian cancer, 24.2% for uterine cancer, 22.2% for bladder cancer, and 30.0% for renal pelvis and ureter cancer. As side effects, myelosuppression, especially leukocytopenia, occurred in 73.6%.

Anorexia (37.1%) and nausea and vomiting (29.7%) occurred but were rather mild. Hair loss and stomatitis were less frequent and milder than with other anthracyclines. The incidence of electrocardiogram (ECG) changes was 2.8%, but the changes were not severe.

Pirarubicin is the generic name of (2″R)-4′-O-tetrahydropyranyladriamycin (THP), is an anthracycline antitumor agent discovered by Umezawa *et al.* in 1979 (*35*). This agent exerts carcinostatic activity similar to or stronger than that of adriamycin (ADM) against various experimental tumors (*33, 34*). In addition, studies using hamsters suggested that pirarubicin has low cardiotoxicity and low skin toxicity (*5*). Thus, clinical studies were started on this agent.

A Phase I study revealed that a major limiting factor of the use of pirarubicin is bone marrow suppression, especially a decrease in the WBC count. The maximum tolerable single dose of pirarubicin was surmised to be 55 mg/m² (*36*). Other side effects were mainly gastrointestinal disorders, but they were mild in severity. No hair loss or abnormal findings of the liver or kidney function were recorded. One case showed transient abnormal electrocardiogram (ECG) findings, but the cause-effect relationship between the findings and pirarubicin administration was unclear. The maximum tolerable dose of pirarubicin was reported by Ogawa *et al.* (*21*) to be 54 mg/m², which is almost the same as that reported by Majima (*14*), *i.e.*, 66.6 mg/m².

Based on experimental and Phase I clinical trial data, the Phase II study was performed by a group of 44 medical institutions throughout Japan, employing patients with solid tumors as the subjects during the period from October of 1982 through March of 1985. During this study period, 7 substudy groups were organized and Phase II studies were performed in relation to head and neck, breast, gastrointestinal, gynecological, and

---

* Kanda 1-8, Chiyoda-ku, Tokyo 101, Japan (斉藤達雄).

urogenital cancers. This paper reports the results of the Phase II studies in which pirarubicin was administered by the intravenous route.

Criteria of Response

The subjects of this study were selected in accordance with the "Criteria for Evaluation of Clinical Effects of Cancer Chemotherapy on Solid Tumors" (*11*) of the Japan Society for Cancer Chemotherapy. However, each of various tumors was selected in accordance with the evaluation criteria or a draft thereof for the effect of chemotherapy on cancers of each organ. Final evaluation was made by the Efficacy Evaluation Committee.

Administration Methods

As a rule, one of the following four dosage regimens was employed.

A-1:   40–60 mg/b.w., once every 3–4 weeks.
A-2:   30–40 mg/b.w., 2 consecutive days every 3 weeks.
B   :   20–30 mg/b.w., once a week.
C   :   10–20 mg/b.w., 5 consecutive days every 3 weeks.

Pirarubicin was dissolved in distilled water for injection or in a 5% glucose solution and administered intravenously or by intravenous drip infusion. Administration of 2–3 courses was decided as the target of each regimen.

In addition to the intravenous administration, intra-arterial administration, intravesical administration or intrapleural administration was also employed in the treatment of some kinds of tumors. Pirarubicin was supplied by Sanraku Ocean Co., Ltd. (currently Sanraku Co., Ltd.) and Meiji Seika Kaisha, Ltd.

Criteria for evaluation of efficacy and adverse reactions

The efficacy of each regimen was evaluated in accordance with the Criteria for Evaluation of Clinical Effects of Cancer Chemotherapy on Solid Tumors by the Japan Society for Cancer Chemotherapy. These criteria are almost the same as those in the WHO Handbook for Reporting Results of Cancer Treatment, 1979 (*26, 27*).

Separate evaluation was made on patients with measurable and evaluable lesions and patients with only malignant pleural or peritoneal effusion. The histopathological effect of each regimen was also separately evaluated in accordance with the criteria established by Shimosato *et al.* (*28*).

While taking into consideration the results of evaluation performed by each investigator, the Efficacy Evaluation Committee (whose members were selected from the medical institutions participating in the Phase II study on pirarubicin) made the final evaluation of the therapeutic efficacy.

Adverse reactions were classified into various grades in accordance with the method of description of adverse reactions provided in the Criteria for Evaluation of Effect of Chemotherapy for Solid Cancers.

Response to Treatment

1. Details of subject patients

The total number of registered patients with solid tumors was 934. The administration method was intravenous injection in 756 cases, intra-arterial injection in 92 cases, intravesical infusion in 50 cases and intrapleural or multiple routes in 36 cases. This report covers the data for the intravenous administration cases (Table I).

TABLE I. Classification of Cases Administered Intravenously

Treated cases	756
Ineligible cases	
Total	198
No evaluable lesions	52
With active multiple cancers	6
Performance status 4	53
With highly damaged bone marrow, liver, kidney, and heart functions	12
With severe complication	1
Insufficient washout period after previous therapy	74
Eligible cases	
Total	558
Excluded cases	4
Drop-out cases	42
Cases impossible to evaluate	6
Evaluated cases	506
Measurable and evaluable	499
Malignant pleural or peritoneal effusion	4
Judged histopathologically	3

TABLE II. Background Factors of Evaluated Cases

Item			Number of cases
Evaluated cases			558
Sex	Male		273
	Female		285
Age	(Years)		15–86
	Average		59.4
P.S.	0		115
	1		161
	2		133
	3		145
	4[a]		4
Previous therapy	Chemotherapy	(+)	291
	(Anthracyclines)		(79)
		(−)	267
	Radiotherapy	(+)	106
		(−)	452
	Operation	(+)	286
		(−)	272
No previous therapy			173

[a] P. S. by bone lesion.

Of the 756 intravenous administration cases, 198 were ineligible, and thus a total of 558 cases were analyzed. There were 4 excluded cases, 42 dropout cases, and 6 unevaluable cases, so that a total of 506 cases were evaluable. Of these, 499 patients had measurable and evaluable lesions. In 4 patients, only malignant pleural or peritoneal effusion was the subject of evaluation, while in 3 patients with bladder cancers, only histopathological evaluation was possible.

2. *Background factors of subjects*

Table II shows background factors of the subjects such as age, sex, performance status (PS) *etc.* Regarding the presence or absence of prior therapy, 173 patients had no prior therapy, while 291 patients had undergone prior chemotherapy. Of the latter group, anthracyclines had been administered to 79.

3. *Clinical efficacy*

Of the total of 506 evaluable cases who underwent intravenous administration, the results of evaluation of the 499 which had measurable and evaluable lesions are shown in Table III.

The response rates (CR+PR) were 18.8% for head and neck cancers, 13.1% for stomach chancer, 21.4% for breast cancer, 22.2% for bladder cancer, 30.0% for renal pelvis and ureter cancers, 26.8% for ovarian cancer, and 24.2% for uterine cancer. PR was seen in 2 cases each of colon/rectal cancer and lung cancer, and in one case each of vaginal cancer, prostate cancer, sarcoma, and tumor of the mesothelium. The time to achievement of a response in the 77 responding cases, consisting of 10 CR cases and 67 PR cases, differed to some degree depending on the kind of cancer, but the mean time was 85.3 days.

In 4 cases in which only a malignant pleural or peritoneal effusion was the subject of the evaluation, one case of lung cancer showed a response to the regimen. In the 3 cases of bladder cancer, which were evaluated on the basis of the histopathological effect, one case showed a response to the regimen.

Table IV shows the response rate as a function of the administration method. The response rate (CR+PR) was 13.7% for the A-1 method, 10.5% for the A-2 method, 17.7% for the B method, and 25.7% for the C method. The response rate tended to increase as the interval between administrations became shorter, but no statistically significant differences were observed among the administration methods.

The response rates for the A-1 method and B method were analyzed as a function of a single dose (Table V). In the A-1 method, a good response appeared beginning from a dose of 40 mg/b.w. The largest number of subjects was in the 60 mg/b.w. group, and the response rate in this group was 20.8%. With the B method, the response rates were 38.9% for 20 mg/b.w., 6.9% for 30 mg/b.w., and 19.2% for 40 mg/b.w.

Looking at the relationship between the total administered dose and the response rate, it is seen that the response rates were 9.2% in the groups given 200 mg or less, 27.8% in the group given 201–300 mg and 49.1% in the group given 301 mg or more.

With regard to the relationship between the presence or absence of prior chemotherapy and the response rate, the response rate was 12.7% in the group with prior chemotherapy, while it was 18.4% in group with no prior chemotherapy (Table VI). When the efficacy of the regimen was analyzed in the group with prior chemotherapy as a function of the presence or absence of prior use of anthracycline agents, the response

TABLE III. Clinical Efficacy

Tumor	Cases treated (A)	Cases evaluated (B)	Response CR	Response PR	Response NC	Response PD	Response rate (%) CR+PR (A)	Response rate (%) CR+PR (B)	Duration of response Average day (Min.–Max.)
Head and neck cancer	67	64	—	12	45	7	17.9	18.8	22.8 (2– 64)
Thyroid gland cancer	2	1	—	—	1	—	—	—	—
Esophageal cancer	4	2	—	—	1	1	—	—	—
Stomach cancer	76	61	1	7	38	15	10.5	13.1	63.3 (28–203)
Colon-rectum cancer	37	33	—	2	15	16	5.4	6.1	69.0 (31–107)
Liver cancer	8	5	—	—	3	2	—	—	—
Bile duct cancer	5	3	—	—	2	1	—	—	—
Pancreatic cancer	4	3	—	—	3	—	—	—	—
Small intestine cancer	1	1	—	—	—	1	—	—	—
Lung cancer	84	82	—	2	68	12	2.4	2.4	70.0 (42– 98)
Breast cancer	87	84	4	14	39	27	20.7	21.4	94.9 (28–338)
Kidney cancer	6	4	—	—	4	—	—	—	—
Bladder cancer	31	27	2	4	11	10	19.4	22.2	52.5 (28–106)
Renal pelvis and ureter cancer	11	10	1	2	3	4	27.3	30.0	169.0 (40–417)
Ovarian cancer	42	41	1	10	21	9	26.2	26.8	168.0 (44–372)
Uterine cancer	34	33	1	7	16	9	23.5	24.2	94.8 (42–343)
Vaginal cancer	2	2	—	1	—	1	50.0	50.0	28
Testicular cancer	1	1	—	—	1	—	—	—	—
Prostatic cancer	17	15	—	1	8	6	5.9	6.7	61
Skin cancer	10	6	—	—	6	—	—	—	—
Sarcoma	8	8	—	1	3	4	12.5	12.5	56
Mesothelioma	3	3	—	1	2	—	33.3	33.3	252
Malignant thymoma	2	2	—	—	1	1	—	—	—
Mikulicz tumor	1	1	—	—	1	—	—	—	—
Unknown primary lesion	7	7	—	3	4	—	42.9	42.9	130.7 (116–149)
Total	550	499	10	67	296	126	14.0	15.4	85.3 (2–417)

NC, no change ; PD, progressive disease.

TABLE IV.   Clinical Efficacy by Administration Regimen

Administration regimen	Cases evaluated	Response				Response rate CR+PR (%)
		CR	PR	NC	PD	
A-1 (once every 3–4 weeks)	291	5	35	173	78	13.7
A-2 (2-day consecutive administration, every 3–4 weeks)	38	2	2	23	11	10.5
B (once a week)	113	2	18	63	30	17.7
C (every day)	35	—	9	25	1	25.7
Others	22	1	3	12	6	18.2
Total	499	10	67	296	126	15.4

TABLE V.   Efficacy Rates by Single Dose

Administration procedure	Single dose (mg)	Cases evaluated	Response				Response rate CR+PR (%)
			CR	PR	NC	PD	
A-1	Less	14	—	—	10	4	—
(Once every 3–4 weeks)	than 40	—	—	—	—	—	—
	40–	58	1	4	34	19	8.6
	50–	64	—	6	41	17	9.4
	60–	125	4	22	69	30	20.8
	Over 70	30	—	3	19	8	10.0
B	Less	2	—	—	2	—	—
(Once a week)	than 20	—	—	—	—	—	—
	20–	18	1	6	8	3	38.9
	30–	58	—	4	36	18	6.9
	40–	26	—	5	12	9	19.2
	Over 50	9	1	3	5	—	44.4

TABLE VI.   Efficacy Rates as Function of Previous Chemotherapy

Previous chemotherapy	Cases evaluated	Response				Response rate CR+PR (%)
		CR	PR	NC	PD	
Yes	260	3	30	149	78	12.7
Anthracyclines	—	—	—	—	—	—
(+)	70	—	10	40	20	14.3
(−)	187	3	20	106	58	12.3
Unknown	3	—	—	3	—	—
No	239	7	37	147	48	18.4

rate was 14.3% in the group with prior use, while it was 12.3% in the group with no prior use of anthracyclines.

4.   *Adverse effects*

Analysis of the 558 subject cases revealed some kind of adverse reaction in 483 cases (86.6%) (Table VII). As subjective symptoms, high incidences were seen of anorexia (37.1%), nausea/vomiting (29.7%), and general malaise (18.5%). In addition, loss of hair (9.7%), fever (7.2%) and stomatitis (5.4%), *etc.* were observed. Of these, adverse reactions of Grade 3 or Grade 4 in terms of severity occurred in 7.2% of the anorexia

TABLE VII. Side Effects

	Grade	Number of cases (%)		Side effect		Number of cases (%)	
Eligible		558					
Number of episodes of side effects		483 (86.6)					
Anorexia	1	88 (15.8)		WBC	3.9–3.0	81 (14.5)	
	2	79 (14.2)	207 (37.1)	(×10³/cmm)	2.9–2.0	156 (28.0)	410 (73.6)/557
	3	26 (4.7)			1.9–1.0	137 (24.6)	
	4	14 (2.5)			Under 1.0	36 (6.5)	
Nausea and vomiting	1	102 (18.3)		RBC	299–250	73 (13.1)	
	2	51 (9.1)	166 (29.7)	(×10⁴/cmm)	249–200	42 (7.5)	126 (11.6)/557
	3	10 (1.8)			199–150	10 (1.8)	
	4	3 (0.4)			Under 150	1 (0.2)	
Stomatitis	1	23 (4.1)		Hb	10.9–9.5	33 (6.4)	
	2	5 (0.9)	30 (5.4)	(g/dl)	9.4–8.0	62 (12.0)	137 (26.6)/516
	3	2 (0.4)			7.9–6.5	33 (6.4)	
	4				Under 6.5	9 (1.7)	
Fever		40 (7.2)		Plt	9.9–7.5	27 (4.9)	
Malaise		103 (18.5)		(×10⁴/cmm)	7.4–5.0	21 (3.8)	85 (15.6)/546
Phlebitis		7 (1.3)			4.9–2.5	22 (4.0)	
Eruption		3 (0.5)			Under 2.5	15 (2.7)	
Diarrhea		18 (3.2)		Changes in ECG		10/361 (2.8)	
Hair loss	1	28 (5.0)		Hepatic dysfunction		29/543 (5.3)	
	2	23 (4.1)	54 (9.7)	Renal dysfunction		8/521 (1.5)	
	3	3 (0.5)		Hemorrhage		5 (0.9)	
	4			Others[a]		18 (3.4)	
				No side effects		75 (13.4)	

[a] Dizziness (2), palpitation (2), gustatory disorder, dry mouth, heart born, uncomfortable feeling, bad breath, somnolentia, staggers, melena, red urine, abdominal pain, numbness, pigmentation, ileus, angialgia, chest pain.

cases and 2.3% of the vomiting cases, while Grade 3 occurred in 0.4% of the stomatitis cases and 0.5% of the hair loss cases; there were no Grade 4 cases of stomatitis or hair loss. As objective symptoms, a decrease in the WBC count to less than 4,000/mm³ was found in 73.6% of all the subjects; on the other hand, a decrease in the platelet count to less than 100,000/mm³ occurred in 15.6%; incidence of a decreased platelet count was thus lower than that of decreased WBC count. The RBC count was decreased in 22.6%, while a decrease in the hemoglobin level occurred in 26.6% of the subjects. Changes in the ECG were seen in 10 (2.8%) subjects, and consisted of 4 cases of abnormalities in the ST-T wave, 2 cases of premature contraction and one case each of sinus tachycardia, low electric potential, arrhythmia, and cardiac ischemia. There were no cases of congestive heart failure. The incidences of hepatic dysfunction and renal dysfunction were 5.3% and 1.5%, respectively.

Evaluation of Response

Progress in the chemotherapy of cancers has been seen in the successive development of various clinically potent carcinostatic agents. Among these, ADM, which has strong carcinostatic activity and a broad antitumor spectrum, is currently widely employed in clinical medicine not only as an agent for the treatment of solid tumors but also as an agent capable of bringing about remission of tumors of the hematopoietic tissues and organs (2–4, 6, 19). On the other hand, however, ADM was found to show cumulative cardiotoxicity, and this drawback constitutes a serious limiting factor to its usage (15, 19, 24, 25). Thus, in Japan and other countries much effort is going into the development of anthracyclines which cause fewer adverse reactions but have antitumor activity similar to or higher than that of ADM (7). Aclacinomycin is one such agent developed in Japan, and it is now widely employed mainly in the treatment of tumors of the hematopoietic tissues and organs (38).

Pirarubicin, a new anthracycline agent, was discovered by Umezawa *et al*. Preclinical studies indicated it to have strong antitumor activity and low cardiotoxicity, and thus clinical studies have been initiated.

We recently carried out a nationwide Phase II study on pirarubicin in patients with solid tumors and obtained a response rate (CR+PR) of 15.4% (77/499). As a function of the type of tumor, a high response rate was obtained in head and neck cancers (18.8%), stomach cancer (13.1%), breast cancer (21.4%), urinary tract epithelial cancer (bladder, renal pelvis, and ureter cancers) (24.3%), ovarian cancer (26.8%), and uterine cancer (24.2%); these cases were also numerous.

Various Japanese research groups have reported that pirarubicin shows clinical efficacy in the treatment of solid tumors: these include head and neck cancers (8, 9, 30), stomach cancer (18, 31, 37), gynecological cancers (10, 29), breast cancer (1, 32), urogenital tumors (17), and lung cancer (16).

Although comparison of these results with those obtained with ADM is difficult, the ADM response rates by Japanese researchers were compiled by Ogawa (20) as follows: stomach cancer, 14.5%; breast cancer, 30.8%; ovarian cancer, 25%; uterine cancer, 25%; *etc*. Thus, it can be said that pirarubicin has an efficacy similar to that of ADM.

In the present study, 3 administration schedules were tested: (1) once every 3 to 4 weeks, (2) once a week, and (3) every day. However, no significant differences in pirarubicin's efficacy were found among these administration schedules. The optimum single dose in each administration schedule was surmised to be as follows, taking into consideration both the response rate and adverse reactions: 40–60 mg/b.w. for the once every 3 to 4 week administration schedule, 20–40 mg/b.w. for the weekly administration schedule, and 10–20 mg/b.w. for the daily administration schedule.

When screening for derivatives of a drug, one of the most important characteristics looked for is the absence of cross-tolerance with the original drug. Kunimoto *et al.* (*12*) reported that cancer cells (*in vitro*) which had acquired tolerance to ADM showed partial cross-tolerance to pirarubicin. However, some researchers have reported positive results of clinical cross-tolerance while others have reported negative results. Thus, no clear conclusion has yet been reached (*13, 22*).

In the present study, no differences were detected in the response rate between patient groups with and without prior chemotherapy using anthracycline agents. However, there were patients who responded to pirarubicin after not having responded to ADM. This finding suggests that pirarubicin has, at least in some cases, no cross-tolerance with ADM.

Subjective adverse reactions of anorexia, nausea/vomiting, general malaise, hair loss, fever, stomatitis, *etc.* were observed. However, all these symptoms were comparatively mild, and the hair loss and stomatitis were especially milder and also less numerous than those observed following administration of ADM. These points are thought to be promising characteristics of pirarubicin. As an objective adverse reaction, suppression of the bone marrow function, represented by a decrease in the WBC count, was striking. This is thought to be a limiting factor in the use of pirarubicin as is true with ADM. The incidence of ECG abnormalities was low at 2.8%.

With respect to the cardiotoxicity of anthracycline agents, their acute toxicity and cumulative toxicity constitute problems. Okuma *et al.* (*23*) reported on the basis of an analysis using a Holter ECG that the acute toxicity of pirarubicin was weaker than that of ADM. Also, to date, there have been no reports of clinical results which suggest that pirarubicin possesses acute cardiotoxicity.

Regarding the cumulative cardiotoxicity of pirarubicin, on the other hand, only transient tachycardia in one patient was seen in the present study of 24 patients to whom the drug had been administered in a dose exceeding 500 mg/b.w., and no myocardiopathy or other sympton was detected. However, more cases must be studied in order to determine the upper limit of pirarubicin corresponding to a 500 mg/m² dose of ADM.

On the basis of the above results, pirarubicin can be concluded to be an agent having a broad antitumor spectrum against solid tumors, exerting potent antitumor activity and causing milder adverse reactions such as hair loss and cardiotoxicity than the serious conditions caused by ADM administration.

Although it is necessary to investigate further for the presence or absence of cross-tolerance with ADM, cumulative cardiotoxicity, advisability of concomitant use with other drugs, *etc.*, pirarubicin is surmised to be a useful drug for the clinical treatment of solid tumors.

Acknowledgments
This report was written with the cooperation of many members and facilities to whom the author expresses his thanks.

REFERENCES

1. Abe, O., Kasei, Y., Soejima, S. *et al.* Phase II study of THP for mammary cancer with collaboration. *Jpn. J. Cancer Chemother.*, **13**, 578–585 (1986) (in Japanese).
2. Arcamone, F., Franceshi, G., Penco, S. *et al.* Adriamycin (14-hydroxydaunomycin), a novel antitumor antibiotic. *Tetrahedron Lett.*, **13**, 1007–1010 (1969).
3. Bonadonna, G. Clinical evaulation of adriamycin, a new antitumor antibiotic. *Br. Med. J.*, **30**, 503–506 (1969).
4. Blum, R. H. and Carter, S. K. Adriamycin, a new anticancer drug with significant clinical activity. *Ann. Intern. Med.*, **80**, 249–259 (1974).
5. Dantchev, D., Paintrand, M., Hayat, M. *et al.* Low heart and skin toxicity of a tetrahydropyranyl derivative of adriamycin (THP-ADM) as observed by electron and light microscopy. *J. Antibiot.*, **32**, 1085–1086 (1979).
6. Di Marco, A., Gaetani, M., and Scarpinato, B. M. Adriamycin, a new antibiotic with antitumor activity. *Cancer Chemother. Rep.*, **53**, 33–37 (1969).
7. Hansen, H. H. Anthracyclines and cancer therapy. Proceedings of a Symposium. Ronneby Brunn, Sweden (1982).
8. Honda, T., Oyama, K., Sonoda, T. *et al.* Experience in therapy of malignant tumors on head and neck with THP-adriamycin. *Jpn. J. Cancer Chemother.*, **10**, 2538–2544 (1983) (in Japanese).
9. Ishii, M., Eikawa, K., Kato, T. *et al.* Experience in therapy with THP-adriamycin [of head and neck cancer]. *Rev. Otorhinolaryngol.*, **27**, 763–768 (1984).
10. Kato, T., Nishimura, H., Umezu, J. *et al.* Phase II study of THP-ADM in patients with gynecological cancer. *Jpn. J. Cancer Chemother.*, **12**, 1962–1967 (1985) (in Japanese).
11. Koyama, Y. and Saito, T. Criteria for evaluation of clinical efficacy in chemotherapy of cancer: Criteria for evaluation of direct efficacy in chemotherapy of solid cancers, Ministry of Welfare. Report of research group by grant-in-aid for cancer research (1977–1980).
12. Kunimoto, S., Miura, K., Umezawa, K. *et al.* Cellular uptake and efflux and cytostatic activity of 4′-O-tetrahydropyranyladriamycin in adriamycin-sensitive and-resistant tumor cell lines. *J. Antibiot.*, **37**, 1697–1702 (1984).
13. Majima, H. Experience in preliminary Phase II study on THP-ADM. *Jpn. J. Cancer Chemother.*, **10**, 805–810 (1983) (in Japanese).
14. Majima, H. Phase I clinical study of 4′-O-tetrahydropyranyldoxorubicin (THP-ADM). *Jpn. J. Cancer Chemother.*, **10**, 134–140 (1983) (in Japanese).
15. Minow, R. A., Benjamin, R. S., Lee, E. T. *et al.* Adriamycin cardiomyopathy—Risk factors. *Cancer*, **39**, 1397–1402 (1977).
16. Negoro, S. Results of therapy of adriamycin and THP-adriamycin for non small cell lung cancer. *J. Jpn. Soc. Cancer Ther.*, **10**, 1163 (1984) (in Japanese).
17. Niijima, T. Phase II collaborative study of (2″R)-4′-O-tetrahydropyranyladriamycin (THP) for urological malignancies. *Jpn. J. Cancer Chemother.*, **13**, 224–231 (1986) (in Japanese).
18. Niimoto, M., Yoshinaka, K., Hattori, T. *et al.* Phase II study on THP patients with gastrointestinal cancer. *Jpn. J. Cancer Chemother.*, **13**, 362–367 (1986) (in Japanese).
19. O'Bryan, R. M., Baker, L. H., Gottlieb, J. E. *et al.* Dose response evaluation of adriamycin in human neoplasia. *Cancer*, **39**, 1940–1948 (1977).
20. Ogawa, M. Adriamycin. *Clin. Cancer*, **21**, 1031–1036 (1975).
21. Ogawa, M., Miyamoto, H., Inagaki, J. *et al.* Phase I study on new anthracycline, 4′-O-tetrahydropyranyladriamycin. *Jpn. J. Cancer Chemother.*, **10**, 129–133 (1983) (in Japanese).
22. Okita, H., Ogawa, M., Miyamoto, H. *et al.* Phase II study on THP-ADM. *Jpn. J. Cancer Chemother.*, **11**, 138–142 (1984) (in Japanese).
23. Okuma, K., Furuta, K., Ota, K. *et al.* Acute cardiotoxicity of anthracyclines—Analysis

using Holter ECG. *Jpn. J. Cancer Chemother.*, **11**, 902–911 (1984) (in Japanese).

24. Okuma, K. and Ota, K. Heart toxicity of anticancer agents—Heart toxicity by adriamycin. *Jpn. J. Cancer Chemother.*, **7**, 917–923 (1980) (in Japanese).

25. Praga, C., Beretta, G., Vigo, P. L. *et al.* Cardiac toxicity from antitumor therapy. *Oncology*, **37** (Suppl. 1), 51–58 (1980).

26. Saito, T. (ed.) "Chemotherapy of Cancer: Criteria for Evaluation of Efficacy in Immunotherapy of Cancer and the Development of Anticancer Bgents" (1981). Science Forum, Tokyo.

27. Saito, T. (ed.) "Development of Medical Treatment of Cancer and Evaluation of Efficacy," pp. 115–127 (1985). Realize Inc., Tokyo.

28. Shimosato, Y., Oboshi, S., and Baba, K. Histological evaluation of efficacy of radiotherapy and chemotherapy for carcinomas. *Jpn. J. Clin. Oncol.*, **1**, 19–35 (1971).

29. Suzuki, M., Yoshihara, A., Hirono, M. *et al.* Experience in therapy of malignant tumors with THP-ADM in the field of obstetrics and gynecology. *J. New Rem. Clin.*, **32**, 1823–1830 (1983).

30. Takeda, C. A Phase II study on (2″R)-4′-O-tetrahydropyranyladriamycin (THP) in patients with head and neck cancers. *Jpn. J. Cancer Chemother.*, **13**, (5), 1970–1979 (1986).

31. Takenaka, K., Tamada, R., Hiramoto, Y. *et al.* Phase II study on THP for gastrointestinal cancer. *Jpn. J. Cancer Chemother.*, **12**, 2155–2160 (1985) (in Japanese).

32. Tominaga, K., Kitamura, M., Hayashi, K. *et al.* Effects of 4′-epi-adriamycin, THP-adriamycin and mitoxantrone for mammary cancer. *Jpn. J. Cancer Chemother.*, **11**, 1669–1674 (1984) (in Japanese).

33. Tsuruo, T. Antitumor activity of tetrahydropyranyl derivatives of adriamycin. *Jpn. J. Cancer Chemother.*, **8**, 179–180 (1981) (in Japanese).

34. Tsuruo, T., Iida, H., Tsukagoshi, S. *et al.* 4′-O-Tetrahydropyranyladriamycin as a potential new antitumor agent. *Cancer Res.*, **42**, 1462–1467 (1982).

35. Umezawa, H., Takahashi, Y., Kinoshita, M. *et al.* Tetrahydropyranyl derivatives of daunomycin and adriamycin. *J. Antibiot.*, **32**, 1082–1084 (1979).

36. Wakui, A., Yokoyama, M., Konno, K. *et al.* Collaborative Phase I study on THP. *Jpn. J. Cancer Chemother.*, **12**, 118–124 (1985) (in Japanese).

37. Wakui, A., Yokoyama, M., Yoshida, Y. *et al.* Phase II study on THP in patients with advanced gastrointestinal cancer. *Jpn. J. Cancer Chemother.*, **13**, 1032–1037 (1986) (in Japanese).

38. Yamada, K., Nakamura, T., Tsuruo, T. *et al.* A Phase II study on aclacinomycin A in acute leukemia in adults. *Cancer Treat. Rev.*, **7**, 177–182 (1980).

FUNDAMENTAL STUDY ON A LOW MOLECULAR IMMUNOMODIFIER, UBENIMEX

Masaaki Ishizuka

Institute for Chemotherapy, Microbial Chemistry Research Foundation[*1]

H. Umezawa and the author searched for low molecular weight immunomodifiers in microbial products to use in cancer therapy from among inhibitors of enzymes located on cell surfaces and succeeded in finding ubenimex.[*2] Ubenimex was found to be an inhibitor of aminopeptidase B and leucine aminopeptidase which are located not only in cells but on cell surfaces. It binds to macrophages, T cells and other cells through its binding activity to leucine aminopeptidase. Ubenimex modulates the immune system and exerts an antitumor effect on syngeneic tumors. Fundamental studies on ubenimex are reviewed.

In 1971 H. Umezawa and the author's group initiated the search for a low molecular weight immunomodifier in microbial products which would be effective in inhibiting tumor growth. At that time, coriolin, a unique antitumor antibiotic produced by a mushroom, was discovered by Takeuchi, Iinuma et al. (*30*), and its synthetic derivative, diketocoriolin B was found to enhance antibody formation in mice (*9, 31*). Kunimoto et al. studied the mechanism of action of diketocoriolin B and found it to be an inhibitor of Na^+-K^+-ATPase located in cell membrane (*16*). Thus, we assumed that the binding of diketocoriolin B to Na-K-ATPase in membranes of lymphoid cells modulated host-mediated events including immune response. Studies on low molecular weight enzyme inhibitors produced by microorganisms were started by Umezawa, Aoyagi et al. (*35*). They found that aminopeptidase B and leucine aminopeptidase exist not only in cells but also on cell surfaces (*4*) and confirmed the location of alkaline phosphatase and esterase on these surfaces. On the basis of these findings, the studies were extended to seek immunomodifiers in inhibitors of these enzymes and ubenimex (Fig. 1), amastatin, arphamemine, forphenicine, and ebelactones were found (*37*). Ubenimex was subjected to detailed study which is reviewed in this chapter.

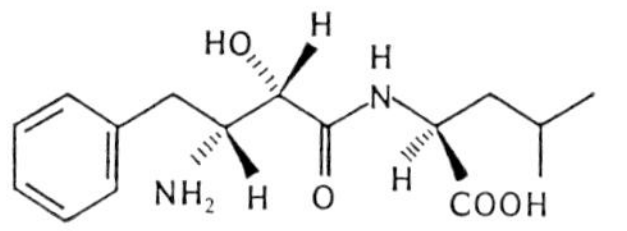

Fig. 1. Structure of ubenimex

Discovery of Ubenimex

Ubenimex was found to be primarily an inhibitor of aminopeptidase B by Umezawa *et al.* (*35*). Aoyagi *et al.* (*4*) reported that aminopeptidases were located not only in cells

---

[*1] Motono 18-24, Miyamoto, Numazu, Shizuoka 410-03, Japan (石塚雅章).
[*2] Ubenimex is currently used against bestatin at the recommendation of WHO.

TABLE I.   Effect of Ubenimex and Its Stereoisomers on DTH Response
in Mice and Their Inhibitory Activities against Aminopeptidases

Stereoisomers	Dose (μg/mouse)	DTH (% of enhancement)	IC$_{50}$ (μM)	
			Aminopeptidase B	Leucine aminopeptidase
(2S, 3R)-AHPA-(S)-Leu[a]	10	55	0.16	0.032
	1	50		
(2S, 3R)-AHPA-(R)-Leu	10	56	18	11
	1	51		
(2R, 3R)-AHPA-(S)-Leu	10	8	320	24
	1	13		
(2R, 3R)-AHPA-(R)Leu	10	24	>800	>800
	1	5		
(2R, 3S)-AHPA-(R)-Leu	10	0	440	>800
	1	2		

[a] [(2S, 3R)-3-amino-2-hydroxy-4-phenylbutanoyl]-(S)-leucine (ubenimex).

but also on the cell surface. To obtain substances binding to the cell surface, inhibitors produced by microorganisms were screened by testing the inhibitory effect of each microbial product (cultured filtrate) on the enzyme, and ubenimex was found in cultured filtrates of a strain classified as *Streptomyces olivoreticuli.*

Ubenimex is obtained as colorless needles. Hydrolysis with 6N HC1 yields L-leucine and (2S, 3R)-3-amino-2-hydroxy-4-phenylbutanoic acid (AHPA). The configuration of the latter amino acid was determined to be 2S and 3R by X-ray crystal analysis, and, based on results of other chemical analyses, the structure was determined to be [(2S, 3R)-3-amino-2-hydroxy-4-phenylbutanoyl]-L-leucine (29). Ubenimex inhibits aminopeptidase B (K_i, 6.0×10^{-8} M) and leucine aminopeptidase (K_i, 2.0×10^{-8} M) but not aminopeptidase A (28).

Ubenimex is well absorbed upon oral administration, more than 85% is excreted into urine and 10% is metabolized to p-hydroxy ubenimex. p-Hydroxy ubenimex, [(2S, 3R)-3-amino-2-hydroxy-4-hydroxyphenylbutanoyl-L-leucine] is an active metabolite with inhibitory activity against aminopeptidases (5).

Ubenimex and its stereoisomers have been synthesized and we confirmed that the inhibitory activity against aminopeptidases and the immunomodulating activity were observed only with 2S isomers (11) (Table I).

Augmentation of Immune Responses

Firstly, it was found that ubenimex augmented immune responses in mice (36). It also augmented delayed-type hypersensitivity (DTH) to sheep red blood cells (SRBC) and to oxazolone over a wide dose range (10). In mice given more than 50 mg/kg, it increased the number of antibody-forming cells in spleen (36). The enhancement of immune responses by ubenimex was more obvious in aged mice (older than 12–14 weeks) (3, 12), and in immunosuppressed mice which were tumor-bearing or were given cyclophosphamide (12) than in normal mice. The administration of ubenimex to these immunosuppressed mice restored the reduced response to an almost normal level, and aged mice augmented the response to that of young mice (6–8 weeks old). Graft *versus* host reaction (GVHR) in X-ray-irradiated and in newborn mice was augmented by ubenimex (3, 39).

In connection with the enhancement of immune responses by this drug its inhibitory activity on suppressors has been reported: administration of ubenimex inhibited the generation of suppressor cells against DTH response. Moreover, ubenimex treatment of mice into which suppressor cells had been transferred enhanced their reduced DTH response markedly, indicating its inhibitory action on suppressor cells (38). The effect of ubenimex on suppressor factors derived from cancer patients has been studied by Noma and Yata (22). They found that the drug inhibited the suppressor action of the sera of these patients on immunoglobulin (Ig) production of peripheral lymphocytes stimulated by pokeweed mitogen (PWM). These results indicate that the enhancing effect of ubenimex on immune responses is partly due to its inhibitory activity on the generation and/or action of suppressors.

Aspects on Lymphocytes, Macrophages, and Bone Marrow Cells

Administration of ubenimex to mice stimulated the proliferation of T cells (11, 18) and bone marrow cells (19). As reported by Müller (19), intraperitoneal injection of ubenimex increased the activity of DNA polymerase α in T cells, but not in B cells, and the terminal deoxynucleotidyl transferase in bone marrow was also stimulated. Concanavalin A (Con A)—or lipopolysaccharide (LPS)-induced mitogenesis of lymphocytes was also stimulated by ubenimex in a dose-dependent manner (11, 20). The drug's effect on proliferation of T cells was observed in the presence of macrophages (11) and, as will be mentioned later, stimulation with ubenimex induced the release of interleukin 1 (IL-1) from the macrophages.

The binding site of ubenimex on cells was studied by Aoyagi et al. (5) and Müller et al. (20). Müller's group reported that macrophages have the most abundant binding sites ($1,459 \times 10^4$ mol/cell), and T cells from spleen and L5178y cells (T-lymphoma) have 254×10^4 mol/cell and 134×10^4 mol/cells, respectively. B cells from spleen have a low number of binding sites, 92×10^4 mol/cell. The number of binding sites per cell paralleled those of leucine aminopeptidase activity. Furthermore, the number of binding sites and the activity of the cell surface binding leucine aminopeptidase during cell cycle were examined by Müller's group using synchronized L5178y cells. The highest number of binding sites was observed during the growth period from S-to G_2-phase (4.8×10^6 mol/cell), while the lowest was during the period between G_1-phase (1.4×10^6 mol/cell) and early S-phase (1.3–2.0×10^6 mol/cell). The highest enzyme activity was determined during S/G_2-phase (151 pmol/10^5 cells) (17). These data thus suggest that the receptor of ubenimex is leucine aminopeptidase, and the observations were confirmed by a study on microdistribution of ubenimex in mice (39).

Ubenimex prevents bone marrow depression caused by cyclophosphamide or mitomycin C in mice. The influence of ubenimex on colony forming unit in culture (CFU/c) production in mouse bone marrow cell cultures was examined in the presence of colony-stimulating factor (GM-CSF). The number of bone marrow stem cells in mice increased when ubenimex was given and the number of CFU/c also increased in bone marrow cell cultures (12). Incubation of bone marrow stem cells with the drug *in vitro* enhanced the production of CFU/c and increased the binding capacity of bone marrow cells to CSF (21). The effect of ubenimex was also confirmed on human bone marrow cells. As reported by Kimura *et al.* (*14*), nucleated cell counts of bone marrow increased in 85% of cancer patients with ubenimex treatment.

Induction and/or Production of Cytokines

As described above, the data indicate that macrophages are necessary for ubenimex-stimulated increase of incorporation of ^{3}H-thymidine into T cells. In a study of the effect of ubenimex on the release of IL-1 from macrophages in mice. Addition of the drug to macrophage cultures was found to stimulate the production of IL-1, and peritoneal macrophages taken from animals given ubenimex released IL-1 into culture supernatant (*27*, *39*).

Ubenimex enhanced the release of interleukin 2 (IL-2) into the cultured supernatant of mouse spleen cells stimulated with Con A, although ubenimex alone could not stimulate IL-2 production in those cultures. In experiments with rat spleen cells, however, incubation with ubenimex alone did stimulate IL-2 release into the culture fluid (*27*). Noma *et al.* showed that ubenimex enhanced the IL-2 release from phytohemagglutinin (PHA)-stimulated human peripheral lymphocytes (*23*). The effect of ubenimex on IL-2 production was also reported by Dunlap *et al.* (*7*) and by Kishter *et al.* (*15*). These actions of ubenimex on the immune system are thus shown due to its binding to macrophages through leucine aminopeptidase, which results in IL-1 induction and the activation of helper T cells and in the release of IL-2.

The effect of ubenimex on interferon production was also investigated. Although ubenimex alone did not induce interferons in sera of normal mice, it enhanced Con A-induced interferon production in mouse spleen cell cultures and LPS-induced interferon production in mice sensitized with BCG (*24*).

Antitumor Effect against Experimental Tumors and Survey of Antitumor Effectors

On the basis of the experimental results reported above, the antitumor effect of ubenimex against animal tumors was tested (Table II). At the start of this study, we employed ascitic type tumors to test the antitumor activity: Ehrlich ascites tumor and L1210 which had been used in screening antitumor antibiotics; ubenimex, however, showed no life span prolongation effect against these tumors. The antitumor activity of the drug was determined against IMC carcinoma which arose spontaneously in CDF_1 mice (*10*, *12*); this tumor can be transferred only through CDF_1 mice. The tumor cells were inoculated subcutaneously and ubenimex was given orally at different intervals before or after the tumor inoculation for 5 consecutive days. Thirty days thereafter, the resulting tumors were weighed. Ubenimex inhibited tumor growth when the administration was begun on day 8 or day 14 after the tumor cell inoculation, but its administration 7 days before or 1 day after the tumor inoculation was less effective. Optimum doses of bestatin (0.05 to 5 mg/kg) exhibiting antitumor activity against IMC carcinoma were required to demonstrate the effect of ubenimex. The antitumor effect was reduced in athymic mice (*1*), in X-ray irradiated and in asialo GM_1 serum-treated mice (*13*). The drug has a low toxicity to mice and shows only a weak cytotoxicity to IMC carcinoma cells *in vitro* at above 100 μg/ml. From these observations, the antitumor effect was thought to be due to host-mediated events; thus, the antitumor effectors generated and activated by ubenimex were investigated (*1*, *13*). After ubenimex therapy, the antitumor

TABLE II. Antitumor Activities against Animal Tumors

Antitumor effect
  By ubenimex alone
    Against transplantable tumors
      IMC carcinoma
      Gardner lymphosarcoma
      C1498 leukemia
    Against autochthonous tumors
    (Carcinogen-induced tumors)
        20-MC induced skin cancer in mice
        MNNG-induced stomach cancer in rats
    Against experimental metastases
      P388 leukemia into lymph nodes
      Melanoma (B16-BL6) into lung
      Lewis lung carcinoma into lung
  In combination with other drugs
    L-1210 leukemia
    Colon 26
    AH66 hepatoma
Activation of effector cells
  Cytotoxic T cells
  NK cells
  Macrophages
  Antibody-dependent killer cells

effect of spleen cells taken from mice treated or untreated with the drug was tested by Winn assay (*13*). Spleen cells taken from ubenimex-treated mice exhibited a marked suppression of tumor growth. The antitumor activity of these cells was reduced by a treatment removing T cells and natural killer (NK) cells, whereas spleen cell preparations enriched in T cells showed the strongest antitumor activity. NK activity measured against YAC-1 cells remained at approximately the same activity as that in normal mice. These facts indicate that the administration of ubenimex to IMC carcinoma-bearing mice generates cytotoxic T cells and NK cells.

Ubenimex inhibited other syngeneic murine tumors. Its administration on days 7 to 11 after tumor inoculation inhibited the growth of myeloid leukemia C1498, and spleen cells taken from mice treated with ubenimex inhibited the tumor growth. In this case, antibody-dependent cellular cytotoxicity and NK activity were enhanced (*1*). The antitumor effect produced by delayed treatment against IMC carcinoma and C1498 might be due to the stimulation of concomitant immunity by ubenimex.

As reported by Blomgren *et al.*, the NK activity of human peripheral blood was also augmented by ubenimex both *in vivo* and *in vitro* (*6*). Cytostatic action of macrophages thus activated against lymphomas and P815 mastocytoma cells has also been reported (*26*).

Ubenimex is effective in inhbiting experimental metastases in mice. Tsuruo *et al.* reported that it suppressed lymph node metastasis of P388 leukemia (*33*); the metastasis of B16-BL6 melanoma cells was also suppressed by ubenimex treatment. In the latter case, the effective doses (50–250 mg/kg) were higher than those against other tumors (*32*). The effector cells against B16-BL6 thus activated were determined to be macrophages. Recently, the effect of ubenimex at 50 mg/kg against metastases of Lewis lung carcinoma has also been confirmed (personal communication).

The combined effect of ubenimex with antitumor drugs was reported. The drug enhanced the antitumor effects of cyclophosphamide and adriamycin against L1210 (*10*, *12*) as well as the effects of 5-fluorouracil, mitomycin C and *cis*-platinum against Colon 26 adenocarcinoma (*2*). In these experiments the timing of ubenimex administration was important; it may be dependent on the mechanism of action of each drug against the tumor and on host-defense mechanisms. Bleomycin is known as an antitumor antibiotic without immunosuppressing activity. The combination of bestatin with bleomycin against AH66 hepatoma in rats showed a marked effect (*2*).

An antitumor substance with immunomodulating activity is desirable to for the inhibition of autochthonous tumors, and the effects of ubenimex against chemical carcinogen-induced tumors were reported. On the induction of skin cancer in mice, the administration of ubenimex (twice a week for 15 weeks starting from the initiation of 20-methylcolanthrene treatment) suppressed tumor growth and prolonged the survival period (*10*). The effect of ubenimex was confirmed on N-methyl-N'-nitro-N-nitrosoguanidine (MNNG)-induced stomach cancer in rats (*8*, *39*). Rats were given MNNG in drinking water for 34 weeks and ubenimex was given by intraperitoneal injection twice a week for 84 weeks or from the 36th week onward. At the 85th week, stomachs were examined macroscopically and histopathologically according to the procedure proposed by the Japanese Society for Gastric Cancer. Ubenimex treatment on both schedules suppressed the frequency of tumor development and the growth of tumors. In this experiment, NK activity was increased in ubenimex-treated rats. These results indicate the effectiveness of ubenimex in inhibiting the development of autochthonous tumors.

The Microdistribution of Ubenimex in Tumor-bearing Mice

The microdistribution of ubenimex in mice bearing IMC carcinoma was reported (*39*). ³H-ubenimex was distributed at high concentrations in macrophages which had infiltrated into solid tumors, whereas in other cells it was detected in only small amounts. In lymphoid organs, ubenimex was also distributed at high concentrations in macrophages. As mentioned above, the binding of ubenimex to leucine aminopeptidase located on the cell surface of macrophages was reported by Müller *et al.* (*20*). In this study the binding to cells through leucine aminopeptidase was confirmed.

CONCLUSIONS

Ubenimex is a dipeptide found in microbial products which has immunomodulating activity and shows an antitumor effect through the activation of the host defense mechanism. It is an inhibitor of aminopeptidase B and leucine aminopeptidase which are located at the cell surface, and binds to macrophages, T cells and bone marrow progenitor cells through its binding activity to leucine aminopeptidase. High concentrations are distributed in macrophages of mice and induce the production of IL-1. In addition, ubenimex enhances the production of IL-2 by T cells stimulated with Con A or in mixed lymphocyte cultures. These results indicate that the actions of ubenimex on the immune system are due to its binding to macrophages which results in IL-1 production, and the activation of helper T cells, in turn, results in the release of IL-2. Moreover, the effect of the drug on enhancement of induction and/or production of cytokines leads to stimulation of the generation and/or the activation of antitumor effector cells, *i.e.* NK cells, cytotoxic T cells and antibody-dependent killer cells. Ubenimex is somewhat effective in inhibiting tumor growth in mice when administration is started 1 or 2 weeks after implantation of tumor cells; it appears to augment the concomitant immunity to the tumor induced in these mice. Therefore, ubenimex may be effective in inhibiting tumor growth in a host in which concomitant immunity to the tumor has been induced.

In bone marrow progenitor cells, ubenimex increases the binding capacity to GM-colony stimulating factors and enhances production of CFU/c. These effects may make it effective in restoring bone marrow depression and in enhancing the antitumor effect of other antitumor drugs.

Ubenimex was found among inhibitors of enzymes on cell membrane during a search for low molecular immunomodifiers by H. Umezawa and the author. Chemically defined low molecular immunomodifiers should have low toxicity and well-characterized biochemical and pharmacological behavior. Ubenimex and others found in future should contribute to an increase in the rate of cure of cancer and other diseases.

REFERENCES

1. Abe, F., Shibuya, K., Uchida, M., Takahashi, K., Horinishi, H., Matsuda, A., Ishizuka, M., Takeuchi, T., and Umezawa, H. Effect of bestatin on syngeneic tumors in mice. *Gann*, **75**, 89–94 (1984).
2. Abe, F., Shibuya, K., Ashizawa, J., Takahashi, K., Horinishi, H., Matsuda, A., Ishizuka, M., Takeuchi, T., and Umezawa, H. Enhancement of antitumor effect of cytotoxic agents by bestatin. *J. Antibiot.*, **37**, 411–413 (1985).
3. Abe, F., Hayashi, M., Horinishi, H., Matsuda, A., Ishizuka, M., and Umezawa, H. Enhancement of graft-versus-host reaction and dealyed cutaneous hypersensitivity in mice by ubenimex. *J. Antibiot.*, **39**, 1172–1177 (1986).
4. Aoyagi, T., Suda, H., Nagai, M., Ogawa, K., Suzuki, J., Takeuchi, T., and Umezawa, H. Aminopeptidase activities on the surface of mammalian cells. *Biochim. Biophys. Acta*, **452**, 131–143 (1976).
5. Aoyagi, T., Ishizuka, M., Takeuchi, T., and Umezawa, H. Enzyme inhibitors in relation to cancer therapy. *J. Antibiot.*, **30** (Suppl.), 121–132 (1977).
6. Blomgren, H., Strender, L.-E., and Edsmyr, F. The influence of bestatin on the lymphoid system in the human. *In* "Small Molecular Immunomodifiers of Microbial Origin–Fundamental and Clinical Studies of Bestatin," ed. H. Umezawa, pp. 71–99 (1981). Japan Scientific Societies Press, Tokyo / Pergamon Press, Oxford.
7. Dunlap, B. E., Dunlap, S. A., and Rich, D. H. Effect of bestatin on *in vitro* response of murine lymphocytes to T cell stimuli. *Scand. J. Immunol.*, **20**, 237–245 (1984).
8. Ebihara, K., Abe, F., Yamashita, T., Shibuya, K., Hayashi, E., Takahashi, K., Horinishi, H., Enomoto, M., Ishizuka, M., and Umezawa, H. The effect of ubenimex on N-methyl-N'-nitro-N-nitrosoguanidine-induced stomach tumor in rats. *J. Antibiot.*, **39**, 966–970 (1986).
9. Ishizuka, M., Iinuma, H., Takeuchi, T., and Umezawa, H. Effect of diketocoriolin B on antibody formation. *J. Antibiot.*, **25**, 320–321 (1972).
10. Ishizuka, M., Masuda, T., Kanbayashi, N., Fukazawa, S., Takeuchi, T., Aoyagi, T., and Umezawa, H. Effect of bestatin on mouse immune system and experimental murine tumors. *J. Antibiot.*, **33**, 642–652 (1980).
11. Ishizuka, M., Saito, H., Sugiyama, Y., Takeuchi, T., and Umezawa, H. Mitogenic effect of bestatin on lymphocytes. *J. Antibiot.*, **33**, 653–662 (1980).
12. Ishizuka, M., Aoyagi, T., Takeuchi, T., and Umezawa, H. Activity of bestatin: enhance-

ment of immune responses and antitumor effect. *In* "Small Molecular Immunomodifiers of Microbial Origin–Fundamental and Clinical Studies of Bestatin," ed. H. Umezawa, pp. 17–38 (1981). Japan Scientific Societies Press, Tokyo / Pergamon Press, Oxford.

13. Ishizuka, M., Masuda, T., Mizutani, S., Takeuchi, T., and Umezawa, H. Antitumor cells found in tumor-bearing mice given ubenimex. *J. Antibiot.*, **40**, 697–701 (1987).

14. Kimura, I., Nakata, Y., and Terao, S. Effect of bestatin on bone marrow. *In* "Small Molecular Immunomodifiers of Microbial Origin–Fundamental and Clinical Studies of Bestatin," ed. H. Umezawa, pp. 119–123 (1981). Japan Scientific Societies Press, Tokyo / Pergamon Press, Oxford.

15. Kishter, S., Hoffman, F. A., and Pizzo, P. A. Production of and response to interleukin-2 by cultured T cells: Effects of lithium chloride and other putative modulators. *J. Biol. Resp. Modif.*, **4**, 185–194 (1985).

16. Kunimoto, T., Hori, M., and Umezawa, H. Mechanism of action of diketocoriolin B. *Biochim. Biophys. Acta*, **298**, 513–525 (1973).

17. Leyhausen, G., Schuster, D. K., Vaith, P., Zahn, R. K., Umezawa, H., Falke, D., and Müller, W.E.G. Identification and properties of the cell membrane bound leucine aminopeptidase interacting with the potential immunostimulant and chemotherapeutic agent bestatin. *Biochem. Pharmacol.*, **32**, 1051–1057 (1983).

18. Müller, W.E.G., Zahn, R. K., Arendes, J., Munsch, N., and Umezawa, H. Activation of DNA metabolism in T-cells by bestatin. *Biochem. Pharmacol.*, **28**, 3131–3137 (1979).

19. Müller, W.E.G. Effect of bestatin on DNA and RNA metabolism in T-cells. *In* "Small Molecular Immunomodifiers of Microbial Origin–Fundamental and Clinical Studies of Bestatin," ed. H. Umezawa, pp. 39–58 (1981). Japan Scientific Societies Press, Tokyo / Pergamon Press, Oxford.

20. Müller, W.E.G., Schuster, D., Zahn, R. K., Maidhof, A., Leyhausen, G., Falke, D., Koren, R., and Umezawa, H. Properties and specificity of binding sites for the immunomodulator bestatin on the surface of mammalian cells. *Int. J. Immunopharmacol.*, **4**, 393–400 (1982).

21. Nemoto, K., Abe, F., Karakawa, K., Horinishi, H., and Umezawa, H. Enhancement of colony formation of mouse bone marrow cells by ubenimex. *J. Antibiot.*, **40**, 894–898 (1987).

22. Noma, T. and Yata, J. Effect of bestatin on the lymphocyte functions of cancer patients. *In* "Immunomodulation by Microbial Products and Related Synthetic Compounds," ed. Y. Yamamura, S. Kotani, and I. Azuma, pp. 480–484 (1981). Excerpta Medica, Amsterdam, Oxford, Princeton.

23. Noma, T., Klein, B., Cuppisol, D., Yata, J., and Serrou, B. Increased sensitivity of IL2-dependent cultured T cells and enhancement of *in vitro* IL2 production by human lymphocytes treated with bestatin. *Int. J. Immunopharmacol.*, **6**, 87–92 (1984).

24. Okura, A., Ishizuka, M., and Takeuchi, T. Effect of ubenimex on the production of murine interferon. *J. Antibiot.*, **41**, 261–263 (1988).

25. Saito, M., Takegoshi, K., Aoyagi, T., Umezawa, H., and Nagai, Y. Stimulatory effect of bestatin, a new specific inhibitor of aminopeptidases, on the blastogenesis of guinea pig lymphocytes. *Cell. Immunol.*, **40**, 247–262 (1978).

26. Schorlemmer, H. U., Bosslet, K., and Sedlacek, H. H. Ability of the immunomodulating dipeptide bestatin to active cytotoxic mononuclear phagocytes. *Cancer Res.*, **43**, 4148–4153 (1983).

27. Shibuya, K., Hayashi, E., Abe, F., Takahashi, K., Horinishi, H., Ishizuka, M., Takeuchi, T., and Umezawa, H. Enhancement of interleukin 1 and interleukin 2 releases by ubenimex. *J. Antibiot.*, **40**, 363–369 (1987).

28. Suda, H., Aoyagi, T., Takeuchi, T., and Umezawa, H. Inhibition of aminopeptidase B and leucine aminopeptidase by bestatin and its stereoisomer. *Arch. Biochem. Biophys.*, **177**, 196–200 (1976).

29. Suda, H., Takita, T., Aoyagi, T., and Umezawa, H. The structure of bestatin [letter]. *J. Antibiot.*, **29**, 100–101 (1976).
30. Takeuchi, T., Iinuma, H., Iwanaga, J., Takahashi, S., Takita, T., and Umezawa, H. Coriolin, a new basidiomycetes antibiotic. *J. Antibiot.*, **22**, 215–217 (1969).
31. Takeuchi, T., Takahashi, S., Iinuma, H., and Umezawa, H. Diketocoriolin B, an active derivative of coriolin B by Coriolus consors. *J. Antibiot.*, **24**, 631–635 (1971).
32. Talmadge, J. E., Lenz, B. F., Pennington, R., Long, C., Phillips, H., Schneider, M., and Tribble, H. Immunomodulatory and therapeutic properties of bestatin. *Cancer Res.*, **46**, 4505–4510 (1986).
33. Tsuruo, T., Naganuma, K., Iida, H., Yamori, T., Tsukagoshi, S., and Sakurai, Y. Inhibition of lymph node metastasis of P388 leukemia by bestatin in mice. *J. Antibiot.*, **34**, 1206–1209 (1981).
34. Umezawa, H. Structures and activities of protease inhibitors of microbial origin. *Methods Enzymol.*, **45**, 678–695 (1976).
35. Umezawa, H., Aoyagi, T., Suda, H., Hamada, M., and Takeuchi, T. Bestatin, an inhibitor of aminopeptidase B, produced by actinomycetes. *J. Antibiot.*, **29**, 97–99 (1976).
36. Umezawa, H., Ishizuka, M., Aoyagi, T., and Takeuchi, T. Enhancement of delayed type hypersensitivity by bestatin, an inhibitor of aminopeptidase B and leucine aminopeptidase. *J. Antibiot.*, **29**, 857–859 (1976).
37. Umezawa, H. Small molecular weight immunomodifiers produced by microorganisms: their screening and discoveries, and the genetics of microbial secondary metabolites. *In* "Small Molecular Immunomodifiers of Microbial Origin-Fundamental and Clinical Studies of Bestatin," ed. H. Umezawa, pp. 1–16 (1981). Japan Scientific Societies Press, Tokyo/Pergamon Press, Oxford.
38. Umezawa, H. Studies on low molecular weight immunomodifiers, bestatin. Discovery and actions. *Drug Exp. Clin.*, **10**, 519–531 (1984).
39. Umezawa, H., Ishizuka, M., Takeuchi, T., Abe, F., and Shibuya, K. Bestatin, a low molecular immunomodifier produced by microorganisms. *Dev. Industr. Microbiol.*, **27**, 31–36 (1987).

REVIEW OF BESTATIN CLINICAL RESEARCH

Kazuo Ota

*Aichi Cancer Center**

A new immunomodulating agent, bestatin (INN: ubenimex) is less toxic even after long-term oral administration and has significant modifications in immunological response, such as increased T-cell population, increased helper/inducer cell number, enhanced natural killer cell activity and increased bone marrow cell proliferation. Randomized Phase III studies to date are reviewed. A cooperative randomized control study of bestatin immunotherapy in combination with remission maintenance chemotherapy for adult acute nonlymphocytic leukemia (ANLL) was performed. After induction of complete remission, patients were randomized to the bestatin group (30 mg/b.w. per os (p.o.) daily) and the control group. The eligible 101 patients (bestatin: 48, control: 53) were analyzed; the bestatin group achieved a longer remission than the control ($p=0.06$) and a statistically significant longer survival ($p=0.007$). Though this prolongation of remission was not significant in the bestatin group compared to the control group in the 15–49 age bracket ($p=0.139$), in the 50–65 bracket it was significantly longer ($p=0.044$). Bestatin is shown as a clinically useful drug for the immunotherapy of adult ANLL, since it prolonged survival and remission, especially in elderly patients, with few side effects. Prospective randomized control studies have been performed in various other cancers including malignant melanoma, carcinoma of the lung, stomach, bladder, head and neck, and esophagus; however, adjuvant bestatin immunotherapy for these cancers should be further investigated to confirm its activity.

Bestatin (INN: ubenimex) is a small molecular weight dipeptide, N-[(2S, 3R)-3-amino-2-hydroxy-4-phenylbutanoyl]-L-leucine, discovered by Umezawa *et al.* (*24*) in the culture filtrate of *Streptomyces olivoreticuli.* Fundamental studies revealed that bestatin shows less toxicity even after long-term oral administration, and demonstrates a modulating activity of cellular immunity, possibly *via* its binding to aminopeptidases located on the cell surface of immune cells, as well as host-mediated antitumor activity against murine tumors (*7*). In this paper I review the clinical research on bestatin.

Phase I and II Studies of Bestatin

The results of Phase I and Phase II clinical trials of bestatin can be summarized as follows (*1, 5, 10–14, 20, 23*). 1) Bestatin is rapidly absorbed following oral administration. 2) Incidence of side effects was very low and no severe adverse reaction was observed. 3) No abnormal laboratory findings due to bestatin were found. 4) Maximal tolerated dose could not be determined but may be at least 900 mg/b.w./day for 4 weeks.

---

* Kanokoden 1-1, Chikusa-ku, Nagoya 464, Japan (太田和雄).

5) Oral administration of 30–100 mg (mostly 30 mg)/b.w./day of bestatin produced the following significant modifications in the immunological response. 1) T-cell population: increased E-rossete forming T-cell number; 2) T-cell subset: increased helper/inducer cell number (OKT4+ cells) and OKT4+/OKT8+ ratio (10); 3) proliferative responses of lymphocytes: enhanced lymphocyte blastogenesis to phytohemagglutinin (PHA); 4) delayed-type hypersensitivity reaction: enhanced skin reaction to purified protein derivative (PPD) and PHA; 5) natural killer (NK) cell activity: enhanced cytolytic activity of NK cells to tumor cells (17); 6) adverse effect on the immunological response at large doses of 300 and 900 mg/b.w./day: suppressed immunological parameter (which was the reason why the oral administration of 30 mg/b.w./day was chosen for further clinical trials); 7) bestatin monotherapy at a dose of 30 mg/b.w./day produced a complete response in a penile cancer patient with minimal residual disease during an interval of one month longer after radiotherapy and a partial response in a patient with recurrent breast cancer (5, 13); 8) effects on bone marrow: increased peripheral and bone marrow neutrophile counts in cancer patients treated with bestatin (8), increased colony forming unit in culture (CFU/c) from the bone marrow of leukemic children under remission (18), and increased CFU/c from the healthy bone marrow with bestatin, possibly mediated by T-lymphocytes (11).

Phase III Studies of Bestatin

Randomized Phase III studies to date are summarized in Table I. Prospective randomized controlled trials have been performed in various malignant diseases including acute leukemia, malignant melanoma, lung cancer, stomach cancer, bladder cancer, head and neck cancer, and esophageal cancer.

1. Acute leukemia

A cooperative randomized control study of immunotherapy with bestatin in combination with remission maintenance chemotherapy for adult acute nonlymphocytic leukemia (ANLL) was performed from 1980 to 1983 (19). Remission induction therapy was given with combination chemotherapy, principally BHAC·DMP, consisting of behenoyl cytosine arabinoside, daunorubicin, 6-mercaptopurine (6-MP), and prednisolone (PRD), or similar active combinations. After complete remission was achieved, a remission consolidation with three administrations of BHAC·DMP was given. Following the induction of complete remission and its consolidation, patients were randomly allocated to the bestatin group or the control group after stratification on the basis of disease type (myeloblastic or monocytic) and age (15–49 or 50–64 years). For remission maintenance chemotherapy, alternating therapy was carried out every 5 weeks using VEMP, consisting of vincristine (VCR), cyclophosphamide, 6-MP, and PRD, and BHAC·DMP. The patients who were allocated to the bestatin group were given bestatin at 30 mg/b.w. per os (p.o.) daily as long as possible concomitantly with maintenance chemotherapy.

Out of the total 115 patients registered, the 101 eligible patients (48 in the bestatin group and 53 in the control group) were analyzed. Various background factors of the patients were compared, but no significant differences were detected between the two groups.

1) Results

After a follow-up period of 2 years to 4 years and 7 months after registration, the

TABLE I. Prospective Randomized Controlled Studies of Bestatin in Cancer

No.	Subject	Principal investigator	No. of eligible patients	Observation period (month)	Remission or no recurrence			Survival		
					Duration (month) control/bestatin	Rate (%) control/bestatin	Difference	MST (month) control/bestatin	Rate (%) control/bestatin	Difference
1.	ANLL	K. Ota	101	<58	12/21	24.2/36.7	$p=0.060$	19/33	25.9/46.1	$p=0.007$
2.	Melanoma	S. Ikeda	69	<40		59.4/77.1	$p<0.05$		61.4/78.3	$p<0.05$
3.	Lung cancer	M. Fukuoka	74	<36	Not evaluated			5.6/9.3		$p<0.05$
4.	Lung cancer	T. Yasumitsu	65	<60	Not evaluated			36/—	43.9/74.1	$p<0.05$
5.	Lung cancer	C. Mouritzen	252	<33	More favorable in the bestatin group		$p=0.3275$	More favorable in the bestatin group		$p=0.1706$
6.	Stomach cancer	T. Hattori	77	<60	Not evaluated			More favorable in the bestatin group		$p=0.411$
7.	Bladder cancer	H. Blomgren	151	<66	More favorable in the bestatin group		$p=0.044$	More favorable in the bestatin group		$p=0.49$
8.	Bladder cancer	Y. Kumamoto	124	24		66.7/81.4	$p=0.08$	Not evaluated		
9.	Head and neck cancer	C. Takeda	325	24		64.2/66.4	$p=0.42$		70.9/80.5	$p=0.096$
10.	Esophageal cancer	H. Sato	145	<29	Not evaluated			More favorable in the bestatin group		$p=0.076$

Remarks:
1. Combined with remission maintenance chemotherapy after induction of complete remission.
2. Combined with post-surgical chemotherapy in stage Ib and II.
3. Combined with chemotherapy and/or radiotherapy in stage III and IV inoperable squamous cell carcinoma.
4. Combined with post-surgical chemotherapy and/or radiotherapy in operated stage I-III squamous cell carcinoma.
5. Operated stage I and III non-small cell carcinoma.
6. Combined with post-surgical chemotherapy in curatively operated stomach cancer.
7. Mostly T 2, 3, post-radiotherapy.
8. Combined with bleomycin intravesical instillation in superficial bladder cancer.
9. Curatively operated or irradiated patients with squamous cell carcinoma.
10. Operated squamous cell carcinoma (mostly stage II, III).

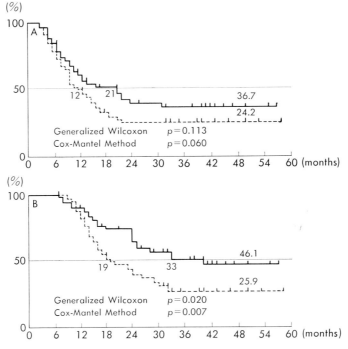

FIG. 1.   Remission duration (A) and survival (B) in ANLL
— bestatin (*n*=48); --- control (*n*=53).

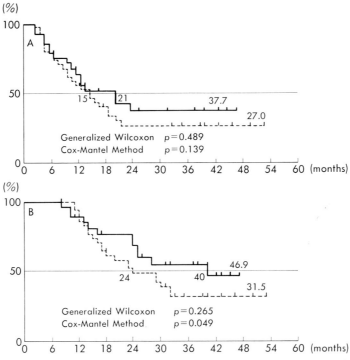

FIG. 2.   Remission duration (A) and survival (B) in ANLL (age: 15–49)
— bestatin (*n*=28); --- control (*n*=34).

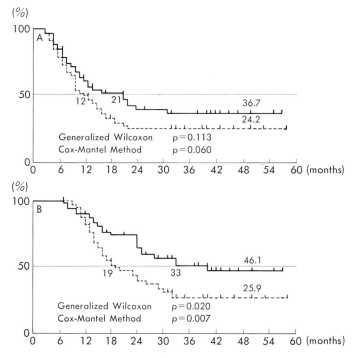

FIG. 3.   Remission duration (A) and survival (B) in ANLL (age 50–65)
— bestatin ($n=20$); --- control ($n=19$).

bestatin group had achieved a longer remission than the control group ($p=0.06$), and also showed a statistically significant longer survival ($p=0.007$) (Fig. 1). In the 15–49 age bracket, the prolongation of remission was not significant in the bestatin group compared to the control group ($p=0.139$), but survival in the bestatin group was significantly longer ($p=0.049$) (Fig. 2). In the 50–65 age bracket, the bestatin group achieved both significantly longer remission ($p=0.044$) and significantly longer survival ($p=0.003$) (Fig. 3).

Recurrence was observed in 58.3% of the bestatin group and 73.6% of the control group, and complete remission was 53.6% in the bestatin group against 30.8% ($p<0.1$) in the control group. Longer survival was achieved in the bestatin group but the differences were borderline ($p=0.068$).

Side effects of bestatin were observed in 5 (9.6%) of 52 patients, 2 patients (3.8%) each with rash and itchiness and one (1.9%) with numbness. However, they were very mild and disappeared when the bestatin therapy was continued or discontinued. There were no abnormalities traceable to bestatin under laboratory examination.

After a follow-up period of 5 years and 10 months following completion of the study, survival in the bestatin group in overall ANLL was still significantly longer than in the control group ($p=0.003$).

2)   *Discussion and conclusion*

There have been a number of reports concerning the use of immunotherapy after achieving complete remission in adult ANLL; however, no consensus has yet been reached with regard to the efficacy of immunotherapy. Foon *et al*. (*4*) analyzed 24 published reports involving immunotherapy with BCG, *Corynebacterium*, or leukemic cells as an adjuvant immunotherapy in acute myeloblastic leukemia (AML). They found that patients who received a combination of immunotherapy with maintenance chemotherapy had no significant prolongation of remission duration, but a significant survival advantage was detected in those patients.

In the present study the survival was significantly longer in the bestatin group than the control group in overall ANLL, and a prolongation of remission duration was also observed in the bestatin group, though the difference was borderline. However, the remission duration was significantly longer in patients in the 50–65 age bracket of the bestatin group than in the control group. It is generally agreed that immune activity is suppressed in elderly patients, and it has been reported that suppressed immune activity in aged animals recovered following bestatin treatment (3). It is therefore reasonable to consider that the immune modulating effects of bestatin would be more strongly manifested in elderly patients than in younger ones.

On the basis of the above findings, it is concluded that bestatin is a clinically useful drug for the immunotherapy of adult ANLL, since it prolonged the survival and remission duration, especially in elderly patients with few side effects.

2.   Malignant melanoma

A cooperative randomized control study of immunotherapy with bestatin in combination with chemotherapy in malignant melanoma was perfomed from 1980 to 1983 (6). Patients clinically diagnosed as malignant melanoma were preoperatively given one course of combination chemotherapy DAV, consisting of dacarbazine, nimustine, and VCR. At the postoperative stage of malignant melanoma, stage Ib and II patients were randomly allocated to the bestatin group or the control group. Both groups were given 2–3 courses of DAV, and the patients of the bestatin group were given bestatin at 30 mg/ b.w. p.o. daily for more than 6 months until recurrence or metastasis was observed.

The 69 eligible patients (35 in the bestatin group and 34 in the control group) were then analyzed, and comparison of the various background factors of those in the two groups revealed no significant biases.

Results

After a follow-up period of 2 years to 3 yesrs and 4 months after registration, both the disease-free interval rate and the survival rate after operation in the bestatin group were significantly higher than in the control group ($p<0.05$). The estimated 40-month disease-free interval was 77.1% for the bestatin group and 59.4% for the control group, and the respective survival rates were 78.3% and 61.4%.

Side effects of bestatin, chiefly consisting of reversible gastro-intestinal disturbances, were observed in 7.1% of bestatin-treated patients.

These findings suggest that bestatin is a useful agent for the immunotherapy of stage Ib and II malignant melanoma patients.

3.   Lung cancer

Three prospective randomized control trials using bestatin were performed in lung cancer cases. One was a study of inoperable advanced lung cancer (22). Patients were given chemotherapy with or without radiotherapy, and randomly allocated either to the bestatin group or the control group. After stratifying on the basis of histology of the cancer, patients in the bestatin group were given bestatin at 30 mg/b.w. p.o. daily as long as possible.

The 231 eligible patients were analyzed. Overall survival was not significantly different between the bestatin group and the control group ($p=0.11$). In 74 squamous cell cancer patients (38 in the bestatin group and 36 in the control group), however, a significantly longer survival time was achieved in the bestatin group than in the controls ($p<0.05$): median survival time (MST) was respectively 9.3 months and 5.6 months.

Another study was an ongoing one of operated stage I-III lung cancer (25). Patients were given postoperative chemotherapy with or without radiotherapy according to the stage and histologic type, and randomly allocated to the bestatin group or the control group. Patients in the bestatin group were given bestatin at 30 mg/b.w. p.o. daily for more than one year. The 65 eligible patients with squamous cell carcinoma (34 in the bestatin group and 31 in the control group) were analyzed, and significantly longer survival was achieved in the bestatin group ($p<0.05$). The survival rate was 74.1% for the bestatin group and 43.9% for the control group 4 years after operation.

The last ongoing study dealt with adjuvant treatment in operated stage I and II non-small cell lung cancer and was performed in 15 European university clinics by the European Lung Cancer Study Group. (16). By April 1st, 1986, 601 patients had entered the study. Patients in the bestatin group were given bestatin at 90 mg/b.w./day p.o. every other for 5 years or until proven recurrence or death. The 252 eligible patients (122 in the bestatin group and 130 in the control group) were included in an interim analysis 33 months after inception of the study. Neither disease-free nor overall survival were significantly different, though the disease-free survival proved more favorable in this group ($p<0.3275$) and overall survival was also better in the bestatin group ($p=0.1706$). A few years must pass before the final conclusions of this study will be available.

4. Stomach cancer

A prospective randomized control study of bestatin was performed in adjuvant chemoimmunotherapy for operated stomach cancer from Novermber 1980 to April 1984. (26).

Patients were given chemotherapy consisting of mitomycin C at 20 mg/b.w. intravenously (i.v.) for surgery, mitomycin C at 10 mg/b.w. i.v. the next day, then tegafur at 1,000 mg/b.w./day as a suppository in the hospital and tegafur at 600 mg/b.w./day p.o. after discharge from the hospital. Patients in the bestatin group were given bestatin at 60 mg/b.w. p.o. daily for as long as possible. The 96 eligible patients (51 in the bestatin group and 45 in the control group) were then analyzed; survival rates in the bestatin group were slightly higher and considerably higher in stage III and IV compared to the control group, but the differences were not significant ($p=0.4119$) and ($p=0.1621$), respectively. However, the effectiveness of bestatin was suggested in postoperative peritoneal recurrence in the cases with positive histological invasion of the stomach wall veins ($p<0.1$).

5. Bladder cancer

Two prospective randomized control trials of bestatin were performed for bladder cancer. One was adjuvant bestatin immunotherapy after full-dose local radiotherapy of 64 Gy in the management of nonmetastatic transitional cell carcinoma of the bladder (2). The 151 eligible patients (75 in the bestatin group and 76 in the control group) were then analyzed for a long follow-up period of 6 years. Disease-free survival of the patients was significantly improved in the bestatin group compared to the control group ($p=0.044$);

however, overall survival was not affected by the bestatin treatment ($p=0.49$). The beneficial effect of bestatin seemed to be more marked in men ($p=0.018$) than women ($p=0.89$), and in the patients with less advanced disease (T1 and T2) ($p=0.10$) compared to more advanced disease (T3 and T4) ($p=0.23$).

The other study involved a randomized control trial to prevent recurrence of superficial bladder cancer using intravesical instillation of bleomycin in combination with or without bestatin (9). The 124 eligible patients (66 in the bestatin group and 58 in the control group) were then analyzed. Patients in both groups were given bleomycin intravesical instillation of 60 mg/b.w./day for 7 days, then 60 mg/b.w./day every month intermittently for 2 years, and patients in the bestatin group were given bestatin of 60 mg/b.w./day for as long as possible. In the 2-year follow-up period the bladder cancer nonrecurrence rate was higher in the bestatin group at 12 months than in the control group ($p=0.08$). This difference was especially significant in patients with a single tumor ($p<0.05$).

6. Head and neck cancer

A cooperative prospective randomized control trial of adjuvant bestatin immunotherapy was performed in curatively operated or irradiated patients with squamous cell carcinoma of the head and neck (15). Patients of the bestatin group were given bestatin at 30 mg/b.w. p.o. daily for 2 years after the radical treatment. The overall 325 eligible patients (165 in the bestatin group and 160 in the control group) were analyzed as to survival at 2 years. Two-year survival rate of the bestatin group was 80.5%, and higher than the 70.9% in the control group ($p=0.096$), Survival was better in the bestatin group in stage III patients ($p=0.010$) and in the group aged over 60 years ($p=0.067$) than in the control group.

7. Esophageal cancer

A cooperative prospective randomized control study of bestatin adjuvant immunotherapy combined with preoperative treatment was performed in esophageal cancer (21). Patients were stratified in preoperative treatment with bleomycin alone at total 45–100

TABLE II.   Overall Incidence of Side Effects

Symptoms		No. of occurrences	Percentage
Hepatic disorders		2	0.21
Skin disorders	Rash, flushing	10	1.06
	Pruritus	4	0.43
	Alopecia (slight)	1	0.11
		15	1.60
Gastrointestinal disorders	Nausea, vomiting	5	0.53
	Diarrhea	2	0.21
	Stools loose, flaculence	1	0.11
		8	0.85
Other disorders	Facial edema	1	0.11
	Strange oral feeling	1	0.11
	Numbness	1	0.11
	Headache	1	0.11
		4	0.43
Total (939 cases)		29	3.09

mg, radiation alone at total 30–40 Gy and the combination of bleomycin and radiation. Patients in the bestatin group were given bestatin at 30 mg/b.w. p.o. daily before and after operation as long as possible. The 145 eligible patients (59 in the bestatin group and 86 in the control group) were then analyzed as to survival. Overall survival was better in the bestatin group compared to the control group ($p=0.076$). In patients treated with preoperative radiation alone the bestatin group showed better results, the difference in survival being significant ($p=0.01$).

Side Effect of Bestatin

The side effects of bestatin are summarized in Table II (27). Among the side effects in 939 patients including Phase I, II, and III studies, the most frequent were skin disorders such as rash and pruritus (15 cases, 1.6%), followed by gastrointestinal disorders including nausea, vomiting and diarrhea (8 cases, 0.85%). The overall incidence of side effects was 3.09%. Most of these were mild and disappeared during administration of bestatin or after its discontinuation.

CONCLUSION

On the basis of the above stated results of Phase III studies, the immunotherapeutic benefits of bestatin were definitely proven in adult ANLL, in combination with remission maintenance chemotherapy after induction of complete remission. However, adjuvant bestatin immunotherapy for various other cancers should be further investigated to confirm its activity.

REFERENCES

1. Arimori, S., Nagao, T., Shimizu, Y., Watanabe, K., and Komatsuda, M. The Effect of bestatin on patients with acute and chronic leukemia and malignant lymphoma. *Tokai J. Exp. Clin. Med.*, **5**, 63–71 (1980).
2. Blomgen, H., Naslund, I., Esposti, P. L., Johansen, L., and Aaskoven, O. Adjuvant bestatin immunotherapy in patients with transitional cell carcinoma of the bladder. *Cancer Immunol. Immunother.*, **25**, 41–46 (1987).
3. Bruley-Rosset, M., Florentin, I., Kiger, N., Schulz, J., and Mathé, G. Restoration of impaired immune functions of aged animals by chronic bestatin treatment. *Immunology*, **38**, 75–83 (1979).
4. Foon, F. A., Smalley, R. V., and Riggs, C. W. The role of immunotherapy in acute myelogenous leukemia. *Arch. Intern. Med.*, **143**, 1726–1731 (1983).
5. Ichikawa, T., Hirokawa, I., and Ishihara, Y. Clinical studies of bestatin on genitourinary cancer. *Jpn. J. Antibiot.*, **38**, 166–178 (1985) (in Japanese).
6. Ikeda, S. and Ishihara, K. Randomized, controlled study by bestatin in the treatment of stage Ib and II malignant melanoma. *Int. J. Immunother.*, **11**, 73–79 (1986).
7. Ishizuka, M., Masuda, T., Kanbayashi, N., Fukasawa, S., Takeuchi, T., Aoyagi, T., and Umezawa, H. Effect of bestatin on mouse immune system and experimental murine tumors. *J. Antibiot.*, **33**, 642–652 (1980).
8. Kimura, I., Ohnoshi, T., Nakata, Y., and Terao, S. Effect of bestatin on the bone marrow. *Jpn. J. Cancer. Chemother.*, **8**, 586–589 (1981) (in Japanese).
9. Kumamoto, Y., Tsukamoto, T., Tamiya, T. *et al.* Clinical research of prevention of recurrence of superficial bladder cancer. Cooperative study of clinical efficacy of bleomycin intravesical instillation and bestatin. *Hinyokiyo*, **31**, 1861–1883 (1985) (in Japanese).

10. Kumano, N., Suzuki, S., Oizumi, K., Konno, K., Himori, T., Mitachi, Y., and Wakui, A. Imbalance of T cell subsets in cancer patients and its modification with bestatin, a small molecular immunomodulator. *Tohoku J. Exp. Med.*, **147**, 125–133 (1985).

11. Maekawa, T., Sonoda, Y., Okamoto, Y., Tsuda, S., Nishida, K., Taniwaki, M., Abe, T., and Takino, T. Effect of bestatin on human granulocyte-macrophage progenitor cells (CFU-c) *in vitro* and its possible mechanism of action. *J. Kyoto Pref. Univ. Med.*, **93**, 1039–1044 (1984) (in Japanese).

12. Majima, H. and Suzuki, M. Phase I clinical study of bestatin. *Jpn. J. Cancer Chemother.*, **8**, 278–284 (1981) (in Japanese).

13. Majima, H., Suzuki, M., and Nakano, M. Phase I and preliminary phase II study of bestatin. *Jpn. J. Cancer Chemother.*, **7**, 89–94 (1980) (in Japanese).

14. Majima, H. Phase I clinical study of bestatin. *In* "Recent Results of Bestatin 1985," ed. H. Umezawa, pp. 67–72 (1986). Japan Antibiotics Research Association, Tokyo.

15. Miyake, H., Takeda, C., Okuda, M. *et al.* Adjuvant therapy with bestatin for squamous cell carcinoma of the head and neck. *Otol. Fukuoka*, **30**, 1142–1151 (1984) (in Japanese).

16. Mouritzen, C. Bestatin as adjuvant treatment in operated stage I and II non-small cell lung cancer. *In* "Recent Results of Bestatin 1986," ed. H. Umezawa, pp. 61–66 (1986). Japan Antibiotics Research Association, Tokyo.

17. Noma, T., Yoshimura, N., and Yata, J. Depressed lymphocyte function of cancer patients and their correction by bestatin (product of *Streptomyces olivoreticuli*). *In* "Current Concepts in Human Immunology and Cancer Immunomodulation," ed. B. Serrou *et al.*, pp. 611–616 (1982). Elsevier Biomedical Press B. V., Amsterdam.

18. Okawa, H., Handa, T., Inada, M., Suzuki, M., Kusaka, H., and Yata, J. Hematopoietic colony stimulating effect of immunopotentiators. *Jpn. J. Cancer Chemother.*, **7**, 2155–2160 (1980) (in Japanese).

19. Ota, K., Kurita, S., Yamada, K., Masaoka, T., Uzuka, Y., and Ogawa, N. Immunotherapy with bestatin for acute nonlymphocytic leukemia in adult. *Cancer Immunol. Immunother.*, **23**, 5–10 (1986).

20. Saito, K., Miyasato, H., Tajima, K., and Ikeda, S. Phase I study of bestatin: (I) A clinical study on determination of an optimal dose of bestatin. *Jpn. J. Cancer Chemother.*, **10**, 211–217 (1983) (in Japanese).

21. Sato, H., Isono, K., Nabeya, K. *et al.* Effect of bestatin on primary tumor and prognosis in patients with esophageal carcinoma. *J. Jpn. Soc. Cancer Ther.*, **19**, 2312–2326 (1984) (in Japanese).

22. Takada, M. and Fukuoka, M. Controlled study of ubenimex on inoperable lung cancer. Bestatin Workshop, 16th International Congress of Chemotherapy, Jerusalem (1989).

23. Takino, T., Sawai, K., Abe, T., Maekawa, T., Okamoto, Y., Inazawa, J., Tsuda, S., Nishida, K., Taniwaki, M., Sonoda, Y., Edagawa, J., Fujii, H., and Ohgawara, Y. A phase II study on immunochemotherapy with bestatin for hematological malignancies. *J. Kyoto Pref. Univ. Med.*, **93**, 405–412 (1984) (in Japanese).

24. Umezawa, H., Aoyagi, T., Suda, H., Hamada, M., and Takeuchi, T. Bestatin, an inhibitor of aminopeptidase B, produced by actinomycetes. *J. Antibiot.*, **29**, 97–99 (1976).

25. Yasumitsu, T., Kotake, Y., Nakano, N., and Ohshima, S. A randomized clinical trial of ubenimex in resected lung cancer. Bestatin Workshop, 16th International Congress of Chemotherapy, Jerusalem (1989).

26. Yoshinaka, K., Tanaka, T., Takagami, S., Saeki, T., Nishiyama, M., Toge, T., Niimoto, M., and Hattori, T. Prospective randomized controlled study on bestatin in gastric cancer surgery. *Jpn. J. Cancer Chemother.*, **15**, 493–498 (1988) (in Japanese).

27. Yugeta, E., Anegawa, H., and Matsuda, A. Japanese NDA application and the current status of bestatin. *In* "Recent Results of Bestatin 1986," ed., H. Umezawa, pp. 101–112 (1986). Japan Antibiotics Research Association, Tokyo.

III. NEW APPROACHES

NEW ANTITUMOR ANTIBIOTICS BASED UPON NOVEL MECHANISM OF ACTION

Nobuo Tanaka[*1],[*2]

Institute of Applied Microbiology, University of Tokyo

We have sought new antitumor antibiotics based upon a novel mechanism of action. A new nucleoside analog, cadeguomycin, has been found from a *Streptomyces*, and the structure, 7-carboxy-7-deazaguanosine, has been determined. The antibiotic stimulates incorporation of pyrimidine nucleosides into K562 and YAC-1 leukemic cells. The mechanism of action has been elucidated: cadeguomycin-5'-monophosphate inhibits dCMP deaminase. The antibiotic markedly enhances the activity of cytosine arabinoside by blocking the conversion of AraCMP to AraUMP. Cadeguomycin also potentiates other cytidine and deoxycytidine analogs. 2-crotonyloxymethyl-4,5,6-trihydroxycyclohex-2-enone (COTC) inhibits adriamycin-, aclarubicin-, and bleomycin-resistant L5178Y lymphoma cells more significantly than the parental cells, while potentiating the activity of aclarubicin against aclarubicin-resistant cells. COTC interacts with sulfhydryl groups and inhibits DNA polymerase α and mitosis. New antitumor antibiotics, lactoquinomycins A and B, have been isolated from a *Streptomyces* and the structures elucidated. Lactoquinomycins inhibit adriamycin-, aclarubicin-, and bleomycin-resistant L5178Y cells more markedly than the parental cells. The mechanism of action has been studied and free radical formation found apparently important for its action.

In our laboratory, we have searched for novel anticancer antibiotics based on a new mechanism of action. Our work on cadeguomycin, 2-crotonyloxymethyl-4,5,6-trihydroxycyclohex-2-enone (COTC), and lactoquinomycins are presented in this publication.

Cadeguomycin

1. Discovery (14)

In 1980, we found that *Streptomyces hygroscopicus* IM7912T produces two substances: one inhibits [³H]thymidine incorporation into K562 human myelogenous leukemia cells and the other enhances it. They were purified from the culture fluid and characterized. The former was identified as tubercidin and the latter a new nucleoside antibiotic. The novel agent was designated cadeguomycin, because the chemical structure is 7-carboxy-7-deazaguanosine and the producing organism belongs to the genus *Streptomyces*.

[*1] Yayoi 1-1-1, Bunkyo-ku, Tokyo 113, Japan (田中信男).

[*2] Present address: Banyu Pharmaceutical Co., Ltd., Nihonbashi Honcho 2-2-3, Chuo-ku, Tokyo, Japan.

2. Structure determination (4, 5, 16)

Cadeguomycin, $C_{12}H_{14}O_7N_4$, FD-MS: m/z 326(M$^+$), is a weakly acidic substance, showing ultraviolet (UV) $\lambda_{max}^{H_2O}(\varepsilon)$ 232 (19677), 272 (6881), and 298 nm (7607), and IR ν_{max}^{KBr} 1650 (C=O) and 3,420 (NH or OH) cm^{-1}. The UV spectrum is similar to other pyrrolo[2,3-*d*]pyrimidines. The structure of cadeguomycin, 2-amino-3,4-dihydro-4-oxo-7-β-D-ribofuranosyl-7H-pyrrolo[2,3-*d*]pyrimidine-5-carboxylic acid, has been elucidated by ^{1}H NMR and ^{13}C NMR and compared with other pyrrolo[2,3-*d*]pyrimidines and their nucleosides, and confirmed by chemical synthesis (Fig. 1).

3. Stimulation of pyrimidine nucleoside incorporation and its mechanism (12, 15)

Cadeguomycin enhances pyrimidine, but not purine, nucleoside incorporation into K562 human myelogenous leukemia cells. Preincubation of K562 cells with cadeguomycin (5 μg/ml) for 18 hr induces 17, 10, and 6 fold increases in uptake of [^{3}H]thymidine, [^{3}H]uridine, and [^{3}H]deoxycytidine, respectively, into acid-insoluble material (Fig. 2). The degree of echnancement is logarithmic with the antibiotic concentrations in a range of 0.2–5 μg/ml. Cadeguomycin also stimulates pyrimidine nucleoside uptake into YAC-1 cells but not into other cells. Cadeguomycin-treated K562 cells show higher activity of pyrimidine nucleoside and/or nucleotide kinases, suggesting that enhancement of pyri-

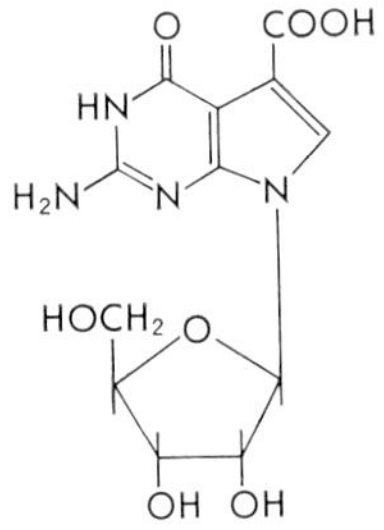

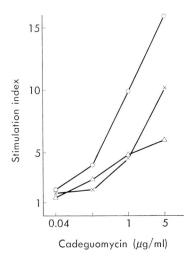

FIG. 1. Structure of cadeguomycin

FIG. 2. Stimulation by cadeguomycin of [^{3}H]thymidine (○), [^{3}H]deoxycytidine (△) or [^{3}H]uridine (×) incorporation in K562 cells after 18 hr preincubation

TABLE I. Analysis of [³H] Ara-C Incorporated into the Acid-soluble Fraction of K562 Cells

Cadeguo-mycin (μM)	Incubation with Ara-C (min)	Ara-C (fmol/10⁶ cells)	AraCMP (fmol/10⁶ cells)	AraCDP+AraCTP (fmol/10⁶ cells)
0	15	2,300±272[a] (89)[b]	203±32 (8)	84±18 (3)
75		620±40 (36)	597±33 (35)	495±51 (29)
0	30	2,040±55 (88)	186±16 (8)	87±10 (4)
75		870±44 (34)	823±165 (33)	839±142 (33)

K562 cells were treated with 75 μM cadeguomycin for 18 hr and incubated with [³H]Ara-C for 15 or 30 min.

[a] Mean±SD.

[b] Numbers in parentheses, percentage of total [³H]Ara-C and its nucleotides.

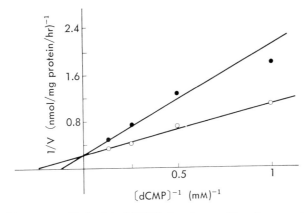

FIG. 3. Lineweaver- Burk plot of dCMP deaminase with cadeguomycin-5′-mono-phosphate (CDM-MP)

● assayed with dCTP at 2 μM+CDM-MP (1.8 μM); ○ control.

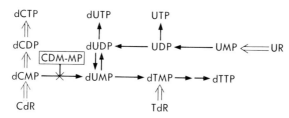

FIG. 4. The interconversion of deoxynucleotides and site of action of cadeguomycin
CDM-MP, cadeguomycin-5′-monophosphate; ⇒ reactions enhanced by cade-guomycin.

midine nucleoside uptake occurs during the phosphorylation process. The mechanism of action has been further studied *in vivo* and *in vitro*. Cadeguomycin-5′-monophosphate has been synthesized and found to inhibit dCMP deaminase: K_i 1.7 μM (Fig. 3). The results suggest that cadeguomycin is phosphorylated *in vivo* and the 5′-monophosphate inhibits dCMP deaminase, resulting in enhancement of pyrimidine nucleoside incorporation (Fig. 4).

4. Potentiation of cytotoxicity of 1-β-D-arabinofuranosylcytosine (Ara-C) and other pyrimidine nucleoside analogs (3, 11, 17)

The cytotoxicity to K562 cells of Ara-C is markedly enhanced by cadeguomycin (Fig. 5). The IC_{50} of Ara-C is 0.35 μM in the absence of cadeguomycin and 0.025 μM in the presence of 0.6 μM cadeguomycin; the degree of potentiation is 14. More significant stimulation of Ara-C activity by cadeguomycin is observed with Ara-C-resistant K562 cells (Fig. 6). Potentiation of Ara-C is also observed in mouse lymphoma YAC-1 cells, with the degree depending upon cadeguomycin concentration. The treatment of K562 cells with 75 μM cadeguomycin for 18 hr increased cellular uptake of [³H]Ara-C and formation of Ara-C nucleotides. The level of AraCDP plus AraCTP, the active form, is *ca.* 10 times higher in the cadeguomycin-treated cells than that in the untreated cells following 30 min incubation with [³H]Ara-C (Table I). Since Ara-C is converted to the active form, AraCTP, and inactivated by dCMP deaminase, the mechanism of potentia-

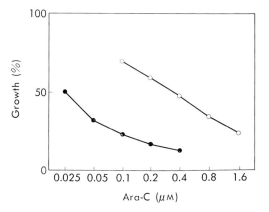

FIG. 5.   Effect of cadeguomycin on Ara-C cytotoxicity for K562 cells
Two ml of cell suspension (2×10⁴/ml) were cultured in a 24-well plastic plate at 37°C with various concentrations of Ara-C in the absence (○) or presence (●) of 0.6 μM cadeguomycin. The viable cells were determined after 5 days, and the average of triplicate determinations is presented.

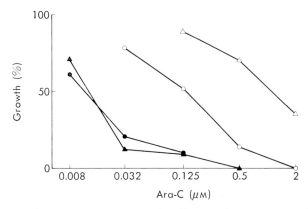

FIG. 6.   Effect of cadeguomycin on Ara-C cytotoxicity for parental and Ara-C-resistant K562 cells
●▲, + CDM 0.6 μM; △ Ara-C-resistant; ○ parent.

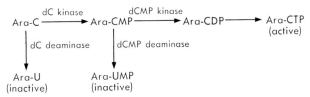

FIG. 7.   Activation and inactivation of Ara-C

TABLE II.   Effects of Cadeguomycin on Cytotoxicity of Pyrimidine
Base and Nucleoside Analogs for Growth of K562 Cells

Analogs	IC_{50} of analogs (μM)		Potentiation ratio
	Cadeguomycin (μM)		
	0	3	
Ara-C	0.35	0.0062	56.4
5-Fluoro CdR	6.2	0.61	10.2
5-Aza CdR	0.10	0.019	5.3
5-Aza CR	1.35	0.45	3.0
5-Fluoro UdR	1.9	1.6	1.2
3-Deaza UR	0.25	0.35	0.71
5-Fluoro Ura	8.2	15	0.55

CdR, deoxycytidine; CR, cytidine; UdR, deoxyuridine; UR, uridine; Ura, uracil.

tion of Ara-C by cadeguomycin may be due to the prevention of conversion of AraCMP to AraUMP in the activation process (Fig. 7). The cytotoxicity of 5-fluorodeoxycytidine (FCdR), 5-azadeoxycytidine, and 5-azacytidine to K562 cells is enhanced by cadeguomycin, although the degree of potentiation is less than that of Ara-C (Table II). On the contrary, the activity of 5-fluorodeoxyuridine (FUdR), 3-deazauridine, 5-fluorouracil (5FU) is not stimulated by cadeguomycin, suggesting the potentiation activity is limited to cytidine and deoxycytidine analogs. The results are in accordance with the assumption that the potentiation is due to the inhibition by cadeguomycin of dCMP deaminase.

2-Crotonyloxymethyl-4,5,6-trihydroxycyclohex-2-enone(COTC)

1. Isolation and characterization (10)

We have been interested in drug-resistance of tumor cells, and obtained drug-resistant sublines of murine T-lymphoblastoma L5178Y cells. We found that the 5′-nucleotide phosphodiesterase activity of the plasma membrane is higher in adriamycin-, aclarubicin-, and bleomycin-resistant cell sublines than that in the parental cell line (1, 2. 9). The drug resistance is due to alteration of membrane transport of the antibiotics in these resistant cells. Based on these observations, we attempted to isolate inhibitors of the enzyme from microorganisms. We isolated an inhibitor from a *Streptomyces*, and identified it with COTC by UV, IR, ¹H NMR, and ¹³C NMR spectrometry (10).

2. COTC blocks 5′-nucleotide phosphodiesterase

IC_{50} was 60 μg/ml by the method employed. Adriamycin-, aclarubicin-, and bleomycin-resistant sublines of L5178Y cells are more sensitive to COTC than to the parental cells: IC_{50} of growth inhibition 3.3, 1.15, 1.55, and 4.4 μg/ml, respectively. Therefore,

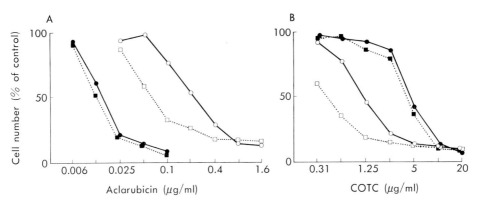

F IG. 8.   Synergistic effects of aclarubicin and COTC on growth of an aclarubicin-
resistant subline of L5178 Y cells
    A: effects of aclarubicin in the presence and absence of a sublethal concentration
of COTC.   B: effects of COTC in the presence and absence of a sublethal concentration of aclarubicin.

	COTC (A) (μg/ml)	Aclarubicin (B) (μg/ml)
● sensitive	0	0
■ sensitive	0.5	0.005
○ resistant	0	0
□ resistant	0.5	0.075

the higher activity of 5′-nucleotide phosphodiesterase seems related to the collateral sensitivity of these cells to COTC.

3.   Potentiation of aclarubicin cytotoxicity by COTC (10)

    We further studied the combined effects of COTC and aclarubicin on the growth of
aclarubicin-resistant cells. The aclarubicin-resistant cells are more sensitive to aclarubicin
in the presence of a sublethal concentration of COTC (0.5 μg/ml) than in the absence of
COTC. The IC_{50} of aclarubicin was 0.062 and 0.2 μg/ml in the presence and absence of
COTC, respectively (Fig. 8A). On the contrary, the parental cells show the same sensitivity to aclarubicin with or without COTC.

    The aclarubicin-resistant cells are more sensitive to COTC in the presence of a
sublethal concentration of aclarubicin (0.075 μg/ml) than in the absence of aclarubicin:
IC_{50} was 0.3 and 0.9 μg/ml, respectively. The parental cells exhibit the same sensitivity
to COTC with or without a sublethal concentration of aclarubicin (0.005 μg/ml) (Fig.
8B).

    The synergistic activity of both antibiotics on aclarubicin-resistant cells suggests
that COTC affects the transport of aclarubicin in the aclarubicin-resistant cells. This
assumption has been confirmed by experiments using [³H]adriamycin. COTC enhances
uptake of [³H]adriamycin or blocks efflux of [³H]adriamycin in the aclarubicin-resistant
cells, but not in the parental cells.

4.   Mechanism of action (10)

    COTC reacts with sulfhydryl groups of 5′-nucleotide phosphodiesterase. We were

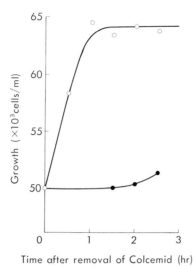

FIG. 9.   Effect of COTC on growth of synchronized L5178 Y cells
COTC was added to the culture 90 min before colcemid removal and was washed
off together with colcemid at 0 hr.   ○ control;   ● COTC 20 μg/ml.

interested in the mechanism by which a sulfhydryl inhibitor causes the lethal effect on
tumor cells, and studied the mechanism of tumoricidal activity of COTC.

COTC preferntially inhibits DNA synthesis over RNA and protein syntheses. The
IC_{50} for thymidine incorporation is approximately 25 μg/ml. The inhibition degree becomes higher by prior incubation for 90 min: IC_{50} is *ca.* 7 μg/ml. COTC blocks DNA
polymerase α, but does not significantly affect DNA polymerases β and γ. The inhibition
degree depends upon concentrations of the enzyme, but not upon those of template DNA,
suggesting that COTC reacts with the enzyme.

The effect of COTC on mitosis has been studied in cultures of L5178Y cells synchronized by Colcemid treatment. As illustrated in Fig. 9, COTC markedly blocks mitosis; complete inhibition was demonstrated at a drug concentration of 20 μg/ml.

In summary, although COTC is a multifunctional drug and can react with various
sulfhydryl substances, the inhibition of DNA polymerase and some mitotic process may
be related directly to its lethal action.

Lactoquinomycins(LQM)

1.   Discovery (8, 13)
In the screening for new antitumor antibiotics using drug-resistant neoplastic cells,
we found that *Streptomyces tanashiensis* IM8442T produces novel substances which inhibit drug-resistant cell sublines of L5178Y murine T-lymphoma more markedly than
the parental cells. The new antibiotics were designated lactoquinomycins(LQM) A and
B, following their chemical structures.

2.   Structure assignment (7, 8)
LQM-A, $C_{24}H_{27}NO_8$, FAB-MS: m/z 458 (MH$^+$), is a basic substance, showing UV
$\lambda_{max}^{H_2O}(\varepsilon)$ 215(37,600), 254(10,700), and 432 nm(4,760), and IR $\nu_{max}^{CHCl_3}$ 1,790 (γ-lactone),

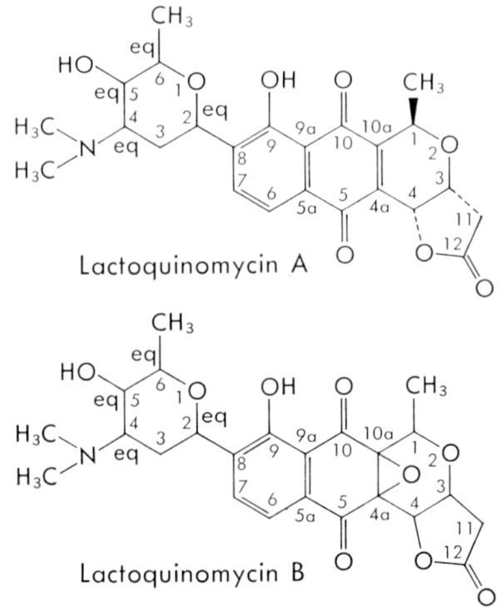

Lactoquinomycin A

Lactoquinomycin B

FIG. 10. LQM-A and LQM-B

TABLE III. Cytotoxicity of LQM-A and -B

Cell line	IC$_{50}$ (ng/ml)	
	LQM-A	LQM-B
K562 human leukemia	33	160
L1210 murine leukemia	13	200
P388 murine leukemia	30	120
L5178Y murine lymphoma		
Parental	20	430
Adriamycin-resistant	6	210
Aclarubicin-resistant	13	430
Bleomycin-resistant	8	190

1,665 and 1,650 (quinone) cm^{-1}. The structure has been elucidated by ^{1}H NMR, ^{13}C NMR and ORD by comparing with that of kalafungin (Fig. 10).

LQM-B, C$_{24}$H$_{27}$NO$_9$, FD-MS m/z 473(M$^+$) is a basic substance showing UV $\lambda_{max}^{H_2O}(\varepsilon)$ 239(15,100), 287(3,450), and 369nm(5,300) and IR $\nu_{max}^{CHCl_3}$ 1,790(γ-lactone), and 1,700 and 1,650 (quinone)cm^{-1}. The structure has been elucidated by ^{1}H NMR and ^{13}C NMR and compared with LQM-A, indicating that LQM-B is a 4a, 10a-epoxide derivative of LQM-A (Fig. 10).

3. Biological activity (8, 13)

Antibiotic-resistant cell sublines of L5178Y T-lymphoblastoma are more significant-ly inhibited by LQM-A or LQM-B than the parental cell line (Table III). LQM-A is more active than LQM-B against K562 human leukemia, L1210 and P388 murine leu-kemia and L5178Y cells. LQM-A is effective against Ehrlich carcinoma in mice.

4. Mechanism of action (6)

LQM-A inhibits biosyntheses of DNA, RNA and protein to a similar extent in adriamycin-resistant mouse leukemia L5178Y cells at concentrations higher than 0.08 μg/ml. It serves as a good electron acceptor when cytochrome c reductase is used as a quinone

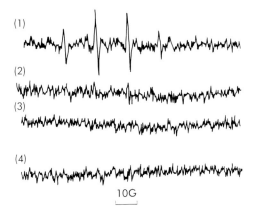

FIG. 11. ESR spectra of the radical produced by LQM-A
    (1)   LQM-A+cyt-*c* reductase+NADH
    (2)   cyt-*c* reductase+NADH
    (3)   LQM-A+NADH
    (4)   LQM-A+DT-diaphorase+NADH

reductase. The treatment of cells with LQM-A significantly reduces cellular NADH and ATP levels. Generation of superoxide radical by LQM-A in cell lysate is observed by reduction of nitro blue tetrazolium, and the production of hydroxyl radical is confirmed by electron spin resonance (Fig. 11). The radical formation is important for the cytotoxicity of LQM-A.

REFERENCES

1. Fukazawa, H., Nishimura, T., Tanaka, N., and Suzuki, H. 5′-Nucleotide phosphodiesterase and alkaline phosphatase in tumor cells: evidence for existence of novel species in the cytosol. *Biochim. Biophys. Acta*, **966**, 99–106 (1988).
2. Fukazawa, H., Suzuki, H., and Tanaka, N. A novel tumor-associated molecular species of 5′-nucleotide phosphodiesterase. *Biochem. Biophys. Res. Commun.*, **130**, 1072–1077 (1985).
3. Kim, S. H., Okabe, T., Tanaka, N., and Suzuki, H. Effects of cadeguomycin on cytotoxicity of cytosine arabinoside and other pyrimidine nucleoside analogs: a comparative study. *J. Antibiot.*, **40**, 1776–1777 (1987).
4. Kondo, T., Goto, T., Okabe, T., and Tanaka, N. Synthesis of cadeguomycin (7-deazaguanosine-7-carboxylic acid). *Tetrahedron Lett.*, **24**, 3647–3650 (1983).
5. Kondo, T., Okamoto, K., Yamamoto, M., Goto, T., and Tanaka, N. A total synthesis of cadeguomycin, a nucleoside antibiotic produced by *Streptomyces hygroscopicus*. *Tetrahedron*, **42**, 199–205 (1986).
6. Nomoto, K., Okabe, T., Suzuki, H., and Tanaka, N. Mechanism of action of lactoquinomycin A with special reference to the radical formation. *J. Antibiot.*, **41**, 1124–1129 (1988).
7. Okabe, T., Nomoto, K., Funabashi, H., Okuda, S., Suzuki, H., and Tanaka, N. Lactoquinomycin, a novel anticancer antibiotic. II. Physico-chemical properties and structure assignment. *J. Antibiot.*, **38**, 1333–1336 (1985).
8. Okabe, T., Nomoto, K., and Tanaka, N. Lactoquinomycin B, a novel antibiotic. *J. Antibiot.*, **39**, 1–5 (1986).
9. Sugimoto, Y., Nishimura, T., Suzuki, H., and Tanaka, N. Alteration of membrane-as-

sociated enzymes in drug-resistant sublines of mouse lymphoblastoma L5178Y cells. *J. Antibiot.*, **34**, 1200–1205 (1981).

10. Sugimoto, Y., Suzuki, H., Yamaki, H., Nishimura, T., and Tanaka, N. Mechanism of action of 2-crotonyloxymethyl-4, 5, 6-trihydroxycyclohex-2-enone, an SH-inhibitory anti-tumor antibiotic and its effect on drug-resistant neoplastic cells. *J. Antibiot.*, **35**, 1222–1230 (1982).

11. Suzuki, H., Kim, S. H., Tahara, M., Okazaki, K., Okabe, T., Wu, R. T., and Tanaka, N. Potentiation of cytotoxicity of 1-β-arabinofuranosylcytosine for K562 human leukemic cells by cadeguomycin. *Cancer Res.*, **47**, 713–717 (1987).

12. Suzuki, H. *et al.* Personal communication.

13. Tanaka, N., Okabe, T., Isono, F., Kashiwagi, M., Nomoto, K., Takahashi, M., Shimazu, A., and Nishimura, T. Lactoquinomycin, a novel anticancer antibiotic. I. Taxonomy, isolation and biological activity. *J. Antibiot.*, **38**, 1327–1332 (1985).

14. Tanaka, N., Wu, R. T., Okabe, T., Yamashita, H., Shimazu, A., and Nishimura, T. Cadeguomycin, a novel nucleoside analog antibiotic. I. The producing organism, production and isolation of cadeguomycin. *J. Antibiot.*, **35**, 272–278 (1982).

15. Wu, R. T., Okabe, T., Kim, S. H., Suzuki, H., and Tanaka, N. Enhancement of pyrimidine nucleoside uptake into K562 and YAC-1 cells by cadeguomycin. *J. Antibiot.*, **38**, 1588–1595 (1985).

16. Wu, R. T., Okabe, T., Namikoshi, M., Okuda, S., Nishimura, T., and Tanaka, N. Cadeguomycin, a novel nucleoside analog antibiotic. II. Improved purification, physicochemical properties and structure assignment. *J. Antibiot.*, **35**, 279–284 (1982).

17. Yuan, B. D., Wu, R. T., Sato, I., Okabe, T., Suzuki, H., Nishimura, T., and Tanaka, N. Biological activity of cadeguomycin. Inhibition of tumor growth and metastasis, immunostimulation, and potentiation of 1-β-D-arabinofuranosylcytosine. *J. Antibiot.*, **38**, 642–648 (1985).

BASIC STUDIES ON SPERGUALINS

Setsuko Kunimoto,[*1] Masaaki Ishizuka,[*2] Hironobu Iinuma,[*1]
and Tomio Takeuchi[*1,*2]

*Institute of Microbial Chemistry[*1] and Institute for Chemotherapy[*2]*

Spergualin (SG) was screened from culture broth of *Bacillus laterosporus* based on its growth-inhibitory activity against chick embryo fibroblasts transformed by Rous sarcoma virus. It exhibits marked antitumor activity against murine leukemias such as L1210, P388, P815, C1489, EL4, and RL male 1. Among SG analogs, 15-deoxyspergualin (DSG) has a stronger antitumor activity than SG itself. Both compounds induce tumor resistance in mice cured of L1210 (IMC) by stimulating interleukin 2 (IL-2) production and enhancing natural killer activity of spleen cells. They are thought to exhibit antitumor activity by cytotoxicity and activation of the immune system. Moreover, they show strong immunosuppressive activity for tumor-free animals, and no severe toxicity. They may have potential usefulness in cancer chemotherapy, organ transplantation, and the control of autoimmune diseases.

During our studies on antitumor antibiotics spergualin (SG) was found in 1981 from a culture filtrate of *Bacillus laterosporus* through its activity to inhibit focus formation in chicken fibroblasts by Rous sarcoma virus (RSV) (*25*). It has a unique structure (*30*) which is not known in many antibiotics (Fig. 1), and was named after the spermidine and guanidine moieties in its structure. Among SG analogs 15-deoxyspergualin (DSG) has a stronger activity than SG itself (*5, 24, 28*). As was expected from the novel structure, SG and DSG showed interesting biological activities in cancer treatment and their immunological effect in animals. The mechanism of action is not yet known, but the antitumor activity is thought to be brought about by their cytocidal and immunostimulating ability. A dose-dependent immunosuppressive effect is also shown by both compounds. Their immunosuppressive activities seem stronger in normal animals than in those in tumor-bearing states. An important characteristic is that they have these activities at a dosage less than one fifth or one tenth of acute toxic dose levels and with very low cumulative toxicity. Phase I clinical trials of DSG are being conducted in Japan and U.S.A.

In this review we will describe the purification of SG, the synthesis of DSG, biological activities of the two compounds, and their structure-activity relationships.

Purification of SG

SG was purified (*25*) from a culture broth of *B. laterosporus* BMG162-aF2 siolated from a soil sample collected at Ohira-san, Tochigi Prefecture, Japan. The bacterium was

[*1] Kamiosaki 3-14-23, Shinagawa-ku, Tokyo 141, Japan (國元節子, 飯沼寛信, 竹内富雄).
[*2] Motono 18-24, Miyamoto, Numazu, Shizuoka 410-03, Japan (石塚雅章, 竹内富雄).

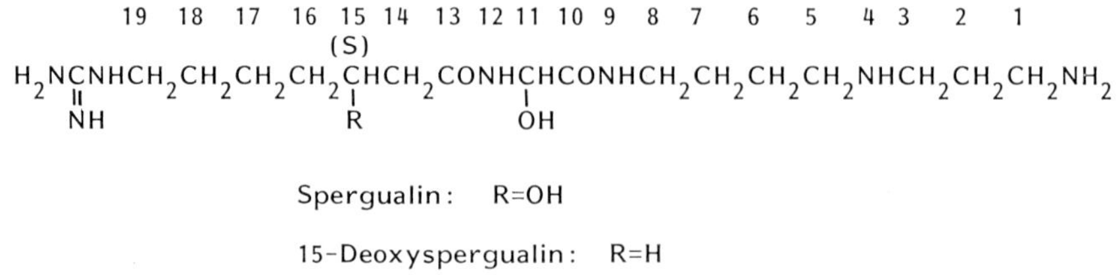

19 18 17 16 15 14 13 12 11 10 9   8   7   6   5   4 3   2   1
(S)
H₂NCNHCH₂CH₂CH₂CH₂CHCH₂CONHCHCONHCH₂CH₂CH₂CH₂NHCH₂CH₂CH₂NH₂
‖ | |
NH   R   OH

Spergualin: R=OH

15-Deoxyspergualin: R=H

FIG. 1.   Structure of SG and DSG

cultured in a medium containing 2.0% glycerol, 2.0% dextrin, 1.0% soy peptone, 0.3% yeast extract, 0.2% ammonium sulfate, and 0.2% calcium carbonate (adjusted to pH 7.4) on a reciprocal shaker at 28°C for 5 days. The antibiotic activity was traced using the cylinder plate method with *Bacillus subtilis* PCI219 as the test organism. SG was purified as trihydrochloride hemihydrate through column chromatography with Amberlite IRC-50, CM-Sephadex C-25, and Sephadex LH-20 from culture filtrate. The compound is a colorless hygroscopic powder and soluble in water and methanol.

The structure of SG was determined to be (11S, 15S)-1-amino-19-guanidino-11,15-dihydroxy-4,9,12-triazanonadecane-10,13-dione (*30*).

SG has weak antibacterial activity against gram-positive and -negative bacteria. *B. subtilis* PCI219, *Staphylococcus aureus*, *Salmonella typhi* T-63, and *Proteus vulgaris* OX19 are fairly sensitive to SG (*25*).

SG inhibited focus formation by RSV in chicken embryo fibroblasts to 50% at 5.5 μg/ml and its cytotoxic effect in these fibroblasts reached 50% at 13 μg/ml. SG showed 2.3 fold more effectiveness to RSV-transformed cells than to normal cells (*25*).

Synthesis of DSG

DSG is an epimeric mixture at C-11. It has been chemically synthesized from diethyl-L-tartrate, N-2-cyanoethylputrescine, and ω-aminoheptanoic acid as shown in Fig. 2 (*26–28*). To explore the relationship between the configuration of C-11 and bioactivity, both (−) and (+)-enantiomers of DSG were synthesized using the combination with asymmetric hydrolysis of the peptide bond by carboxypeptidase P from *Penicillium*

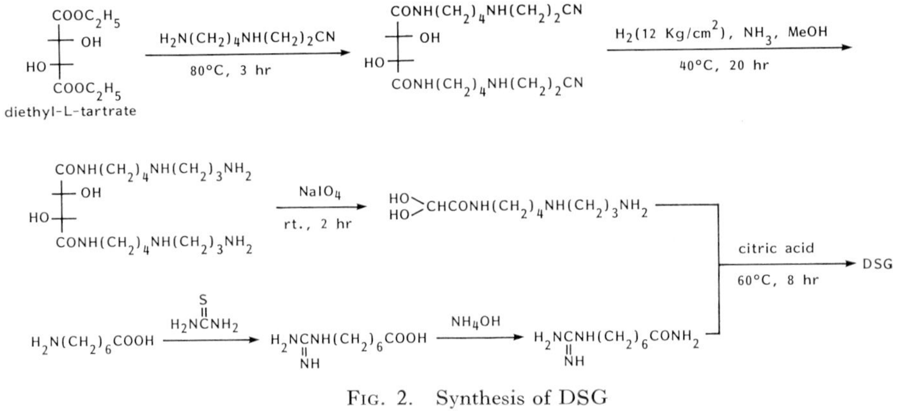

COOC₂H₅
    + OH   H₂N(CH₂)₄NH(CH₂)₂CN   CONH(CH₂)₄NH(CH₂)₂CN
HO +   ──────────────────→   + OH   H₂(12 Kg/cm²), NH₃, MeOH
    COOC₂H₅   80°C, 3 hr   HO +   ──────────────────────→
diethyl-L-tartrate   CONH(CH₂)₄NH(CH₂)₂CN   40°C, 20 hr

        CONH(CH₂)₄NH(CH₂)₃NH₂
            + OH   NaIO₄   HO
HO +   ──────────→   >CHCONH(CH₂)₄NH(CH₂)₃NH₂ ──────────┐
        CONH(CH₂)₄NH(CH₂)₃NH₂   rt., 2 hr   HO   │
                                                                                    citric acid │
                                                                                    60°C, 8 hr   ──→ DSG
                           S
                           ‖
                        H₂NCNH₂   NH₄OH
H₂N(CH₂)₆COOH   ──────────→ H₂NCNH(CH₂)₆COOH ──────→ H₂NCNH(CH₂)₆CONH₂ ─┘
                                          ‖   ‖
                                          NH   NH

FIG. 2.   Synthesis of DSG

janthinellum or carboxypeptidase W from wheat bran. The antitumor activity of DSG depended on the ($-$)-enantiomer (S-configuration at C-11). ($+$)-Enantiomer was almost totally inactive (*26*).

Antitumor Activity

Antitumor activities of SG against 14 experimental tumors are summarized in Table I (*21*). SG was effective the all of 7 leukemias transplanted intraperitoneally (i.p.) or subcutaneously (s.c.) to mice; it was especially effective against L1210 (IMC) tumors. This is a leukemic cell subline which has been maintained in CDF_1 mice at the Institute of Microbial Chemistry in Tokyo since 1965. Mice inoculated by L1210 (IMC) in both i.p. and s.c. forms were completely cured at an optimal drug dosage. SG exhibited activity against M5076 fibrosarcoma, AH66 and AH66F rat hepatomas among other non-leukemic tumors, but not against Meth-A fibrosarcoma, B16 melanoma, Lewis lung carcinoma (LL) or C26 colon adenocarcinoma. The antitumor activity of SG against L1210 (IMC) is shown in Table II with that of DSG (*2*). DSG was more active at lower dosage levels than SG. The antitumor activity of SG against L1210 was dependent on the length of the period of exposure to SG. Continuous infusion for 7 days using an osmotic mini-pump Alzet 2001 and daily administration for 9 days showed the strongest activity (Table III). Plowman *et al.* (*24*) also demonstrated good antitumor activity of DSG against L1210 implanted through i.p. and s.c. with daily i.p. administration of the drug over a wide dosage range. The best therapeutic response was achieved by infusion of 179 mg/kg/day for 3 days using s.c.-implanted Alzet osmotic pumps. This 72-hr infusion produced an approximately 7 log_{10} reduction in the viable tumor cell population. DSG exhibited anti-leukemic activity against N-butyl-N-nitrosourea-induced autochthonous leukemia of rats (*4*), which seemed more relevant to human leukemia than other experimental transplantable leukemias.

During treatment of L1210 (IMC) with SG or DSG we found that 60 day survivors subjected to daily i.p. administration of these drugs rejected a second inoculation of L1210 (IMC) cells (*2, 21, 31*) (Table IV). These mice were resistant only to L1210 (IMC), but not to Meth-A fibrosarcoma, Ehrlich ascites (*2*) or P388 tumor (*31*). In the Winn tumor neutralization assay and the ^{51}Cr-release assay, T-cell fraction prepared from spleens of cured mice had higher cytotoxic activity against L1210 (IMC) than whole spleen cells (*2, 31*). The cytotoxic activity of spleen cells was diminished by treatment with anti-Thy 1.2 or anti-Lyt-2.1 antibody and complement (*2, 31*). The effector cells in the immunological rejection, therefore, were determined to be cytotoxic T-cells. Involvement of the immunological action in the antitumor activity was confirmed through the fact that the antitumor activities of SG and DSG against L1210 (IMC) were much lower in T-cell-deficient athymic mice (*31*) and immunodeficient mice produced by X-ray irradiation (Fig. 3) (*2*), respectively. The induction of antitumor resistance is thought to be due to the stimulation of interleukin 2 (IL-2) production from mixed lymphocyte culture with DSG (*2*). Natural killer activity of spleen cells from surviving mice was enhanced by treatment with SG or DSG after the transplantation of L1210 cells (*2*). Their antitumor activity, however, cannot be explained by enhancement of cellular immunity alone, because spermidine and glyoxylspermidine, partial components of SG, enhance delayed type hypersensitivity and induce IL-2 as do SG and DSG (*3*), in spite of the fact that they do not have antitumor activity themselves. The antitumor activity and the

TABLE I. Antitumor Effect of SG against Various Transplantable Tumors in Mice and Rats[a]

Tumor		Host	Inoculum		max T/C[b]	Optimal dose[c]	Index[d]
			Site	Size			
L1210	Lymphoid leukemia	CDF₁, female	i.p.	10^5	222	50	71
			s.c.	10^5	238	12.5	27
L1210 (IMC)	Lymphoid leukemia	CDF₁, female	i.p.	10^5	>448 (10/10)[e]	6.25	132
			s.c.	10^5	>345 (5/5)	12.5	30
P388	Lymphocytic leukemia	CDF₁, female	i.p.	10^6	183	50	45
P815	Mastocytoma	DBA/2, female	i.p.	10^6	202	50	25
C1498	Myeloid leukemia	C57BL/6, male	i.p.	10^6	206	50	83
EL-4	Thymoma	C57BL/6, male	i.p.	10^6	212	50	217
RLmalel	X-ray induced leukemia	BALB/c, male	i.p.	10^6	167	50	45
AH66	Hepatoma	Donryu, female	i.p.	10^6	170	100	4.4
AH66F	Hepatoma	Donryu, female	i.p.	10^6	224	50	125
M5076	Fibrosarcoma	C57BL/6, female	i.p.	2×10^5	155	50	2.9
Meth-A	Fibrosarcoma	BALB/c, female	i.p.	2.5×10^5	104	25	—
B16	Melanotic melanoma	BDF₁, male	i.p.	10^5	97	6.25	—
LL	Lung carcinoma	BDF₁, male	i.v.	10^5	115	50	—
C26	Colon adenocarcinoma	CDF₁, female	i.p.	5×10^5	94	50	—

[a] SG was administered intraperitonealy (i.p.) daily for 9 days from day 1.

[b] max T/C, maximum value of T/C (%). T/C (%), mean survival period of treated/mean survival period of controls×100.

[c] Dose producing the max T/C (mg/kg/day ×9)

[d] Index = (lethal dose)/(minimum effective dose)

[e] Number in parentheses shows survivors 30 days after inoculation.

i.v., intravenously.

TABLE II. Antitumor Effect of SG and DSG on L1210 (IMC)[a]

mg/kg/day	SG		DSG	
	T/C%[b]	60-Day surivior	T/C%[b]	60-Day survivor
25	250	1/5	273	0/5
12.5	359	2/5	298	0/5
6.3	274	2/5	298	1/5
3.1	160	0/5	382	2/5
1.6	113	0/5	311	3/5
0.8	96	0/5	122	3/5
0.4	96	0/5	145	3/5
0.2	82	0/5	104	0/5

[a] Drug was injected i.p. daily for 9 days starting from day 1 after the i.p. inoculation of 10^5 L1210 (IMC) cells to CDF_1 mice.
[b] Excluding 60–day suvivors.

TABLE III. Effect of Administration Schedules on Antitumor Activity of SG against L1210

Schedule	Dose (mg/kg)		T/C (%)
	Single	Total	
Once	100	100	Tox.[a]
	50	50	105
	12.5	12.5	102
	3.13	3.13	98
q3h×6	50	300	114
	12.5	75	107
	3.13	18.75	107
q4d×2	50	100	107
	12.5	25	107
	3.13	6.25	102
q3h×6–q4d×3	50	900	129
	12.5	225	152
	3.13	56.25	136
q1d×9	50	450	206
	12.5	112.5	199
	3.13	28.13	163
	0.78	7.03	145
Alzet 2001	—	1,800	256
	—	450	210
	—	112.5	185

SG was administered i.p. from day 1. Treatment schedules were as follows: single treatment (once); 6 times at intervals of 3 hr (q3h×6); twice every 4 days (q4d×2); 3 cycles of 6 times a day every 4 days q3h×6-q4d×3); 9 daily treatments (q1d×9); continuous infusion for 7 days using an osmotic mini-pump (Alzet model 2001). Each dosing group was composed of at least 5 mice.
[a] Mice died within 15 min after single administration of 100 mg/kg of SG.

enhancement of IL-2 production and natural killer activity in tumor-bearing mice were observed upon the administration of DSG at below 12.5 mg/kg daily for 9 days. Beyond this dosage, mice died due to tumor. This phenomenon is thought to be due to the im-

TABLE IV.   Antitumor Effect of SG and DSG on L1210 and Rejection of
the Second Inoculation of L1210 in Cured Mice[a]

1st inoculation				2nd inoculation	
Treatment		60-Day survivors[b]		40-Day survivors[c]	
mg/kg×g	Route	SG	DSG	SG	DSG
25	i.p.	1/6	—	1/1	—
12.5	i.p.	9/17	3/8	9/9	3/3
6.2	i.p.	6/11	2/8	6/6	2/2
3.1	i.p.	6/11	4/9	6/6	4/4
1.6	i.p.	—	10/13	—	10/10
0.8	i.p.	—	9/13	—	9/9
0.4	i.p.	—	8/13	—	8/8
400	p.o.	3/6	—	3/3	—
200	p.o.	8/10	5/6	8/8	4/5
100	p.o.	—	7/10	—	7/7
50	p.o.	—	8/10	—	8/8

[a] CDF$_1$ mice were inoculated with 10^5 L1210 (IMC) cells i.p. (the 1st inoculation) and treated with SG or DSG daily for 10 days from 1 day after the inoculation of L1210 (IMC) cells. Sixty days thereafter, the number of survivors (cured mice) were assessed and reinoculated with 10^5 L1210 (IMC) cells i.p. (the 2nd inoculation). After the 2nd inoculation, mice were not treated with SG or DSG and the number of 40-day survivors was assessed.

[b] Number of cured mice/total number of mice treated.

[c] Number of tumor-free mice/total number of cured mice.

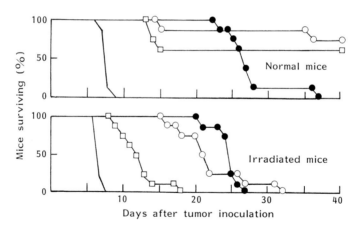

FIG. 3.   Reduction of antitumor activity of DSG on L1210 (IMC) by X-ray irradiation

CDF$_1$ mice were inoculated i.p. with 10^5 L1210 (IMC) cells without or after irradiation of 400 rad of X-ray. Drug was injected 1 day after tumor inoculation daily for 9 days. — control; □ 0.78 mg/kg; ○ 3.12 mg/kg; ● 12.5 mg/kg.

munosuppression activity of the drug. Immunosuppression was observed below that dosage as described in next section. The immunosuppressive activity seems to be stronger in normal animals than in tumor-bearing animals.

Immunosuppressive Activities

SG and DSG have strong suppressive effects on both humoral and cell-mediated immune responses in rodents and dogs (*11, 12, 15, 18, 29*) in a dose-dependent manner. DSG suppressed antibody formation in mice at dosages above 0.4 mg/kg/day for 3 days and establishment of delayed-type hypersensitivity at dosages above 1.6 mg/kg/day for 4 days (*12*). This immunosuppressive activity has caused SG and DSG to be recognized for their efficacies on experimental transplantation systems and autoimmune disease models. They prolong allograft survival in skin-transplantation in rats (*1, 12, 15, 29*) (Table V). Prolongation of graft survival by DSG was observed in pancreatic islets, heart and kidney transplantation in rats (*1*). DSG has a stronger immunosuppressive activity than SG, as is true of its antitumor activity (*15*). These drugs can prevent graft-*versus*-host disease in mice irradiated with a lethal dose of X-ray followed by grafting of allogeneic bone marrow and spleen cells (*16, 19*). Also, both compounds are valuable in models of autoimmune disease such as experimental allergic encephalomyelitis in guinea pigs immunized with isogenic spinal cord (*14*), systemic lupus erythematosus-like lesions developing spontaneously in MRL/MpJ-lpr/lpr(MRL/l) (*10, 17*), male BXSB (*14*) and

TABLE V.   Suppression of Rejection of Skin Allograft by DSG[a]

mg/kg/day	Daily for 10 days		Every other day for 20 days	
	M.S.D.[b]	30-Day survivors	M.S.D.[b]	30-Day survivors
0	9.5±2.5	0/10	8.4±3.2	0/10
3.1	13.4±4.1*	0/10	9.0±2.6	0/10
6.3	15.8±6.4*	0/10	11.5±4.3*	2/10
12.5	17.4±4.9**	0/10	12.1±5.5*	2/10
25.0	Not tested	—	7.8±3.4	5/10

[a] Tail skin taken from SHR rats was grafted onto the abdomen of F344 rats. DSG was given i.p. from 1 day after the transplantation.
[b] Mean survival days of allograft (M.S.D.±S.D.). Excluding 30-day survivors.
* $p<0.05$, ** $p<0.01$.

TABLE VI.   Effect of SG on Enlargement of Lymphoid Organs in MRL/l Mice

Schedule	Dose (mg/kg)	n	Lymph node (g)		Spleen (%)
			Mesenteric	Axillary	
Daily from week 7 through 21	0	10	1.47±0.57	0.85±0.22	0.57±0.08
	2.5	10	0.83±0.41	0.74±0.22	0.31±0.07**
	5	10	0.50±0.23**	0.42±0.17**	0.19±0.05**
	10	9	0.10±0.07**	0.11±0.08**	0.10±0.02**
Daily from week 13 through 27	0	6	1.22±0.23	0.79±0.29	0.70±0.14
	2.5	8	0.90±0.42	1.02±0.43	0.49±0.26
	5	9	0.60±0.42**	0.51±0.27*	0.23±0.05**
	10	7	0.18±0.05**	0.15±0.05**	0.13±0.04**

SG was administered i.p. daily for 4 weeks to male MRL/l mice. The mice were sacrificed 1–2 days after completion of SG administration and lymph nodes, spleens, blood, and kidneys were removed. Blood and kidneys were treated as shown in Table VII. Data are shown as mean±S.D.
* $p<0.05$, ** $p<0.01$.

TABLE VII.   Therapy of Lupus Nephritis in MRL/l Mice by SG

Schedule	Dose (mg/kg)	Anti-DNA titer (A_{405} nm)	BUN (mg/dl)	Degree of glomerular damage (score)
Daily from week 7 through 21	0	0.48±0.24	38.7±9.0	1.8±0.5
	2.5	0.43±0.31	35.8±8.6	1.6±0.2
	5	0.18±0.06*	21.1±2.5*	0.9±0.3*
	10	0.12±0.06*	16.2±2.3*	0.3±0.2*
Daily from week 13 through 27	0	0.58±0.30	43.0±9.7	2.7±0.5
	2.5	0.49±0.27	38.8±7.9	2.1±0.5*
	5	0.26±0.09*	28.0±5.5*	1.6±0.5*
	10	0.17±0.07*	25.9±8.0*	0.7±0.6*

After the treatment shown in the legend of Table VI anti-DNA antibody and urea nitrogen (BUN) in serum were determined. Kidneys were fixed, sectioned, and stained. Glomerular damage was indicated by a pathological score based on the severity of change where 0=none, 1=minimal, 2=slight, 3=moderate, and 4=severe.

[a] MRL/+mice of the same age did not have detectable anti-DNA titer ($A_{405} \leq 0.1$) in 1/100 dilution of their sera. Data are shown as mean±S.D.

* $p < 0.01$.

[NZB×NZW]F$_1$ (23) mice, and streptozotocin-induced diabetic mice (20). The result with MRL/l mice (14) is shown in Tables VI and VII. One group of mice received SG prophylactically from 7 to 21 weeks of age. The other group received it curatively from 13 to 27 weeks of age. In both groups lupus lesions characterized by enlarged lymphoid organs, high anti-DNA titer and blood urea nitrogen and severe glomerular nephritis were significantly suppressed (17).

The study on the immunosuppressive mechanism of SG and DSG is under way. DSG does not reduce functions of zymosan-activated macrophages such as the release of lysosomal enzymes and the production of superoxide anions (12). On the other hand, it does suppress the production of macrophage activating factor mediated by T-cells in the mixed lymphocyte reaction between popliteal lymph node cells from mice inoculated with allogeneic spleen cells in the footpad and the same allogeneic cells treated with mitomycin C (32). In this experiment the administration of DSG increased the numbers of popliteal lymph node cells after inoculation of allogeneic spleen cells, and the response to exogenous IL-2 of these popliteal lymph node cells was inhibited by DSG in spite of an enhancement of IL-2 production in the mixed lymphocyte culture (20). The blastogenic response of concanavalin A (Con A) of spleen cells obtained from rat skin allograft recipients administered DSG was highly stimulated but that of lipopolysaccharide (LPS) was not affected (13). Thus, these drugs show no evidence of suppressing T-cell functions *in vitro*, but seem to stimulate T-cell proliferation. More detailed studies on B- and T-cell subsets are necessary to understand the mechanism of SG and DSG in the immune responses.

Cytotoxicity

Cytotoxicities of SG and DSG on cultured leukemia cells were dependent on the kind of serum contained in the culture media (7–9). Calf serum abundant in amine oxidase gave a strong cytotoxic effect and horse or human serum poor in amine oxidase or calf serum with amine oxidase inhibitors gave weaker cytotoxicities in cultures of leukemia cells. The latter type of cytotoxicity was detected at lower dosage than amine oxidase-dependent cell-kill with a moderate dose dependency but with a strong dependency on incubation time (9). SG and DSG were incorporated into L5178Y cells by a carrier-mediated transport system of polyamines (8). They had higher affinity to amine-oxidase in calf serum than to their transport carrier with inhibition constants (K_i's) of 70 μM and 7.8 μM, respectively (8). So, if amine oxidase is rich in culture media, amine oxidase-dependent cell-kill may be preferentially found and no intracellular event can be observed. The significance in antitumor activity of these two types of cell-kill, one dependent on and the other independent of amine oxidase is not clear.

From the unique structure of SG and DSG, a unique mechanism of action has been expected of these drugs, although at present this mechanism remains a mystery. The syntheses of nucleic acids and protein in intact cells were only slightly inhibited (7), assuring that the compounds are not mitotic poisons. Rate-limiting enzymes of polyamine biosynthesis, ornithine decarboxylase, and S-adenosylmethionine decarboxylase, were not inhibited and very weakly inhibited, respectively (7). Spermidine synthase and spermine synthase were inhibited by DSG with K_i's of 340 μM and 215 μM, respectively (H. Hibasami, personal communication). The induction of ornithine decarboxylase by medium exchange of HTC cell culture was not affected (S. Hayashi, personal communication). Studies on intracellular targets of these drugs must be continued.

Structure-activity Relationship

The structure-activity relationship of SG and its analogs has been studied on a correlation between antitumor and immunosuppressive activities (22, 26–28). Briefly, immunosuppressive activity is related to antitumor activity and DSG is the strongest in both activities among many analogs (Table VIII). The substitution of the amino or methyl-guanidino group for the guanidino group results in loss of the activity (28). Removal of spermidine and substitution of other polyamines for spermidine or acylation or alkylation of the terminal amine of spermidine deprived SG of the antitumor activity. Even when spermidine was connected in the inverse direction antitumor activity was lost (27). SG has two hydroxyl groups with S configuration at the 11 and 15 positions (6, 26). As shown in Table VIII, DSG is more active than SG and acylation of the 15-hydroxyl group with long-chain fatty acids and benzoic acid decreased the activity. Hence, the 15-hydroxyl group is not only unnecessary for antitumor activity, but it also diminishes the activity. The hydroxyl group in the 11 position requires S configuration (26). 11-Deoxy, 11-hydroxymethyl, and 11-methoxy analogs of DSG are active but their activities are inferior to DSG. Though the role of the hydroxyl group in the 11 position is not clear, this structure is important for the activity. The hexamethylene chain next to the guanidino group can be replaced by octamethylene but cannot be displaced by hepta or shorter chains than hexa-methylene (28). This guanidinofattyacyl moiety can be replaced by 4-guanidinophenylbutyric acid but not by 4-guanidinophenylpentanoic, 4-gunidinophenyl-hexanoic or 4-guanidinopropylbenzoic acid (22). So in the guanidinofattyacyl group the length of hexamethylene chain and its flexibility is important for the activity.

Antitumor and immunosuppressive activities require strictly limited structures on guanidino moiety. Somewhat limited structures are required in heptanamide and glyoxylspermidine moieties. The reasons for these requirments develop may be understood if the mechanism of action and the target of the drugs is clarified.

TABLE VIII. Antitumor and Immunosuppressive Activities of SG Analogs

$$\underset{\text{A}}{\text{NH}_2\text{CNH}}-\underset{\text{NH}}{\overset{\text{B}}{(\text{CH}_2)_4}}\text{CHCH}_2\text{CO}-\underset{\text{R}_1}{\text{NHCHCO}}-\underset{\text{R}_2}{\overset{\text{C}}{\text{NH}(\text{CH}_2)_4}}\text{NH}(\text{CH}_2)_3\text{NH}_2}$$

Analogs	Antitumor activity[a]	Inhibition of DTH[b] response	Inhibition of Antibody[b] production
SG (R₁=R₂=OH)	0.78–50	+	+
DSG (R₁=H, R₂=OH)	0.20–25	++	++
ω-Guanidino (A) derivatives (R₁=R₂=OH)			
NH₂	—	—	
CH₃NHCNH‖NH	—		
Derivatives of D (R₁=R₂=OH)			
NH(CH₂)₃NH(CH₂)₄NH(CH₂)₃NH₂	—		
NH(CH₂)₄NH(CH₂)₃NHCOCH₃	50	—	
NH(CH₂)₄NH(CH₂)₃NHC₂H₅	—	—	
NH(CH₂)₃NH(CH₂)₄NH₂	25–50	—	
15-Hydroxy (B) derivatives (R₂=OH)			
R₁=OCO-n-C₁₃H₂₇	6.25–25		
R₁=OCO—◯	—		
Derivatives of C (R₁=H)			
R₂=CH₂OH	0.39–25	+	++
R₂=H	0.39–25	++	++
R₂=OCH₃	0.32–12.5		
Derivatives of B (R₂=OH)			
(CH₂)₈CO	0.1 –12.5		
(CH₂)₇CO	6.25–25	—	
(CH₂)₅CO	—	—	
Derivatives of B (R₂=CH₂OH)			
—◯—(CH₂)₃CO	0.39–25	+	++
—◯—(CH₂)₄CO	3.13–12.5	±	—
—◯—(CH₂)₅CO	—		—
(CH₂)₃—◯—CO	—		—

[a] Antitumor activities against L1210 (IMC) are shown as dosages giving more than 125% of T/C (%) upon i.p. administration daily for 9 days from day 1. — means inactive.

[b] Inhibition of dealayed type hypersensitivity (DTH) response and antibody production in mice of analogs were indicated by comparing with that of SG as follows: −, inactive; ±, active but less than SG; +, approximately the same level as SG; ++, more active than SG.

Toxicity

SG has low toxicity: intravenous injection of 80 mg/kg did not cause the death of mice. The LD_{50} through intraperitoneal injection was about 150 mg/kg (*25*). LD_{50} of

DSG administered intravenously is 12.3 mg/kg in mice, 20.8 mg/kg in rats and 20–30 mg/kg in dogs. The LD_{50}'s seem to fluctuate markedly depending on injection speed. For example, dogs injected with 45 mg/kg through 3 hr intravenous infusion survived. A subacute toxicity study found that the main toxicities of DSG in rats and dogs are atrophy of thymus and spleen, myelosuppression and deficiency of spermiogenesis, atrophy of thymus, myelosuppression and disturbance of gastrointestinal tract, respectively. These toxicities are usually repaired in 35 days after 91 day administration in rats and dogs.

DSG was developed to the stage of preclinical trial by the National Cancer Institute, U.S.A. in 1984. In 1986 Phase I clinical trials started in Memorial Sloan-Kettering Cancer Center, New York, and the University of Texas, San Antonio Health and Science Center, San Antonio. The Phase I protocol is a repetition of 120 hr constant infusion and 4 weeks rest in which the dosage is increased from 80 mg/m²/day×5 days using the modified Fibonacci method. In Japan the clinical trial of DSG as an antitumor or immunosuppressive agent has been ongoing since 1987.

REFERENCES

1. Dickneite, G., Schorlemmer, H. U., Walter, P., Thies, J., and Sedlacek, H. H. The influence of (±) 15-deoxyspergualin on experimental transplantation and its immunopharmacological mode of action. *Behring Inst. Mitteilung.*, **80**, 93–102 (1986).
2. Ishizuka, M., Masuda, T., Mizutani, S., Osono, M., Kumagai, H., Takeuchi, T., and Umezawa, H. Induction of antitumor resistance to mouse leukemia L1210 by spergualins. *J. Antibiot.*, **39**, 1736–1743 (1986).
3. Ishizuka, M., Takeuchi, R., and Umezawa, H. Studies of the effect of spermidine in enhancing cellular immunity. *Proc. Jpn. Acad.*, **58**, Ser. B, 327–330 (1982).
4. Ito, J., Yamashita, T., Takahashi, K., Horinishi, H., Nakamura, T., Takeuchi, T., and Umezawa, H. Anti-leukemic activity of 15-deoxyspergualin against *N*-butyl-*N*-nitrourea-induced autochthonous rat leukemia. *J. Antibiot.*, **39**, 1488–1490 (1986).
5. Iwasawa, H., Kondo, S., Ikeda, D., Takeuchi, T., and Umezawa, H. Synthesis of (−)-15-deoxyspergualin and (−)-spergualin-15-phosphate. *J. Antibiot.*, **35**, 1665–1669 (1982).
6. Kondo, S., Iwasawa, H., Ikeda, D., Umeda, Y., Ikeda, Y., Iinuma, H., and Umezawa, H. The total synthesis of spergualin, an antitumor antibiotic. *J. Antibiot.*, **34**, 1625–1627 (1981).
7. Kunimoto, S., Miura, K., Iinuma, H., Takeuchi, T., and Uemzawa, H. Cytotoxicity of spergualin and amine oxidase activity in medium. *J. Antibiot.*, **38**, 899–903 (1985).
8. Kunimoto, S., Nosaka, C., Xu, C.-Z., and Takeuchi, T. Serum effect on cellular uptake of spermidine, spergualin, 15-deoxyspergualin, and their metabolites by L5178Y cells. *J. Antibiot.*, **42**, 1–7 (1989).
9. Kuramochi, H., Hiratsuka, M., Nagamine, S., Takahashi, K., Nakamura, T., Takeuchi, T., and Umezawa, H. The antiproliferative action of deoxyspergualin is different from that induced by amine oxidase. *J. Antibiot.*, **41**, 234–238 (1988).
10. Makino, M., Fujiwara, M., Aoyagi, T., and Umezawa, H. Immunosuppressive activities of deoxyspergualin. I. Effect of the long-term administration of the drug on the development of murine lupus. *Immunopharmacology*, **14**, 107–114 (1987).
11. Makino, M., Fujiwara, M., Watanabe, H., Aoyagi, T., and Umezawa, H. Immunosuppressive activities of deoxyspergualin. II. The effect on the antibody responses. *Immunopharmacology*, **14**, 115–122 (1987).
12. Masuda, T., Mizutani, S., Iijima, M., Odai, H., Suda, H., Ishizuka, M., Takeuchi, T.,

and Umezawa, H. Immunosuppressive activity of 15-deoxyspergualin and its effect on skin allografts in rats. *J. Antibiot.*, **40**, 1612–1618 (1987).

13. Nemoto, K., Abe, F., Nakamura, T., Ishizuka, M., Takeuchi, T., and Umezawa, H. Blastogenic responses and the release of interleukins 1 and 2 by spleen cells obtained from rat skin allograft recipients administered with 15-deoxyspergualin. *J. Antibiot.*, **40**, 1062–1064 (1987).

14. Nemoto, K., Abe, F., Takita, T., Nakamura, T., Takeuchi, T., and Umezawa, H. Suppression of experimental allergic encephalomyelitis in guinea pigs by spergualin and 15-deoxyspergualin. *J. Antibiot.*, **40**, 1193–1194 (1987).

15. Nemoto, H., Hayashi, M., Abe, F., Nakamura, T., Ishizuka, M., and Umezawa, H. Immunosuppressive activities of 15-deoxyspergualin in animals. *J. Antibiot.*, **40**, 561–562 (1987).

16. Nemoto, K., Hayashi, M., Fujii, H., Ito, J., Nakamura, T., Takeuchi, T., and Umezawa, H. Effect of 15-deoxyspergualin on graft-*v*-host disease in mice. *Transplant. Proc.*, **19**, 3985–3986 (1987).

17. Nemoto, K., Hayashi, M., Ito, J., Abe, F., Takita, T., Nakamura, T., Takeuchi, T., and Umezawa, H. Effect of spergualin in autoimmune disease mice. *J. Antibiot.*, **40**, 1448–1451 (1987).

18. Nemoto, K., Ito, J., Abe, F., Nakamura, T., Takeuchi, T., and Umezawa, H. Suppression of humoral immunity in dogs by 15-deoxyspergualin. *J. Antibiot.*, **40**, 1065–1066 (1987).

19. Nemoto, K., Ito, J., Hayashi, M., Abe, F., Ohtaka, Y., Nakamura, T., Takeuchi, T., and Umezawa, H. Effects of spergualin and 15-deoxyspergualin on the development of graft-versus-host disease in mice. *Transplant. Proc.*, **19**, 3520–3521 (1987).

20. Nemoto, K., Sugawara, Y., Takita, T., Nakamura, T., and Takeuchi, T. Assessment of the anti-diabetic activity of deoxyspergualin in low-dose streptozotocin-induced diabetic mice. *J. Antibiot.*, **41**, 145–147 (1988).

21. Nishikawa, K., Shibasaki, C., Takahashi, K., Nakamura, T., Takeuchi, T., and Umezawa, H. Antitumor activity of spergualin, a novel antitumor antibiotic. *J. Antibiot.*, **39**, 1461–1466 (1986).

22. Nishizawa, R., Takei, Y., Yoshida, M., Tomiyoshi, T., Saino, T., Nishikawa, K., Nemoto, K., Takahashi, K., Fujii, A., Nakamura, T., Takita, T., and Takeuchi, T. Synthesis and biological activity of spergualin analogues. I. *J. Antibiot.*, **41**, 1629–1643 (1988).

23. Okubo, M., Inoue, K., Umetani, N., Sato, N., Kamata, K., Mizukoshi, M., Uchiyama, T., and Shirai, T. Long-term therapy of lupus nephropathy in New Zealand Black / White F_1 hybrid mice by 15-deoxyspergualin. *Proc. Jpn. Soc. Immunol.*, **17**, 722 (1987).

24. Plowman, J., Harrison, S. D., Jr., Trader, M. W., Griswold, D. P., Jr., Chadwick, M., McComish, M. F., Silveira, D. M., and Zaharko, D. Preclinical antitumor activity and pharmacological properties of deoxyspergualin. *Cancer Res.*, **47**, 685–689 (1987).

25. Takeuchi, T., Iinuma, H., Kunimoto, S., Masuda, T., Ishizuka, M., Takeuchi, M., Hamada, M., Naganawa, H., Kondo, S., and Umezawa, H. A new antitumor antibiotic, spergualin: Isolation and antitumor activity. *J. Antibiot.*, **34**, 1619–1621 (1981).

26. Umeda, Y., Moriguchi, M., Ikai, K., Kuroda, H., Nakamura, T., Fujii, A., Takeuchi, T., and Umezawa, H. Synthesis and antitumor activity of spergualin analogues. III. Novel method for synthesis of optically active 15-deoxyspergualin and 15-deoxy-11-O-methylspergualin. *J. Antibiot.*, **40**, 1316–1324 (1987).

27. Umeda, Y., Moriguchi, M., Kuroda, H., Nakamura, T., Fujii, A., Iinuma, H., Takeuchi, T., and Umezawa, H. Synthesis and antitumor activity of spergualin analogues. II. Chemical modification of the spermidine moiety. *J. Antibiot.*, **40**, 1303–1315 (1987).

28. Umeda, Y., Moriguchi, M., Kuroda, H., Nakamura, T., Iinuma, H., Takeuchi, T., and Umezawa, H. Synthesis and antitumor activity of spergualin analogues. I. Chemical modi-

fication of 7-guanidino-3-hydroxyacyl moiety. *J. Antibiot.*, **38**, 886–898 (1985).

29. Umezawa, H., Ishizuka, M., Takeuchi, T., Abe, F., Nemoto, K., Shibuya, K., and Naka-mura, T. Suppression of tissue graft rejection by spergualin. *J. Antibiot.*, **38**, 283–284 (1985).

30. Umezawa, H., Kondo, S., Iinuma, H., Kunimoto, S., Ikeda, Y., Iwasawa, H., Ikeda, D., and Takeuchi, T. Structure of an antitumor antibiotic, spergualin. *J. Antibiot.*, **34**, 1622–1624 (1981).

31. Umezawa, H., Nishikawa, K., Shibasaki, C., Takahashi, K., Nakamura, T., and Take-uchi, T. Involvement of cytotoxic T-lymphocytes in the antitumor activity of spergualin against L1210 cells. *Cancer Res.*, **47**, 3062–3065 (1987).

32. Yoshikawa, Y., Uchida, H., Kuroda, H., Nakamura, T., Obayashi, A., Fujii, A., and Takeuchi, T. *In vivo* effects of deoxyspergualin (NKT-01) on lymphocyte activation in response to alloantigens. *J. Antibiot.*, **41**, 1675–1680 (1988).

ANTIBIOTICS INHIBITING ONCOGENE FUNCTIONS

Makoto HORI,[*1] Yoshimasa UEHARA,[*2] and Tomio TAKEUCHI[*3]

*Showa College of Pharmaceutical Sciences,[*1] National Institute of Health,[*2]
and Institute of Microbial Chemistry[*3]*

Evidence has been accumulating that malfunctioning of cellular oncogenes is a major cause of human cancer. From the viewpoint of cancer
chemotherapy, it seems important to find drugs that are preferentially
active against tumor cells where abnormal cellular oncogenes are manifested. For this purpose, we chose rat kidney cells (NRK) which had an
integrated temperature sensitive oncogene, either src^{ts} or ras^{ts}, because
the cells shift between the tumorous state and the non-tumorous state
simply with the change in culture temperatures. Using these cells, screening was conducted to find antibiotics which inhibited cell growth more
strongly at 33°C than at 39°C (Effect A) and those which altered the transformed morphology of the cells to the normal morphology at 33°C (Effect B). Oxanosine, a guanosine analog, showed "Effect A" on both src^{ts}
and ras^{ts} cell lines while it should "Effect B" on ras^{ts} NRK. Herbimycin,
a benzenoid ansamycin, showed "Effect B" on src^{ts} NRK. The molecular
basis for these effects was also studied. An independent approach to find
inhibitors of *erb*-B product-associated tyrosine kinase activity led to the
isolation of a new compound, erbstatin.

Chemotherapy is based on differential effects of a drug on the host and the parasite.
In this sense, an ideal antitumor drug should be one that is active against tumor cells
but not active against normal cells. Therefore, it is desirable to determine effects of a
potential antitumor compound on an appropriate pair of tumor cells and normal cells
early a screening program. For this purpose, we chose rat kidney cells (NRK) which had
an integrated temperature sensitive oncogene, either src^{ts} *(4)* or ras^{ts} *(19)*, because these
cells shift between the tumorous state and the non-tumorous state simply with the change
in culture temperature. For brevity, cells grown at low temperature and those grown at
high temperature are referred to as tumor and normal cells, respectively. The use of
these cells seemed especially attractive because of the accumulating evidence that malfunctioning of some cellular oncogenes is a major cause of human cancers *(6, 11)*. With
these cells, we conducted two types of screening: one was to find antibiotics which would
preferentially inhibit the growth of tumor cells, *i.e.*, antibiotics causing stronger inhibition at 33°C than at 39°C (Effect A). The other was to find antibiotics which would alter
the tumor cell morphology to normal cell morphology at 33°C, a permissive temperature
(Effect B). Compounds with "Effect A" would be expected to reveal the differences in
cell properties caused by expression of the activated oncogenes, while those with "Effect
B" would be expected to inhibit certain functions of the oncogene products. A number

---

[*1] Tsurumaki 5-1-8, Setagaya-ku, Tokyo 154, Japan (堀　誠).
[*2] Kamiosaki 2-10-35, Shinagawa-ku, Tokyo 141, Japan (上原至雅).
[*3] Kamiosaki 3-14-23, Shinagawa-ku, Tokyo 141, Japan (竹内富雄).

or fresh culture supernatants, mostly actinomycetes, and various known compounds were tested using these criteria. As an alternative approach, inhibitors of the tyrosine kinase activity of *erb*B protein were also sought.

Effect of Oxanosine on the Growth of src-expressed NRK Cells

Oxanosine is a guanosine analogue (Fig. 1), originally isolated by Shimada *et al.* at the Institute of Microbial Chemistry, Tokyo, in 1981 for its antibacterial and antitumor activities (*20*). It prolongs the life span of mice inoculated with L1210 leukemic cells. We found that this antibiotic inhibited the growth of *src*-expressed tumor cells more strongly than that of the normal counterparts. For 50% inhibition, normal cells required about a 10 times higher concentration level of oxanosine than did tumor cells. The molecular basis for this selective effect was studied (*23, 24*). DNA synthesis and RNA synthesis were inhibited by oxanosine in a dose-dependent manner. Here again, tumor cells were about 10 times more sensitive than were normal cells. Therefore, the inhibition of DNA and RNA syntheses was thought to be closely correlated with cell growth inhibition.

The structural similarity between oxanosine and guanosine suggested that oxanosine inhibited some step of the biosynthesis of guanine nucleotides. As expected, oxanosine inhibited the conversion of hypoxanthine to guanine nucleotides, but not to adenine nucleotides, in a dose-dependent manner. Here again, oxanosine showed about a 10 times stronger effect on tumor cells than on normal cells. We concluded, therefore, that the inhibition of guanine nucleotides was the major cause of cell growth inhibition by oxanosine. Two enzymes are involved in the conversion from IMP to GMP. The first enzyme is IMP dehydrogenase and the second is GMP synthetase. We found that oxanosine-5′-phosphate, a putative metabolite of oxanosine, inhibited the former enzyme, either from tumor cells or from normal cells, but not the latter enzyme. IMP dehydrogenase from tumor cells and that from normal cells showed some differences in their kinetic parameters. Most notably, the smaller K_i of the tumor cell enzyme than that of normal cell enzyme indicated a higher sensitivity of the tumor cell enzyme to oxanosine-5′-phosphate. This alteration appeared to be a major cause for the higher susceptibility of tumor cells to oxanosine than that of normal cells.

The alteration of the target enzyme, described above, did not seem to be the sole cause for the selective effect of oxanosine on tumor cells, however. The membrane transport of thymidine, among other nucleoside transports, was elevated in tumor cells (*27*). Oxanosine competed with the thymidine transport, suggesting that oxanosine entered into cells at least in part through the thymidine-specific transport system which was activated in the tumor cells (*23*).

Fᴵɢ. 1. Oxanosine

In summary, the selective toxicity of oxanosine to *src*-expressed tumor cells is based on the sensitization of its target enzyme and on its enhanced transport into the cells. Both alterations are evidently among terminal events of the signal transmission cascade originating from the expression of v-*src* oncogene.

Effect of Oxanosine on the Growth and Morphology of ras-expressed NRK Cells

The effect of oxanosine on K-*ras*ts NRK was very different from that on *src*ts NRK. Oxanosine altered the cell morphology from the tumor cell type to the normal cell type at 33°C (Fig. 2), in addition to its selective inhibition of tumor cell growth. Photomicrographs (a) and (c) are of the tumor cell morphology and normal cell morphology which are ordinarily observed at 33°C and 39°C, respectively. Oxanosine at a concentration near its 50% inhibitory concentration (IC_{50}) altered the tumor cell morphology (a) into what is shown in (b) which closely resembles (c), the normal cell morphology. Mycophenolic acid, another inhibitor of IMP dehydrogenase, also caused a similar alteration of cell morphology. The molecular basis for this phenotypic alteration was studied (9). The *ras* oncogene product p21 is known to bind to GTP or GDP and the complex is believed to function as a signal transducer (1, 3). We presumed, therefore, that depletion of guanine nucleotides was responsible for the dysfunction of p21 and, in turn, resulted in a difficulty in maintaining the transformed morphology. When oxanosine was added to a culture of tumor cells, intracellular concentrations of guanine nucleotides rapidly decreased in contrast to the nearly unchanged level of ATP during as long as 6 hr of incubation. We speculated that this rapid decrease in the guanine nucleotide concentrations must trigger inactivation and/or dysfunction of p21. It is known that p21 is palmitylated at a cysteine residue near the C terminus and is bound to the inner surface of the cytoplasmic membrane through the lipid side chain. This intracellular localization is essential for the function of p21 (33). To determine possible changes in the stability of palmitylated p21, cells were labeled with either [35S]methionine or [3H]palmitic acid for 1 hr and chased for 2 hr or 6 hr in the presence or absence of oxanosine. The cells were harvested and lysed, then p21 was immunoprecipitated from the lysates and electrophoresed. The result indicated that oxanosine accelerated the degradation of p21 and more markedly promoted the release of the palmityl group from the protein. Possible inhibi-

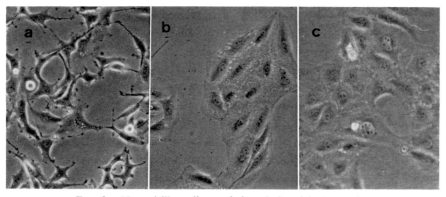

FIG. 2. Normal-like cell morphology induced by oxanosine

Cells were grown at 33°C (a) or 39°C (c) without any test materials. Cells were grown with 3 μg/ml of oxanosine at 33°C (b).

tion by oxanosine of biosynthesis and palmitylation of p21 was also determined in another experiment where cells were first incubated with oxanosine for 2 hr, then labeled with either [^{35}S]methionine or [^{3}H]palmitic acid for 2 hr and processed as described above. Oxanosine only moderately inhibited biosynthesis of p21 while strongly inhibiting palmitylation of the protein.

The mechanism for the morphological alteration of K-*ras*[ts] NRK caused by oxanosine can be summarized as follows. The inhibition of IMP dehydrogenase leads successively to depletion of guanine nucleotides, instability of p21, especially of palmitylated p21, and difficulty in maintaining the tumor phenotypes. Oxanosine never caused such morphological alteration to v-*src*-integrated cells.

Effect of Herbimycin A on the Morphology of src-expressed NRK Cells

Herbimycin A (Fig. 3) was originally isolated for its herbicidal activity by Omura *et al.* (*15*). We found that a fermentation broth of a *Streptomyces* sp. (MH237-CF8) isolated at the Institute of Microbial Chemistry altered the transformed cell morphology of *src*[ts]-NRK cells to the normal morphology at 33°C (Effect B). The active component was identified as herbimycin A (*25*). The fermentation broth or purified herbimycin converted the tumor cell morphology at 33°C to a morphology indistinguishable from cells grown at 39°C (Fig. 4). Removal of the antibiotic allowed the cells to revert to the transformed morphology, indicating that the action of herbimycin A to the cells is reversible.

Herbimycin A as an Inhibitor of src Oncogene Function

The tyrosine kinase activity of p60[src] (product of the v-*src* oncogene), localized at the plasma membrane, is essential for inducing and maintaining the transformed state of Rous sarcoma virus (RSV)-infected cells in culture (*10*). We found that herbimycin did not alter the localization of p60[src] but caused inactivation of p60[src] in cells. The immune complex prepared by mixing the herbimycin-treated cell extracts with antibody against p60[src] was found inactive *in vitro* in phosphorylating the complex itself. The reduced kinase activity was not due to a reduction in the amount of p60[src] protein in the complex because a parallel experiment conducted with [^{35}S]methionine-labeled cell extracts showed only a slight decrease in the radioactivity associated with the complex (*26*). This indicated that the antibiotic inactivated the *src* gene product, leaving a catalytically inactive but still immunoreactive protein.

The major phosphorylation sites of RSV p60[src] are serine at position 17 and tyrosine at position 416 (*16, 22*). Since the kinase activity of p60[src] seems to be modulated by phosphorylation of amino acids in the p60[src] molecule, we examined whether herbimycin

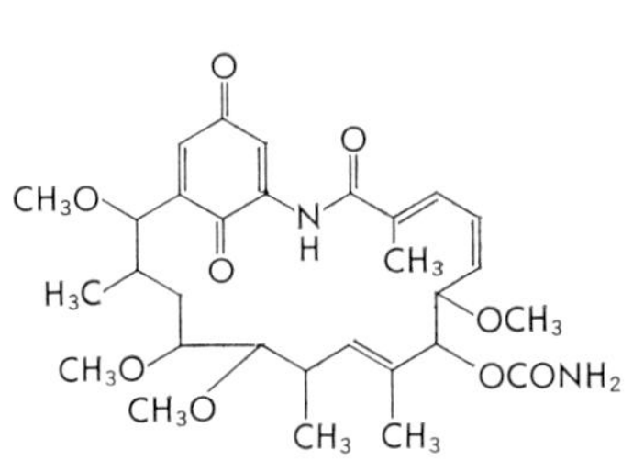

FIG. 3.   Herbimycin A

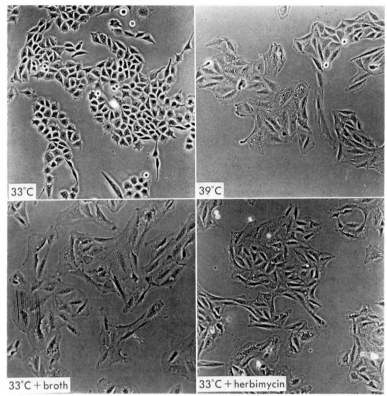

FIG. 4. Normal-like cell morphology induced by herbimycin
Cells were grown at 33°C (top left) or at 39°C (top right) without any test materials. Cells were grown at 33°C with 0.5% (v/v) of a fermentation broth of *Streptomyces* sp. MH237-CF8 (bottom left) or 0.5 μg/ml of herbimycin (bottom right).

inhibited intracellularly the phosphorylation of p60^{src} at any specific site. Herbimycin
induced significant reduction in ^{32}Pi incorporation into p60^{src} (26). Analysis by partial
proteolytic mapping technique using *Staphylococcus aureus* V8 protease revealed that the
loss of phosphorylation occurred selectively in the carboxyl-terminal V2 (26K) fragment
which should contain tyrosine 416 as the major phosphorylated amino acid in the protein
(29). Since this amino acid phosphorylation appears to be the result of autophosphorylation by p60^{src} itself (17), the decreased phosphorylation of tyrosine 416 in herbimycin-
treated cells may be due to the reduced kinase activity. However, the possibility that herbimycin directly interfered with the phosphorylation at this site cannot be excluded. We
previously reported that herbimycin did not inhibit p60^{src} kinase activity *in vitro* and the
molecular events leading to the inactivation were not clear (26). However, we have made
an improvement in the *in vitro* assay system for p60^{src} kinase activity in which phosphorylation of p60^{src} and exogenous substrates were measured and it has been found recently
that herbimycin itself inhibits the kinase activity. Therefore, the antibiotic may interact
directly with p60^{src} in cells.

Reversal of Various Transformed Phenotypes by Herbimycin

Malignant transformation of cultured cells by RSV leads to a variety of alterations

M. HORI ET AL.

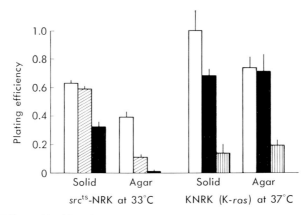

FIG. 5. Effects of herbimycin on colony formation of *src* or *ras* oncogene-expressed NRK cells

Cells were plated at 200 cells/60-mm dish either on a solid support or in soft agar in the absence or presence of indicated concentrations of herbimycin. Number of colonies was counted after 14 days of incubation at 33°C (*src*ts-NRK) or after 10 days culture at 37°C (KNRK). Bars indicate averages of three plates while thin lines at the top of the bars indicate SD.

of cell characteristics including changes in the cell morphology and the structure of cytoskeletons, loss of fibronectin from the cell surface, enhanced glucose uptake, and growth in soft agar medium (*8*). Some of these parameters have been reported to be dissociated in the cells infected with various temperature-conditional mutants of RSV (*32*). Therefore, we tested whether herbimycin changed, even if reversibly, other transformed pheonotypes than the cell shape.

Herbimycin rebuilt the cytoplasmic organization of cytoskeletal proteins, actin (*26*), and reversed various other neoplastic properties such as reduced fibronectin gene expression (*31*), increased glucose uptake, and lowered serum requirement for cell growth (*12*). Among these characteristics, growth in the absence of a solid support (anchorage independence) is thought to be well correlated with *in vivo* tumorigenicity (*21*). Therefore, it was important to know whether herbimycin interfered with colony formation of *src*-transformed cells in soft agar, especially in connection with a possible use in chemotherapy (*12*). As shown in Fig. 5, herbimycin inhibited the colony formation in the soft agar medium more strongly than on a solid support. No such differential effects were observed with KNRK cells in which v-K *ras* oncogene is expressed. These results suggest that herbimycin specifically acts on cells expressing the *src* oncogene and reverses various transformed characteristics to the normal ones.

Effects of Herbimycin on the Transforming Activity of Various Oncogenes

More than 50 oncogenes and oncogene related genes have been identified to date and they are classified into several groups according to their structures and functional similarities (*2*). We examined the effectiveness of herbimycin to reverse the morphologies of chicken and mammalian cells transformed by various oncogenes (*28*). We found that the antibiotic was effective against the cells transformed by tyrosine kinase oncogenes, *src*, *yes*, *fps*, *abl*, *ros*, *erb*B, but did not reverse the transformed morphologies induced by

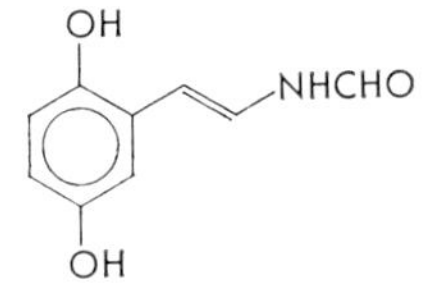

FIG. 6.   Erbstatin

oncogenes *raf*, *ras*, and *myc*. Moreover, we found significant decreases in phosphotyrosine contents of the total cellular proteins and in 36K protein, one of the cellular targets of tyrosine kinase oncogene products (*7*, *18*). The results gave supporting evidence for the selective inhibition by herbimycin of transforming activities of tyrosine kinase oncogenes. It remains to be studied whether the molecular basis for the action to these oncogene products is analogous to the one in *src* as described above.

Erbstatin, an Inhibitor of erbB Product-associated Tyrosine Kinase

As an independent approach, a cell-free assay system including *erb*B product-associated tyrosine kinase was employed to find potential antitumor compounds. The screening led us to the discovery of erbstatin (Fig. 6), a new tyrosine analogue, from a culture supernatant of *Streptomyces* sp. MH435-hF3 (*13*, *30*). Erbstatin was shown to inhibit the *in situ* enzyme activity as well and, furthermore, to prolong the life span of mice inoculated with L1210 leukemic cells, when administered with a Fe^{3+}-chelator. The finding is encouraging, although the molecular basis of the malignancy of L1210 is not yet known. Inhibitors of oncogene product-associated tyrosine kinase have been sought by other research groups also. Genistein (*14*) and amiloride (*5*) are among those reported to inhibit the enzyme.

Are Inhibitors of Oncogene Products Useful in Cancer Chemotherapy?

As shown in the cases of herbimycin *vs. src*-expressed cells and oxanosine *vs. ras*-expressed cells, inhibition and/or inactivation of oncogene products could alter the cell phenotype from "malignant" to "normal". The effect should be reversible because the oncogenes remain intact and should not cause cell death on its own. In fact, herbimycin or oxanosine was only partially cytocidal under conditions which allowed the antibiotics to alter the cell morphology of almost 100% of the cell population. Then what would be the merit of inhibitors of oncogene products? Our latest finding that *src*-integrating cells in a densely populated culture became contact-inhibited in the presence of herbimycin and resumed growth in a synchronized state after removal of the antibiotic seems to shed light on the possible usefulness of these inhibitors (*22b*). The synchronism suggests a possible use of herbimycin for cancer chemotherapy in combination with a delayed administration of 5-fluorouracil, cytosine arabinocide, and so on, which are selectively toxic to DNA synthesizing cells. This strategy seems to be promising because tumor cells in the body are thought to be confronted with physical barriers of surrounding tissues and, therefore, to become contact-inhibited and synchronized when they are exposed to herbimycin for a certain period of time.

REFERENCES

1. Barbacid, M. *ras* Gene. *Annu. Rev. Biochem.*, **56**, 779–827 (1987).
2. Bishop, J. M. Viral oncogenes. *Cell*, **42**, 23–38 (1985).
3. Carmela, C., Hancock, J. F., Christopher, J. M., and Hall, A. The cytoplasmic protein GAP is implicated as the target for regulation by the *ras* gene product. *Nature*, **332**, 548–551 (1988).
4. Chen, Y. C., Hayman, M. J., and Vogt, P. K. Properties of mammalian cells transformed by temperature-sensitive mutants of avian sarcoma virus. *Cell*, **11**, 513–521 (1977).
5. Davis, R. J. and Czech, M. P. Amiloride directly inhibits growth factor receptor tyrosine kinase activity. *J. Biol. Chem.*, **260**, 2543–2551 (1985).
6. Duesberg, P. H. Activated proto-oncogenes: sufficient or necessary for cancer? *Science*, **228**, 669–677 (1985).
7. Erikson, E. and Erikson, R. L. Identification of a cellular protein substrate phosphorylated by the avian sarcoma virus transforming gene product. *Cell*, **21**, 829–836 (1980).
8. Hanafusa, H. Cell transformation by RNA tumor viruses. *Compr. Virol.*, **10**, 401–483 (1977).
9. Itoh, O., Kuroiwa, S., Atsumi, S., Umezawa, K., Takeuchi, T., and Hori, M. Induction by the guanosine analogue oxanosine of phenotypic reversion towards the normal phenotype of K-*ras* transformed rat kidney cells. *Cancer Res.*, **49**, 996–1000 (1989).
10. Jove, R. and Hanafusa, H. Cell transformation by the viral *src* oncogene. *Annu. Rev. Cell Biol.*, **3**, 31–56 (1987).
11. Klein, G. and Klein, E. Evolution of tumors and the impact of molecular oncology. *Nature*, **315**, 190–195 (1985).
12. Murakami, Y., Mizuno, S., Hori, M., and Uehara, Y. Reversal of transformed phenotypes by herbimycin A in *src* oncogene expressed rat fibroblasts. *Cancer Res.*, **48**, 1587–1590 (1988).
13. Nakamura, H., Iitaka, Y., Imoto, M., Isshiki, K., Naganawa, H., Takeuchi, T., and Umezawa, H. The structure of an epidermal growth factor-receptor kinase inhibitor, erbstatin. *J. Antibiot.*, **39**, 314–315 (1986).
14. Ogawara, H., Akiyama, T., Ishida, J., Watanabe, S., and Suzuki, K. A specific inhibitor for tyrosine protein kinase from pseudomonas. *J. Antibiot.*, **39**, 606–608 (1986).
15. Omura, S., Iwai, Y., Takahashi, Y., Sadakane, N., Nakagawa, A., Oiwa, H., Hasegawa, Y., and Ikai, T. Herbimycin, a new antibiotic produced by a strain of *Streptomyces*. *J. Antibiot.*, **32**, 255–261 (1979).
16. Patschinsky, T., Hunter, T., Esch, F. S., Cooper, J. A., and Sefton, B. M. Analysis of the sequence of amino acids surrounding sites of tyrosine phosphorylation. *Proc. Natl. Acad. Sci. U.S.A.*, **79**, 973–977 (1982).
17. Purchio, A. F. Evidence that pp60[src], the product of the Rous sarcoma virus *src* gene, undergoes autophosphorylation. *J. Virol.*, **41**, 1–7 (1982).
18. Radke, K. and Martin, G. S. Transformation by Rous sarcoma virus: effects of *src* gene expression on the synthesis and phosphorylation of cellular polypeptides. *Proc. Natl. Acad. Sci. U.S.A.*, **76**, 5212–5216 (1979).
19. Shih, T. Y., Weeks, M. O., Young, H. A., and Scolnick, E. M. p21 of Kirsten murine sarcoma virus is thermolabile in a viral mutant temperature sensitive for the maintenance of transformation. *J. Virol.*, **31**, 546–556 (1979).
20. Shimada, N., Yagisawa, N., Naganawa, H., Takita, T., Hamada, M., Takeuchi, T., and Umezawa, H. Oxanosine, a novel nucleoside from Actinomycetes. *J. Antibiot.*, **34**, 1216–1218 (1981).
21. Shin, S-I., Freedman, V. H., Risser, R., and Pollack, R. Tumorigenecity of virus-trans-

formed cells in *nude* mice is correlated specifically with anchorage independent growth *in vitro. Proc. Natl. Acad. Sci. U.S.A.*, **72**, 4435–4439 (1975).

22. Smart, J. E., Oppermann, H., Czernilofsky, A. P., Purchio, A. F., Erikson, R. L., and Bishop, J. M. Characterization of sites for tyrosine phosphorylation in the transforming protein of Rous sarcoma virus (pp60[v-src]) and its normal cellular homologue (pp60[c-src]). *Proc. Natl. Acad. Sci. U.S.A.*, **78**, 6013–6017 (1981).

22b. Suzukake-Tsuchiya, K., Moriya, Y., Hori, M., Uehara, Y., and Takeuchi, T. Induction by herbimycin A of contact inhibition in *v-src*-expressed cells. *J. Antibiot.*, **42**, 1831–1837 (1989).

23. Uehara, Y., Hasegawa, M., Hori, M., and Umezawa, H. Differential sensitivity of RSV[ts] (temperature-sensitive Rous-sarcoma virus)-infected rat kidney cells to nucleoside antibiotics at permissive and non-permissive temperatures. *Biochem. J.*, **232**, 825–831 (1985).

24. Uehara, Y., Hasegawa, M., Hori, M., and Umezawa, H. Increased sensitivity to oxanosine, a novel nucleoside antibiotic, of rat kidney cells upon expression of the integrated viral *src* gene. *Cancer Res.*, **45**, 5230–5234 (1985).

25. Uehara, Y., Hori, M., Takeuchi, T., and Umezawa, H. Screening of agents which convert "transformed morphology" of Rous sarcoma virus-infected rat kidney cells to "normal morphology": Identification of an active agent as herbimycin and its inhibition of intracellular *src* kinase. *Jpn. J. Cancer Res. (Gann)*, **76**, 672–675 (1985).

26. Uehara, Y., Hori, M., Takeuchi, T., and Umezawa, H. Phenotypic change from transformed to normal induced by benzoquinoid ansamycins accompanies inactivation of p60[src] in rat kidney cells infected with Rous sarcoma virus. *Mol. Cell. Biol.*, **6**, 2198–2206 (1986).

27. Uehara, Y., Hori, M., and Umezawa, H. Specific increase in thymidine transport at a permissive temperature in the rat kidney cells infected with *src*[ts]-Rous sarcoma virus. *Biochem. Biophys. Res. Commun.*, **125**, 129–134 (1984).

28. Uehara, Y., Murakami, Y., Mizuno, S., and Kawai, S. Inhibition of transforming activity of tyrosine kinase oncogenes by herbimycin A. *Virology*, **164**, 294–298 (1988).

29. Uehara, Y., Murakami, Y., Sugimoto, Y., and Mizuno, S. Mechanism of reversion of Rous sarcoma virus-transformation by herbimycin A: Reduction of total phosphotyrosine levels due to reduced kinase activity and increased turnover of p60[v-src]. *Cancer Res.*, **49**, 780–785 (1989).

30. Umezawa, H., Imoto, M., Sawa, T., Isshiki, K., Matsuda, N., Uchida, T., Iinuma, H., Hamada, M., and Takeuchi, T. Studies on a new epidermal growth factor-receptor kinase inhibitor, erbstatin, produced by MH435-hF3. *J. Antibiot.*, **39**, 170–173 (1986).

31. Umezawa, K., Atsumi, S., Matsushima, T., and Takeuchi, T. Enhancement of fibronectin expression by herbimycin A. *Experientia*, **43**, 614–616 (1987).

32. Weber, M. J. and Friis, R. R. Dissociation of transformation parameters using temperature-conditional mutants of Rous sarcoma virus. *Cell*, **16**, 25–32 (1979).

33. Willumsen, B. M., Norris, K., Papageorge, A. G., Hubbert, N. L., and Lowy, D. R. Harvey murine sarcoma virus p21 *ras* protein: biological and biochemical significance of the cystein nearest the carboxy terminus. *EMBO J.*, **3**, 2581–2585 (1984).

AUTHOR INDEX

SUBJECT INDEX

206